THE FAMILY GUIDE TO SURVIVING STROKE AND COMMUNICATION DISORDERS

SECOND EDITION

Dennis C. Tanner, PhD
Professor
Department of Health Sciences
Northern Arizona University
Flagstaff, Arizona

JONES AND BARTLETT PUBLISHERS
Sudbury, Massachusetts
BOSTON   TORONTO   LONDON   SINGAPORE

World Headquarters

Jones and Bartlett Publishers	Jones and Bartlett Publishers Canada	Jones and Bartlett Publishers International
40 Tall Pine Drive	6339 Ormindale Way	Barb House, Barb Mews
Sudbury, MA 01776	Mississauga, Ontario L5V 1J2	London W6 7PA
978-443-5000	CANADA	UK
info@jbpub.com		
www.jbpub.com		

Jones and Bartlett's books and products are available through most bookstores and online booksellers. To contact Jones and Bartlett Publishers directly, call 800-832-0034, fax 978-443-8000, or visit our website www.jbpub.com.

Substantial discounts on bulk quantities of Jones and Bartlett's publications are available to corporations, professional associations, and other qualified organizations. For details and specific discount information, contact the special sales department at Jones and Bartlett via the above contact information or send an email to specialsales@jbpub.com.

The authors, editor, and publisher have made every effort to provide accurate information. However, they are not responsible for errors, omissions, or for any outcomes related to the use of the contents of this book and take no responsibility for the use of the products and procedures described. Treatments and side effects described in this book may not be applicable to all people; likewise, some people may require a dose or experience a side effect that is not described herein. Drugs and medical devices are discussed that may have limited availability controlled by the Food and Drug Administration (FDA) for use only in a research study or clinical trial. Research, clinical practice, and government regulations often change the accepted standard in this field. When consideration is being given to use of any drug in the clinical setting, the health care provider or reader is responsible for determining FDA status of the drug, reading the package insert, and reviewing prescribing information for the most up-to-date recommendations on dose, precautions, and contraindications, and determining the appropriate usage for the product. This is especially important in the case of drugs that are new or seldom used.

Library of Congress Cataloging-in-Publication Data

Tanner, Dennis C., 1949-
    The Family guide to surviving stroke and communication disorders / Dennis C. Tanner.
      p. cm.
    Includes bibliographical references and index.
    ISBN-13: 978-0-7637-5105-0
    ISBN-10: 0-7637-5105-7
    1.   Cerebrovascular disease—Patients—Rehabilitation—Popular works.   2.   Cerebrovascular disease—Patients—Family relationships—Popular works.   3.   Communicative disorders—Patients—Rehabilitation—Popular works.   4.   Communicative disorders—Patients—Family relationships—Popular works.   I. Title.
    RC388.5.T36 2008
    616.8'105—dc22   2007008000
    6048

Production Credits

Executive Editor: David Cella	Manufacturing and Inventory Coordinator: Amy Bacus
Editorial Assistant: Lisa Gordon	Cover Design: Kristin E. Ohlin
Production Director: Amy Rose	Composition: ATLIS Graphics
Production Editor: Renée Sekerak	Printing and Binding: Malloy Incorporated
Associate Marketing Manager: Jennifer Bengtson	Cover Printing: Malloy Incorporated

Printed in the United States of America
11 10 09 08 07   10 9 8 7 6 5 4 3 2 1

In loving memory of my mother, Elizabeth Tanner.

Contents

Acknowledgments

The author gratefully acknowledges the editorial and production assistance provided by Adam Bast, Margarette Cook, William Culbertson, Rebecca Davis, Anita S. Halper, Elizabeth Sperry, and Jody M. Tanner. I am especially indebted to my teaching assistants, Molly Murphy and Cortney Elwood, for their help in the preparation of this *Second Edition*.

Preface

I began writing the first edition of *The Family Guide to Surviving Stroke and Communication Disorders* in 1997. Since then, much has changed in the world of medicine. The Human Genome Project was largely completed at the turn of the century. It identified and mapped all of the approximately 25,000 genes in human DNA, the genetic instructions for cellular development. Stem cell research, controversial though it is, promises a renewable source of replacement cells to treat diseases and spinal injuries. New cancer therapies are giving hope to patients in arresting the growth and spread of this devastating disease. Surgeries using lasers are common, and more medicines are available than ever before to treat all that ails humans. New brain scanning devices can detect the site and extent of brain damage with far better precision than was available only a decade ago. There have also been advances in stroke prevention, diagnosis, and treatment.

Although stroke remains the third leading cause of death in the United States, the vast majority of strokes are preventable. Research has shown that persons who do not smoke, or who quit the habit, are less likely to suffer a stroke. Drinking alcoholic beverages in moderation is an important stroke prevention measure. Regular exercise, so important to an overall healthy life, also prevents strokes. There are new generations of medications to treat high blood pressure and to reduce the amount of negative blood cholesterol. New surgeries and improvements on old ones are available to open narrowed arteries to the brain.

Knowing the warning signs of stroke is even more important today because when medical treatment is initiated early, the effects of stroke can be minimized. The warning signs include numbness or weakness in the face, leg, or arm; confusion; blindness, blurriness, or other vision problems; and sudden dizziness and headache. One of the most important danger signs is a problem communicating. Slurred speech, problems remembering names of people and objects, difficulty stringing words together to make sentences, and an inability to understand what others are saying are all warning signs of stroke and require immediate medical attention. New medications and other treatments are reducing the severity of strokes, especially when they are given early. Advances in physical and occupational therapies are helping stroke survivors deal with problems walking and other activities of daily living. Since I began writing the first edition of *The Family Guide to Surviving Stroke and Communication Disorders*, there has been an increased understanding about stroke-related communication disorders and their treatment.

While it may seem that therapies and other treatments for stroke-related communication disorders improve at a snail's pace, scientific and clinical understanding of these communication disorders marches on. New therapies are discovered, and there are refinements of existing ones. Each day, thousands of speech-language pathologists evaluate and provide therapies to tens-of-thousands of stroke survivors. The collective clinical understanding of these disorders increases as clinicians communicate informally with other therapists and formally in journals, scientific presentations, workshops, and at conventions. Scientists conduct research on evaluation and treatment procedures and reach scientific conclusions about the merits of clinical procedures. During the past 10 years, scientists and clinicians have concluded that while speech and language therapies are beneficial in the treatment of stroke-related communication disorders, the psychological support provided by friends, family members, and therapists is of the utmost value.

There have been several additions, corrections, and changes to this edition of *The Family Guide to Surviving Stroke and Communication Disorders*. I have changed some illustrations to better show the brain and its parts. These illustrations are more detailed and informative. I have also updated the resource section with current information and resources for the United States, Canada, and other countries.

I have also added a new chapter to this edition: Profiles in Recovery. In this chapter, I profile several stroke survivors and their families and detail their successes in dealing with one or more aspects of the communication disorder. These are inspiring success stories showing these remarkable individuals' courage, determination, and resourcefulness in coping with stroke and the loss of the ability to communicate normally. They are informative case studies about how these patients and their families handle living with stroke and communication disorders.

Over the years, I have had people tell me that *The Family Guide to Surviving Stroke and Communication Disorders* helped them adjust to stroke and the communication disorders resulting from it. People have been especially generous with their praise of the short story, "Murphy's Inner World of Aphasia." However, some have commented that there was little written about his wife, Beth, and her perspectives of this life-altering event. Therefore, I have included "Murphy's Inner World of Aphasia: Beth's Story" in Chapter 13 to bring closure and to give Beth's perspectives about the ordeal.

I am pleased that a major medical publisher, Jones and Bartlett, is doing this *Second Edition*. They show their commitment to quality publishing throughout this book. Most importantly, I hope you, the reader, find this book helpful in dealing with the challenges facing you and your loved ones. After all, that has always been my goal.

Dennis C. Tanner, PhD

About the Author

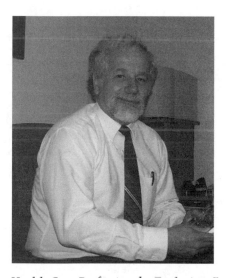

Professor Dennis C. Tanner received the Doctor of Philosophy degree in Audiology and Speech Sciences with a minor in Psychiatry from Michigan State University. Dr. Tanner's published papers on the psychology of neurogenic communication disorders have addressed loss, grief, chronic depression, nursing considerations, culture care issues, Wernicke's aphasia, loss of verbal coping skills, and disorientation in brain-injured persons. Books currently in print by Dennis Tanner include *The Forensic Aspects of Communication Sciences and Disorders*, *The Psychology of Neurogenic Communication Disorders: A Primer for Health Care Professionals*, *Exploring Communication Disorders: A 21st Century Introduction Through Literature and Media*, *The Forensic Aspects of Speech Patterns: Voice Prints, Speaker Profiling, Lie and Intoxication Detection* (with M. Tanner), *Anatomy and Physiology Study Guide for Speech and Hearing* (with W. Culbertson and S. Cotton), *Case Studies in Communication Sciences and Disorders*, *An Advanced Course in Communication Sciences and Disorders*, and *Medical-Legal and Forensic Aspects of Communication Disorders, Voice Prints, and Speaker Profiling*. He has presented two minicourses on the psychology of aphasia and related disorders at conventions of the American Speech-Language-Hearing Association and has been named "Outstanding Educator" by the Association of Schools of Allied Health Professions. Dr. Tanner serves as an expert witness in legal cases involving patients with communication and swallowing disorders and is currently Professor of Health Sciences at Northern Arizona University in Flagstaff, Arizona.

Murphy's Inner World of Aphasia: A Short Story

He liked to be called "Murph," which was short for Murphy. Three years into retirement, he and Beth, his wife of 45 years, were well adjusted to the leisure life. Well, it was not exactly a life of leisure; the chores continued. Some days, it seemed retirement was more demanding and more active than the work world. To Murph, if retirement was not the life of leisure he had always dreamed it would be, at least he set his own pace. And that meant a lot. Today was to be a typical day in the world of the retired, and it was typical, except for one thing. In the next few hours, Murph's life would change forever. Murph would have a stroke.

The Great Cross-Country Journey was scheduled to begin next week. The preowned Bounder motor home had set them back a pretty penny. But what a great machine. Two televisions, a microwave, CD player, and plenty of storage. Murphy would have preferred a diesel rather than the gas engine, but gas was relatively cheap. At seven miles to the gallon, it needed to be.

They had owned the machine two weeks, and Murph did not have buyer's remorse. In fact, he had buyer's glee over the best-looking recreational vehicle he'd ever seen, let alone owned. The Bounder had made Murph happier than he'd been in years. When Beth was out shopping, he would climb up into the driver's seat and just sit. Murph felt like he was on top of the world. He knew what people said about men and boys and the price of their toys. He also didn't care.

Murph knew he had a lot to do before embarking on the great adventure. The Bounder was in good shape but needed some TLC to be brought up to his high standards. Murph had always been a perfectionist. His son, Matt, had offered to help with the preparations, but Murph didn't like to impose on anyone, especially Matt. He knew Matt's twins were a handful, and his free time was limited, what with overtime and all. The birth of the twins had stretched Matt's finances to the limit. Matt's wife, Andrea, had to return to work much too soon after the birth of Murph and Beth's only grandchildren. Murph felt a pang of guilt about spending so much money on the Bounder, but as they say in old beer commercials, "You only go around once."

As Murph got into his pickup to go to the auto-parts store to buy road flares he hoped they would never need, a twinge of tightness gripped his right arm. For a moment, he could not open the door. The aging pickup had always had a sticky door, but this seemed unusual. "Oh well," he thought to himself, "I'll buy some oil for the hinges when I get to the store."

Driving to the store, Murphy tuned in to his favorite radio station. "The Country Voice of the Valley," they liked to proclaim. The nasal country tunes and the late morning sunshine made his increasing anxiety about the tightness in his arm dissolve. He had always liked country music. It was honest and all that. He couldn't imagine listening to anything else. As Murph pulled into the auto-parts store, he hit the curb with too much force. The jolt was enough to test the strength of the seat belt. "Damn," he thought, "There goes the front-end alignment. Now I'll have to get . . . to get . . . What's that called . . ."

Murphy stepped out of the pickup and started walking to the entrance of the store. As he opened the door, again his right arm wouldn't do as he wanted. He stood there for a minute in confusion. "What's wrong with my arm?" he said to no one in particular.

On the way home, Murph was again at peace with the world. The guilt pangs about spending too much money on the Bounder still nudged at his conscience, but the confusion and anxiety slipped away. "Ah, the curative effects of country music," thought Murph.

Murph had always been one to ignore fear. He realized that during the war he had been more lucky than invincible and more lonely than fearful. Like most of his generation, the war had made him realize a lot. Whenever fear reared its ugly head, he was able to kick it back where it belonged. This method of coping had worked well throughout his life. Murph had the gift. If it bothers you, ignore it; it'll go away.

When Murphy got home, Beth was gone. She probably was visiting Matt, Andrea, and the twins. He didn't mind. He'd make one of his world-class sandwiches for lunch. Today, the sandwich would consist of three slices of ham, Swiss cheese, a dollop of horseradish sauce, a pickle, and a tad of mustard. There was no wheat bread, so he settled for the last two slices of white. Had Beth been home, she would have objected to the sandwich. She spent way too much time worrying about blood pressure, cholesterol, and salt intake. The sandwich was delicious, and as the last bite was swallowed, Beth walked through the door. That afternoon, Murph mentioned the problems with his arm and hand. He managed to work it into the conversation while complaining about the usual aches and pains. He minimized the event, more to protect himself from the disturbing thoughts than to prevent her from overreacting.

Murph and Beth spent an uneventful evening together. After dinner, they talked about little things. She pretended to be interested in the playoffs, and he listened to more concerns about the grandchildren. There was a comfortable routine to their lives. It wasn't exciting, but it was predictable and secure. After the television was turned off, they retired to the bedroom. Murph's last words to Beth were, "Did you lock the doors?" As usual, he was asleep within minutes of his head hitting the pillow.

Murph was an early riser. It was hard for him to sleep when the sun was up. He had always considered himself a hard worker. Hard workers get up early, work hard, and go to bed tired. At 5:30 AM, Murph opened his eyes. He felt the warm, comforting presence of Beth next to him. He heard her quiet snore—well, not a snore exactly, more of a muffled buzz. Beth was quite adamant about the fact that ladies do not snore. He quietly got up, always careful not to awaken his mate. If Murph was an early riser, Beth was the consummate night owl. A lark married to an owl. Of course, Murph needed and always received that little catnap during the day. It was one of the perks of retirement. He silently planned the day's activities, careful to schedule that all important catnap. His biggest concern was a problem with the Bounder's air conditioning. "This could be an expensive day," he thought to himself.

As Murph walked toward the bathroom, he felt the strange sensation in his right arm again. His first reaction was one of irritation. He didn't have time for this nonsense. Only this time, it was not limited to his arm; the whole right side of his body felt strange. Suddenly, for the first time in a long time, Murphy was afraid. As Murph reached the bathroom door, his right side gave way and he tumbled into the dresser. He tried to catch himself, but to no avail. The family pictures carefully aligned on the dresser crashed to the floor, causing Beth to say, "What's wrong, Murph?" Murph didn't answer. He didn't understand the question. "Who's on?" he thought.

Murph tried to get up, but it was no use. The entire right side of his body would not budge. Try as he would, Murph could not make his body move. Not his leg, arm, or hand. "This can't be happening," he thought. "What a strange dream," was his last coherent thought.

Beth was awakened by the startling early morning noise. Why would Murph knock the family pictures to the floor? It took only an instant for the events to register completely: Murphy was having a stroke. Maybe he was dying. She should have seen it coming. Strangely, Beth's immediate concern was the pictures on the floor and the broken glass. "Someone could get cut," she thought. Then she had the presence of mind to ask Murphy, "What's wrong?" There was no reply.

Beth dialed 9-1-1 on the bedroom telephone. "Nine, one, one. What's your emergency?" came the matter-of-fact voice on the other end. Within 20 minutes, 20 long minutes, the paramedics arrived. The flashing lights woke the neighbors. There were sounds of police and ambulance radios. A stretcher was brought to the bedroom.

"It's clear the shush is," Murphy slurred.

"He's delirious," thought Beth. She knelt down and tried to comfort him. Murph kept saying the strangest things. "It's shush, beyond." The utterances turned into unintelligible sounds and finally silence as Murphy gradually slipped into unconsciousness. Beth couldn't get the image of Murph lying on the bedroom floor out of her mind. It seemed so odd.

Beth saw the ambulance rush Murph off to the hospital. She was sure that this was just a minor and temporary problem. No way could this be happening to her. Murphy was too strong to fall victim to something like this. A feeling of calm surrounded her as she got into the car to drive to the hospital. There was relief in blotting from her mind the terrible things that were happening to her and Murphy.

Apparently, one of the neighbors had called Matt and Andrea. They met Beth at the hospital's main waiting room. It was good to see familiar faces. They hugged and talked grimly in low voices about the early morning shock. Beth was on the verge of tears. It was hard for her to stay in control. She was afraid of what this day would bring.

Murphy was brought into the emergency room. He became aware of the hustle and bustle, and it frightened him. It was too intense, too hectic. He was placed on heart, oxygen, and blood pressure monitors. Blood was taken for the lab tests, and oxygen tubes were placed in his nose. He was awake during most of the chaotic activities but had little understanding of what was happening. It was like a movie, a bad movie. A catheter was inserted to help with urination.

Twice, Murphy asked for Beth. Unfortunately, to the triage nurse it sounded like, "Care for mother." Murphy couldn't understand why the nurses, technicians, and doctors didn't seem to understand his perfectly normal speech. He then drifted into the sanctuary of sleep. Later that morning, Murphy had a vague sensation of claustrophia while the CT (computerized axial tomography) brain scan was being conducted. He wanted to express his fear but was too tired to do so. He did not like being slid into the small tube. One thing bothered Murphy more than the claustrophia—the shouting. Everyone felt the need to shout instructions. They would move their heads close to his ear and shout things Murphy was incapable of understanding. Apparently, they felt Murphy had lost his hearing.

Dr. William Tobbler, a board-certified neurologist, had been on call all night. It had been a long night. He had been called in to evaluate a youngster with a severe head injury. Seizure after seizure had shaken the little fellow's body. The seizures were finally under control, at least for now. As he watched the elderly man being wheeled into intensive care, he wondered if his services would be required. The man was pale, obviously paralyzed on the right side, and he heard the nurse say he couldn't communicate; he was aphasic.

He saw the hospital's oldest staff physician, John Foster, trailing after the new patient. John had his usual sour look and permanent frown plastered on his face. He liked Foster and the old-fashioned "country doctor" role he played. John was considered a medical jack-of-all-trades.

The intensive care unit (ICU) is a strange place. Technology rules supreme, and the patients, the ones with the illnesses and injuries, appear to be an afterthought. The incessant beeping, clicking, and humming of the expensive machines are constant companions to staff and patients alike. In this hospital, there were 12 intensive care rooms. Murphy was placed in ICU-3. He lay on his back, a stiff sheet covering his body and a multitude of tubes and cords leading to and from him. The curtains were drawn, and the mute images of television flashed in the dimly lit room. Murphy had drifted in and out of sleep during most of the hours spent in the emergency room. He felt like an observer of the strange events occurring to him. It was easier to be an observer than a participant because it was all so unreal.

The first permanent memory Murph had of the ICU was the odor: disinfectant. There was no question is his mind that he was in a hospital; nothing smelled as clean and sterile as alcohol, and hospitals are drenched in it. Murph looked around. He recognized a few of the machines and most of the room's objects. He noted the tubes and lines attached to his body. He felt the irritation of the patches securing the sensors to his chest and arm. His mouth was dry and felt like cotton was stuffed in it. The oxygen tubes in his nose bothered him; he wanted to pull them out. Suddenly, panic gripped him; his hands were tied to the bed. He struggled, but it was no use. In hospital terminology, he was restrained, and restrained well. He couldn't scratch an itch if his life depended on it.

As Murph lay back, succumbing to the restraints, he felt calm; a sense of well-being surrounded him. As he stared at the hospital ceiling, he simply denied what had happened. He convinced himself that nothing bad was happening and if it was, it wasn't happening to him. He welcomed the break from reality, and he slipped into the sanctuary of sleep.

When he awoke, Murph sensed he was in trouble. Something bad had happened. Hospital rooms like this were for people on the verge of death. From deep within his mind, thoughts of escaping from this dangerous place welled up. But strangely, he had no words to carry the thoughts. All that was present was the overwhelming need to escape. "Get me out of here!" was vocalized as nothing. No words came to mind and no movements came to his lips. If Murph could have talked, he would have shouted: "I can't talk, help me!"

Beth met with Dr. Foster in the coffee shop. "It's serious, Beth," Dr. Foster pronounced. "He's had a serious stroke and he might not make it. Even if he does pull through, his speech and ability to walk have been affected." This declaration was no surprise to Beth. She knew it was bad and Dr. Foster had only confirmed it. A wave of sadness washed over her. It was the kind of feeling you get when a loved one is in serious trouble. Her first thought was to share this sad feeling with Murph. He'd understand the depth of it. He'd be strong.

Many doctors would have said to this anxious woman, "The CT scan showed an infarct in the left frontal region of the cortex without a midline shift." Not Dr. John Foster. He had decided a long time ago that this type of medico jargon was a form of verbal abuse. He would never talk to family members, and especially his old friend Beth, like that. He simply said, "The X-ray showed damage on the left side of the brain where speech is found. It is also the area that controls the right arm and leg. In fact, in Murph's case, the entire right side of his body may be paralyzed. It appears to be a clot and not a broken blood vessel."

Dr. Foster took the time to explain as much as he could to Beth.

"Yes, it's early."

"No, he's asleep now."

"Yes, his heart is strong."

"Yes, the stroke could get worse."

"No, brain cells do not grow back."

"No, he's not in a coma."

"Yes, he'll recognize you."

"No, he's not in physical pain."

"Our first goal is to get him stabilized, and then we'll begin thinking about re-habilitation," Dr. Foster planned aloud. He wanted to go into more detail but felt the buzz of his cell phone. He checked the number and politely ended the conver-sation. As he walked off, Beth felt angry as the realities of the situation set in. She was angry with Dr. Foster for confirming the bad news and mad at herself for not doing something to prevent the stroke. She was also mad at Murphy for not taking better care of himself. All she could think was, "Why did this have to happen?" Beth was left alone in the crowded room, more alone than she had ever been.

Back in ICU, Murph saw Beth, Matt, and Andrea enter the room. Their grim faces triggered another bout of anxiety. He imagined their sad faces at his funeral. "Where are the twins?" he wondered in wordless thought. Their young, identical faces always brought a smile. Murph did not like the forlorn faces on the three peo-ple he loved. He tried to say that it was all right and that things were going to be just fine, but there were no words, no sounds, no nothing. All that was present were im-ages and sensations; there was no language to bring order to thought. He heard one and only one word surface to his mind's ear: "Weird." As he attempted to verbalize it, nothing happened. As he tried again and again to express the weirdness of it all, his lips, tongue, and voice box suppressed it. The harder he tried, and the more force he brought to bear, the harder it was to command the movements of speech. With every increased effort to say, "W—eer—d," there was a corresponding increase in the resistance to program it. There were so few words he could remember, and when they did come to mind, they were too complicated to utter. Weird indeed.

Beth was careful not to disrupt the IV needle when she took Murph's hand. Her warm, firm hand in his was the first pleasant, comforting sensation Murph had experienced since his swan dive into the dresser. Tears swelled in his eyes and uncontrollable sobbing followed. Murph found himself crying like a baby. The crying was way out of proportion to the feelings he was experiencing. He wasn't that emotional or that sad. Talk about embarrassing. The nurse observing the family meeting made a mental note that Murphy was "emotionally labile." She had heard the doctors use those terms to indicate a patient who has exaggerated emotions due to brain damage.

Matt and Andrea were at a loss for words. They made small talk about the twins and other things, but it didn't take long for them to realize that the conversation was one-sided. Murph saw the tears in Andrea's eyes, and once again he cried. The embarrassment he felt was incredible. He tried to explain, but once again, all that came out was blathering nonsense. Murph had never felt so out of control, so utterly helpless. On a nonverbal level, he knew that if this was to be his future, death would be a welcomed event.

As chance would have it, Dr. Tobbler arrived to consult on the patient in ICU-3 when Beth, Matt, and Andrea were there. He shook hands with the family and began to explain the medications Murphy was taking. The results of the CT scan were explained in frightening detail. Apparently, Murph was scheduled for an MRI (magnetic resonance imagery) to further help pinpoint the site of the brain damage. Dr. Tobbler said that Murph's stroke was no longer in evolution, which Beth deduced was a good thing. It wouldn't get worse. In a day or two, Murph would be transferred to a regular hospital room.

Day two for Murph was as bad as day one. In fact, it was worse. The lunch tray was placed in front of him, and the nurse helped make the food manageable for a man with movement only on his left side. It was a puree diet, one obviously meant for stroke patients. Murph could barely manage the movement of the spoon to his mouth with his left hand, so a nurse's aide was sent in to help him. Murph knew the reputation of hospital food but it did taste good. In fact, the smell, texture, and taste were welcome, familiar sensations. The nurse's aide was careful to keep the gray, brown, and yellow spoonfuls confined to the general area of his mouth. More embarrassment and more blows to his self-esteem. Murph had an image of himself as an ugly, overgrown baby with food smeared all over his mouth. But the real embarrassment was yet to come.

During the night, Murph's bowels moved. He felt the sensations and tried to call for the nurse but was unsuccessful. He knew he needed to call for a bedpan or to get up and go to the bathroom, but he didn't have the words to plan the acts. He wasn't confused; he knew what was going on. He was perplexed; he couldn't organize himself well enough to push the call light. He couldn't remember how to shout for the nurse.

He lay in his own waste, the smell overwhelming. On the most basic of levels, Murphy knew this was absolutely the worst thing that had ever happened to him. A kind nurse's aide came to his rescue. She cleaned him and the mess. Murph watched her face carefully for any indication of scorn or ridicule. None was detected, and Murph was glad for that. There were few things to be glad about. As she was preparing to leave, Murph tried to utter something, anything, to lessen the embarrassment. Of course, even if he had been the most eloquent speaker in the world, nothing would have eased the awkwardness. Murph had the lowest image of himself he had ever had. The stroke had turned him into a babbling, drooling child, lying in his own waste. A little later, Beth entered the room and quietly sat down.

More words were becoming available to Murph. Fragments of complete inner statements occasionally came to mind. However, his verbal thoughts and visual imagery rarely connected. Occasionally, Murph understood the words of others. He had the most difficulty when people spoke rapidly or strung long sentences together. Dr. Foster asked him if he felt pain, and Murphy was convinced that the good doctor was informing him of the needed rain. Beth brought in a pencil and paper, hoping Murph could write his thoughts. Another blow to Murph's self-esteem: He wrote like a child. All he could muster were scribbles and a few lines that resembled his name. Everyone who saw the scribbles thought he was writing something profound. Matt saw the Bounder, Andrea saw the twins, and one nurse hurriedly brought him a bedpan. His writing was a makeshift inkblot test.

Dr. Linda Curzon was a 34-year-old physiatrist. She had been out of medical school only a few years, but she was more certain than ever that physical medicine and rehabilitation was the right specialty for her. She knew her trade and knew it well. The consult on the stroke patient in ICU-3 came early in the day. The attending physician was Dr. Foster. She'd had problems with Dr. Foster in the past. Old docs often tried to be one-man shows and resisted seeking her, or any other specialist's, opinion. She was director of rehabilitation and vice president of the medical staff, and it just might be that Dr. Foster was resentful of her age or specialty. That was his problem. She was a busy woman. She performed her usual thorough evaluation for rehabilitation potential on Murphy. There was a gleam in his eyes that she liked. The spark of life was still there.

During the course of her examination, Dr. Curzon became angry. A tray had been ordered for this patient, and the nurses had eagerly fed the poor fellow. His face sagged, his tongue deviated on protrusion, his vocal cords would not close completely, and the gag reflex was absent. A first-year intern would have known he was at risk for aspiration pneumonia. His temperature had spiked, and a person had to be deaf not to hear the gurgle in his lungs. Murph was sick and getting sicker. She placed him on NPO (nothing orally) status and ordered a chest X-ray and a speech and swallowing evaluation. She also ordered physical and occupational therapy. Her most pressing concerns were the swallowing problems and the potential for aspiration pneumonia.

Wendy, a certified speech-language pathologist, loved the interaction with the patients but hated the paperwork. The almighty paperwork. It wasn't even paperwork anymore, because the hospital had been computerized. Most notes were entered into the central computer, and you had to request a printout to even see paperwork. Documentation, documentation, and more documentation. Sometimes she felt she spent more time satisfying the needs of the bureaucrats and HMOs than the needs of the patients. As Wendy walked out of the therapy suite, the secretary pulled a slip of paper from her mailbox. Apparently, there was a new speech evaluation in ICU-3. A stroke patient of Dr. Foster's with aspiration pneumonia.

When Wendy walked into the ICU, she saw a nurse's aide leave the patient's room. The lingering odor spoke volumes of what had just happened. "The poor guy," Wendy thought. She said hello to one of the familiar faces in the unit and received a forced, obligatory nod. "They ought to rename this the insensitive care unit," Wendy thought as she typed her personal identification code into the unit's computer. Quickly, a complete history of the medical life and times of the patient was made available. She read his history, procedures, and consults with care. "Rather young to be losing so much," she thought. In her business, young was relative.

She walked into Murph's room and surveyed the situation. The woman sitting next to the bed was probably his wife, but Wendy had learned a long time ago not to make assumptions about relationships. Murph had his eyes closed, but she suspected he was not asleep. Many patients kept their eyes closed, especially after embarrassing events. It was a basic method of escape and avoidance. Gray, thinning hair, thick eyebrows, and a bit on the heavy side. Murph was definitely the grandfather type.

Wendy greeted the woman seated next to the bed. She offered the details expected of her by providing her name and profession. She explained that her job was to evaluate Murph's speech, voice, language, and swallowing abilities. When that was completed, she would provide therapy to help the patient recover as much as possible. Beth had heard the same kind of speech from the physical and occupational therapists; only the names and faces changed. Wendy was careful to project both professionalism and empathy in this first contact. The negativity often associated with strokes could interfere with the working relationship if the clinician was not careful.

"Good afternoon" were the first words Wendy said to Murph. He opened his eyes and saw a young woman standing by his bed. He recognized the two words as a greeting but didn't know if she was bidding him good morning, good day, or good night. He smiled and nodded his head. Murph had already been stung too often with the pain of verbal impotence to attempt speech. Murph had learned quickly that it was a verbal crapshoot every time he opened his mouth. Occasionally, he said the correct word, but more often than not, nothing came out or he blurted out the unexpected. Murphy sensed that this woman was responsible not for his blood, urine, walking, dressing, or breathing; she was here for his speech. He felt his first vague sense of hope.

Each time Murph tried to talk to Wendy, he fought to remember the word or struggled to program it. Even when he remembered the word and programmed it into existence, he produced it with a slur, a distortion caused by weak speech muscles. So far, all of his speech had been whispered. The familiar buzz of his voice box was absent. As Wendy tested his understanding of words, ability to sequence strings of sounds and syllables, and strength of speech muscles, Murph did his best to comply. After all, Murph had always been a hard worker and prided himself on that fact. Murph was glad that someone in this hospital understood the problems he was having with his speech. Wendy really understood. You could tell. She had seen other people adrift in this verbal confusion. Then Murph had another realization: He was not the only person who had ever had this problem. Wendy finished her evaluation and was talking to Beth about him. Beth nodded her head and asked questions. Occasionally, they both looked in Murph's direction.

Murph felt like a visitor in a strange, technologically advanced country. He didn't speak or understand the language of these foreigners. He recognized the objects, utensils, pictures, and uniforms as objects, utensils, pictures, and uniforms. The problem was that the names were different, or completely absent, in this strange foreign country.

The next morning, Murph was lifted from his bed to a wheelchair. He tried to help with the transfer but found that he was dead weight. So many times in his life he had gotten out of bed, and so often he had taken it for granted. He would never take easy movement for granted again.

As he was wheeled to the radiology section of the hospital, the people he passed in the halls and elevator greeted him in an uneasy manner. All he could do was nod his head and produce a slanted smile with his partially paralyzed face. He suspected that he looked a sight and wished they had combed his hair before leaving the room.

One of the signs on the entrance read "Nuclear Medicine." Murph recognized and understood the word "Medicine." After a short wait in the X-ray room, yet another doctor, another specialist, introduced himself. The technicians lifted Murph from the wheelchair to the examining table and tilted him into a nearly vertical position. A long tube was pointed at his head and chest. Everyone donned lead aprons; everyone but Murph, that is. Again, Murph felt frightened. As he looked around, he saw Wendy enter the room. Her smile and friendly manner were comforting. To the technicians, Murph was 190 pounds of human mass to be held firmly in position. But to Wendy, he was a person, an individual. At least, that was what Murphy sensed.

Liquid chalk; that's what it tasted like. The barium was a white substance swallowed while a video X-ray was taped. Wendy and the radiologist watched as Murph, Murph's skeleton really, swallowed the liquid. Most of it shot down to the stomach, but a small amount pooled on the vocal cords. When Murph took another breath, it went directly into his lungs. Murph did better with the barium paste and a cookie soaked in the stuff. But there was no question that Murph breathed the liquid. Wendy noted that, for now, Murph would not be able to eat or drink by mouth and that she would recommend that enteral, or tube-feeding, should be started.

The tube was coated with K-Y Jelly and slipped through his nose. The nurse kept telling Murphy to "Swallow." Actually, she was shouting the word. Once again, Murph wondered if there were something wrong with his hearing. Why would so many people feel the need to shout at him? His nose and throat hurt as the tube went down. Correction. Things don't hurt in a hospital; the patient feels some discomfort. Well, this discomfort hurt! When the end of the tube was finally resting in Murph's stomach and an X-ray was taken, the nurse started feeding Murph through the tube. A white liquid began to flow. This wasn't one of Murph's world-class sandwiches, but it was dinner. What was more important, it provided needed liquid and protein. After a while, Murph felt satisfied; not full, but satisfied.

The next day, Murph was moved to the intermediate care unit. In hospital-speak, this is known as a *step-down* unit. It's not as intense as intensive care, but it's more intense than the acute floor. Murph was beginning to sense that there was a definite hierarchy in the hospital world.

Wendy and the other therapists visited him regularly in the intermediate unit. His right arm, leg, and hand were exercised, splinted, ultrasounded, and massaged. He was taught to stand, sit, and dress differently. Two days later, Murph was moved to the third floor acute care ward. After learning to chew and swallow more carefully, the tube was pulled from his nose. What a wonderful sensation, almost as good as the taste of the soft foods he was given. Soon after that, Murph was transferred to the rehabilitation section of the hospital. Murph knew something was up when Wendy jokingly said, "The vacation is over."

The fall that Murph had taken into the family pictures a few days ago seemed like a distant nightmare. Murph's life had changed permanently. From Murph's perspective, all of the changes were unwanted. In an instant, he was transformed into a dependent, verbally impaired patient in a large, impersonal institution. Although he could see and touch Beth, his mate of 45 years, a wedge had been driven between them. He still felt the love, the fondness for her, but all but the most basic expressions of his feelings were lost. Matt, Andrea, and the grandchildren visited him regularly, but there were painful silences and a lack of friendly chatter. He missed his old life sorely, and it angered him that so much had been taken from him. He certainly had not asked for the stroke, but he felt anger at himself for having it. He was angry at the whole situation. He was frustrated at being unable to change the situation, and that frustration also angered him.

The new relationships he had with the hospital staff were even less satisfying. Between exams, punctures, transfers, and drills, communication was a shadow of what it should have been. Murphy felt isolated, lonely, and depressed. Who wouldn't? His depression worsened as the reality of life after stroke set in. The trigger, setting the depressive spiral into motion, was when Murph overheard that the Bounder was for sale. He couldn't understand the details, but it was clear from Beth and Matt's discussion that his Bounder was for sale. Murph slipped deeper and deeper into depression.

Some of Murph's speech and language had returned on its own. This was called *spontaneous recovery*. Within three weeks of the stroke, Murph's comprehension had returned to the extent that he could understand most of what was spoken to him, as long as people spoke clearly and slowly and avoided complex words. It irritated Murph that some people talked to him like he was retarded. He wasn't and didn't appreciate being talked to like that. It contributed to his depression. Murph could read short sentences and do some simple arithmetic problems. Each day he was getting better. Most patients who survive a stroke improve, at least somewhat. Words were still forced and slurred when he could find the correct ones, but his speech was now functional, meaning he could express his wants and needs. Murph was able to write about as well as he could speak. Wendy told him this is typical for most stroke patients.

Wendy wanted Murph to be put on an antidepressant because he was too devastated by the recent events beyond a normal grief reaction. The injury to the cells of the brain and his inability to adjust to the unwanted events had combined to create a spiral of negativity. The poor guy just couldn't see the light at the end of the tunnel. Wendy would talk to Dr. Curzon about it.

The weekly rehabilitation meetings were highly structured, intense, and always interesting. The physiatrists ran the show and were quite democratic.

Each doctor would provide a case history of the patient to be discussed and then call on the respective professionals for their ideas. Wendy sat quietly during the discussion of an 86-year-old woman with a fractured hip and diabetes. Murph was up next, and she wanted to make certain she covered everything in the brief time allotted to her.

Dr. Curzon matter-of-factly reviewed Murph's history. "The patient is a 68-year-old male who was transferred to the rehabilitation unit three days ago. He is stable and on antibiotics. The thrombosis interrupted blood flow of the middle cerebral artery to the left hemisphere. It was a relatively dense stroke. The patient had hemiparalysis, dysphagia, and was incontinent. He had aspiration pneumonia that is now under control and responding well to the medications."

The physical therapist reported that Murph was doing well. He was still at an "assist level," meaning that he was far from being able to walk by himself. Murphy was having trouble transferring from bed to wheelchair and back again. Wendy was delighted to hear that some movement was returning to Murph's right hand. She recalled a lecture long ago in which the professor reported that speech recovery often correlates with return of function to the right hand.

The occupational therapist reported that Murph was unable to dress himself but was learning self-sufficiency at the expected rate. She noted that Murph was not very motivated lately. She explained how Velcro was substituted for zippers and buttons, and that Murph was improving in other ADLs. Activities of daily living were always called ADLs. Wendy was impressed with the tricks of the trade the occupational therapists had. They were quite clever in teaching patients alternate ways of dressing and eating.

The report from the dietitian was relatively standard for a stroke patient. Wendy often chuckled to herself when the dietitian reported that a particular patient was 10 to 15 pounds over his or her ideal weight. "Who isn't?" she thought.

The social worker reported that Murph's finances were good. He was in a designated Medicare bed and had supplemental insurance. Out-of-pocket expense would still be considerable, but apparently the family resources could handle it. She noted that Beth was a concerned, caring spouse and was adjusting well to Murph's disabilities. As an aside, she reported that Matt tended to be too protective and somewhat anxious about his father. The social worker's final statement was a good introduction to Wendy's presentation. She said that Murphy was depressed and becoming more so.

Wendy reviewed Murph's swallowing status. He was on a soft diet and tolerating it well. As long as he took a deep breath before each swallow and paced himself, there were no occurrences of choking or coughing. She was going to advance his diet and stop the Thick-it. Thick-it is a substance put in the patient's liquids to provide more texture. It helps the patient manage thin liquids during swallowing. Thin liquids such as juices and coffee tend to be the most difficult for patients with swallowing problems.

Wendy noted that Murph's receptive abilities had improved considerably since her first visit with him in ICU. She reported the results of the Token Test, in which the patient follows commands by pointing to or rearranging differently colored and shaped objects. "Murph can understand the majority of speech. Writing seems to be the modality of communication least improving," she reported.

Wendy noted that programming of the words seemed to be the main difficulty. "Murph," she reported, "has more problems sequencing and planning the utterances than he does retrieving the words." Both finding the correct name and then being able to plan and program it into existence were problematic. This was the nature of his type of aphasia. She condensed it into the professional jargon everyone at the conference table would understand: "The patient has Broca's aphasia with a predominance of apraxia of speech. He also has mild dysarthria."

Wendy then asked Dr. Curzon if she would consider prescribing an antidepressant for Murphy. She stated that he was extremely depressed, and it was not resolving on its own. She was also concerned at his listlessness and lack of motivation. She thought the antidepressant would help increase his motivation and ability to benefit from therapy. That was the professional rationale provided to Dr. Curzon. Wendy knew the main reason was that Murph was in pain—psychological pain— and it hurt her to see him suffer. In a few days, the antidepressant would kick in and Murph's spirits would elevate. Then, along with the return of more function, he would likely find the strength to adjust to his communication disorders. Too much had gone wrong in this guy's life: too much, too rapidly. Antidepressants provided many patients a leg up on the adjustment process. As a psychologist once told the staff at the rehabilitation meeting, "It's hard to learn to navigate in a storm. The medications calm the seas."

Wendy had been right—the time spent in ICU, intermediate, and acute care was a vacation compared to the rehabilitation ward. Everything was structured from morning to night. He was dressed and ready to go by 7:15 AM. Breakfast was usually taken in his room, although lunch and dinner were held in the communal dining room. By 8:30 AM., Murph was in the physical therapy gym learning to walk with the assistance of a walker. Things were not going well with the walker. He just couldn't keep his balance. If it weren't for the help of the aide, he would have fallen more than once. Occupational therapy was helping him become more independent in dressing and feeding himself. He was learning to transfer from his wheelchair to the toilet without falling. Murph had therapy with Wendy twice a day. He eagerly anticipated the morning and afternoon sessions. The exercises, drills, and games were helping him remember words and ease their production. His facial muscles were becoming stronger; his speech was more precise. The most difficult hurdle to overcome was the tendency of his mouth to have a mind of its own. Some sequences of sounds and certain words were unavailable to him. Try as he would, he just couldn't get the sounds to come out correctly.

"Automatic speech" was a strange phenomenon. Some words and phrases were impossible to speak when he tried to do so. However, when his mind was elsewhere and he wasn't trying to force speech, those words and phrases were spoken easily and articulately. His daughter-in-law's name was a good example. Once in the

any sort of communication is good
reward communication, don't discourage it.

morning session, Murph was trying to say her name. As he practiced her name, all that came out was "dan rea," "san vea," "dorn a hea." The harder he tried, the more thought he put into it, the further he got from the word. Then, as if in some bizarre magic show, he turned to Wendy and said, "Can't seem to say Andrea today." The automatic utterances were quite frequent and, much to Murph's dismay, readily present on swear words. Murph had never been one to swear much. He was not a crude man. But, boy, the swear words were easy to say since the stroke. They would pop out at the worst times, too. He had to work to forget the first words he accidentally said to the minister during his visit. In some ways, automatic speech was a curse.

Wendy had prepared Murph for group therapy. She had managed to explain to him that he was going to be provided therapy at the same time as some of the other patients. She wheeled Murphy into the large room and placed the locks on the wheelchair when he was in position at the table.

Across from Murph sat a young man. His head had been shaved and a curious question mark scar was prominent next to his ear. Murph said, "Good morning. My name is Murphy." Actually, Murph said, "Should Morning. . . . name, Murph." He wanted to correct the errors, but Wendy had been clear that the best strategy was to keep going forward in these situations. Too many patients spent too much time revising and correcting, struggling and fighting to make the output perfect. In the world of aphasia, perfection is rarely attainable. She was right. The question mark kid had understood what Murph said and replied in a slurred, distorted way.

To Murphy's left was another man. He was about Murph's age. Like Murphy's, his arm was also secured to his chest. He nodded when they made eye contact and burst into tears. Murphy knew what was happening; he'd been there, done that. In fact, he was still there, still doing that as he fought to stop his own tears.

Across from the crying man was a woman in her mid 50s. She was a pleasant looking woman who smiled at Murph and said, "Hello, my name is Helen. Welcome to our kroop, stroop." She then opened her mouth widely and carefully said, "group." Murph nodded.

Next to the woman was another man, clearly older than anyone at the table. He just stared out of the window; he didn't acknowledge anyone or anything. He had a blanket wrapped around him, and a tube was running from his nose up to a plastic bag hung on a steel hanger attached to his wheelchair.

Another man walked into the room. At first Murph thought he might be one of the doctors. He waved and nodded to everyone at the table, then turned to Wendy and precisely said, "The chitters have arranged." Now Murph was still having a problem understanding the speech of others, but this was clearly an odd thing for anyone to say. Then the man turned to Murph and followed his observation about the chitters with the statement, "A new chit. Gone a hafta depend on it?" Then the man looked directly into Murph's eyes and awaited a response.

Murph heard a strange sound coming from his throat. It had been a long time since he had last heard it. He was laughing. Laughing out loud. It wasn't Murphy's style to laugh at other people, but this was just too funny. He looked around and all of the patients, except the man in the blanket, were laughing. Wendy seemed to enjoy it the most. When the laughter subsided, Wendy carefully explained to Murph that Mr. Skinner had jargon aphasia. Apparently, the understanding centers of his brain were damaged and he couldn't monitor his output. He talked clearly but made little sense. He also had a degree of denial about the communication disorder. Mr. Skinner believed that he was talking normally and that people just needed to take the time to understand him. Murphy had a vague recollection of experiencing a similar feeling in the emergency room.

Murph looked forward to group. As time passed, he became friends with Mr. Skinner and the question mark kid. He met the pretty woman's family and tried to build a bridge to the blanket man. But the blanket man was too distant, too alone. Murph hoped he would come around and someday become a participant in the group. Murphy learned to accept the group members for who they were, for what they had become. They were all travelers on a difficult road. They all had lost so much. But they were all gaining, too. New friends, new skills.

Beth helped Murph into the old pickup. He noted that she had trouble opening the door. He'd have to remember to get some oil for the hinges. With the wheelchair in the back, they drove to their home of 40 years. It was good to be home. He had forgotten how pleasant and predictable a home could be. He managed to get around, mostly in the wheelchair. Matt had made the house wheelchair accessible by building ramps and making two doors wider. Murph still saw Wendy for outpatient therapy three times a week, but at least he was home. Although his speech was far from perfect, he got by. Each day, more words came to him. Just like before the fall into the dresser, each new day was an unknown. There would be the good and the bad, the positive and the negative. The stroke had changed many things, but the days continued.

Beth watched Murph playing with the twins in the yard. Murph would count and the twins would run from the fence to a tree. She enjoyed hearing the laughter and the screams from the twins. She thought about the Bounder and the trip they would never take. Her thoughts about the motor home and the great cross-country journey were interrupted by the sight of the twins, both of them, hugging their grandpa. Murph was home.

CHAPTER 1
Stroke and the Ability to Communicate

Everything must be made as simple as possible but not one bit simpler.
—ALBERT EINSTEIN

You are probably reading this book because someone close to you, a relative or a friend, has suffered a stroke, and a communication disorder has resulted. The fact that you are seeking more information is good. Studies have shown that when family and friends have more information, patients are not confronted with too many demands, and their loved ones are able to deal with the disability more realistically.

My purpose in writing this book is to remove as much of the mystery, confusion, and complexities from strokes and the communication disorders that result from them as possible. Strokes are major medical events, and you may feel that they are too complex, too "medical" for you to understand. Sometimes family members and friends believe they must be graduates from medical school to understand what has happened to their loved one. These feelings, while normal, are absolutely unnecessary. There is no need for you and other family members to feel intimidated and overwhelmed. You do not need to be a genius or medical specialist to understand what is going on. What you do need is a simple, straightforward explanation of what can happen to communication abilities when a person has a stroke. That is the goal of this book. When technical medical terms must be used, they will be defined, and examples or descriptions will be provided. As Dr. Foster realized in the short story "Murphy's Inner World of Aphasia," medico-jargon sometimes can confuse more than clarify.

My intent is to provide you with current and relevant information about stroke-related communication disorders. Because there are many types of strokes and so many individual reactions to them, by necessity most of the information provided here is general. Some of what you read will not relate to your particular situation. Other information may be too detailed. Strokes vary a great deal, ar the communication disorders resulting from them can range from mild to severe. Mild communication disorders are often dramatically different from severe ones. A mild communication disorder may be just a nuisance, whereas a severe one may render an individual mute and unable to read, write, or understand the speech of others. A severe communication disorder can leave a person isolated from loved ones and psychologically devastated. Of course, a wide range of stroke-related communication disorders falls between these extremes.

Throughout this book, you will find that although the subject matter appears complex and technical, it can be reduced to simple, understandable information about communication disorders and the people who have them. You will see that some stroke-related communication disorders are the result of a reduction in language, especially vocabulary. Other communication disorders occur because of problems getting the words to come out. What we know about the marvels of the brain, and the damage that can be done to it, can be presented without overly technical or complex terminology. Even the activities of the many specialists involved in your loved one's medical care and rehabilitation can be presented in a straightforward and understandable way. After all, although doctors, nurses, psychologists, therapists, and other health care professionals are well educated and skilled in their trades, they are simply people using available technology, therapeutic principles, and common sense to reduce the effects of the stroke. A common link among most health care professionals is that they are in these professions because they want to help people. They want to do all they can to reduce suffering and minimize the disabilities that can result because of a stroke.

If the stroke occurred recently, you probably feel anxious about the uncertainty of the situation and unsure of what to expect. If the loved one is in a hospital, you may be intimidated by the technology. Hospitals are wonderful places; the best medical care usually is available in them. But hospitals tend to be intense and impersonal, and everyone seems to be in a hurry. Unfortunately, most hospitals often do not provide enough specific information to the patients or their family members about what to expect. Survey after survey has shown that the biggest complaint by patients and their family members is: "I wasn't provided with enough information."

One reason for the lack of information concerns the changing nature of illnesses, especially strokes. In many stroke cases, accurate and firm information about how a patient will ultimately fare is difficult to give because the professionals simply do not know what the course or outcome of the stroke will be. No two strokes are identical, and a variety of influences can affect them. The most common response given to family members and friends is that it is "too soon to tell." While frustrating and frightening, this is often the reality of the situation. If the stroke has just occurred, it *may* be too early to tell what the outcome will be.

It is common for family and friends to feel fearful. Hospitals can be scary places because they deal with life and death situations. Feeling a dose of frustration and anger can also be expected. These feelings are only natural given the difficult and stressful situation. Strokes are powerful events in the lives of both the patients and the people close to them. They often bring many unwanted changes that require major adjustments. Perhaps the worst part of having a stroke with a resulting communication disorder is the lack of ability to communicate with your loved one. Especially when the communication disorder is severe, both the patient and the family often feel a deep sense of isolation. It is not just the patient who is affected by the communication disorder; the whole family suffers.

You should always discuss specific issues with the patient's doctor or other health care professionals. Most professionals will find the time to answer your questions, and it is important that you be direct and to the point when asking them. You might find that keeping a notebook of questions and concerns will help you be focused during these meetings with the health care team. It is frustrating to remember an important question after the meeting with the doctor or other health care professional has concluded.

The Talking Animal

Before embarking on a discussion of strokes and communication disorders, I want to say a few words about our crowning glory as humans—our ability to communicate. Human communication is a broad topic. From the words used to order a hamburger to the directions given to land a jumbo jet, communication permeates our existence. We rely on it to greet acquaintances, and we blame failed marriages on the lack of it. Communication is the reason friendships satisfy and businesses boom. Literature is the art of communication. Without communication our educational, political, and legal systems would limp to a halt. The role of communication in religion is apparent; after all, in the beginning was the "Word." Humans delight when communication is at its best and suffer untold consequences when it fails. Babies are born with the natural ability to learn to communicate, but, sadly, strokes can erase or diminish that same ability.

Like many aspects of our lives, sometimes we recognize just how important the ability to communicate is only when it is taken from us. People with amputated legs often comment on how they took ordinary things for granted, such as getting out of a chair or walking to a car. Insignificant things once done with little thought and no appreciation suddenly become of considerable value to the amputee. Similarly the stroke survivor may suddenly be deprived of chitchat and other discourse. Similar to the way an amputee misses a limb, the stroke survivor sorely misses the easy acts of social interaction. And to the stroke patient completely deprived of the ability to communicate, it feels as though a big part of being human has been taken. The loss of the ability to communicate needs and wants, to plan for business and family activities, and to understand simple goings-on of life renders an individual socially disabled.

The ability to communicate is not a uniquely human skill. Not too long ago, we believed that only humans had the power of language and that animals used only "call and warning signals." A chimpanzee by the name of Washoe changed that. Named after a county in Nevada, Washoe was taught a version of sign language. Much to the amazement of the researchers, he used the signs in a very humanlike way. Washoe taught us that other animals have more highly developed levels of communication than previously thought. Other researchers confirmed the presence of what appears to be language in other chimps and primates, and research is currently being done on dolphins and whales. Whether "true" language exists among other species is still controversial, and research into the subject continues.

Our ability to use language and to engage in high-level communication did not develop rapidly or recently. Anthropologists believe that language developed from a survival need. Because humans were capable of using language, we were more adaptable than other species to our environment. We engaged in communicative acts that increased the probability of survival, and we passed this ability on to our children. Over tens of thousands of years, we have continued to develop this powerful survival skill. Currently, there are about 10,000 languages and dialects. The existence of so many languages in the world is probably related to the isolation of various prehistoric tribes. They were far removed from one another and so developed unique words and sentence structures. Creationists believe that the development of language is a relatively recent event. The Bible explains the variety of languages by the parable of the Tower of Babel, which is where we get the word *babbling* to describe the stage of language development in which a child produces sounds without apparent meaning.

The study of human communication crosses many disciplines. Linguists study the origin and nature of language in various societies and describe and record the languages of the world. During the past 50 years, they have discovered many aspects of how ancient and remote civilizations communicated among themselves and with others. Interestingly all language systems have a common structure—a grammar—that can be compared and analyzed. Although humans communicate in many different languages, they share a common thread of form and structure.

Most universities have communication departments or even whole colleges de-
d to the study of human communication. Research is conducted, and students

learn about rhetoric, public speaking, interpersonal communication, group dynamics, and mass communication.

Speech and hearing sciences and speech-language pathology and audiology are two branches of the study of human communication. These disciplines are based on the scientific method. Both fields conduct and rely on scientific research to build their knowledge base. Speech and hearing sciences look at the way the brain and body work during communication. The muscles, nerves, and chemicals used to communicate are systematically studied, as are speech sound waves. Scientists use powerful instruments to break the speech sound wave into tiny parts that can be analyzed. Speech-language pathology and audiology are branches of both education and the health professions. In this field, professionals are trained to evaluate and treat a multitude of communication disorders, including those resulting from stroke.

The human ability to communicate is remarkable. From the intimate conversations between a mother and her infant to a presidential address, humans value, study, and exercise language—the hallmark of human evolution. We communicate on multiple levels, and we do it all of the time. In fact, it has been said that we cannot *not* communicate. Even our silence is a message.

The Brain and the Power of Speech

The human brain has been studied for centuries. Written accounts about brain function go back thousands of years. The human heart, not the brain, was originally thought to house the soul and memories of life. Over the years, people gradually realized that the brain is the seat of the mind, that the brain, not the heart, is where awareness, or consciousness, is found. The Egyptians, Greeks, and Romans all studied the brain. In fact, they wrote about speech disorders resulting from brain injuries. Some of these writings were detailed. During the past 50 years, however, more research has been conducted about how the brain works than during all of the preceding centuries of recorded history. Even the U.S. Congress designated the 1990s as the "Decade of the Brain." Although the brain still remains a mystery in many ways, there have been great leaps in our knowledge of how it works.

Research into brain functioning continues at a heated pace; new discoveries are made every week. The results of studies come out in technical journals and at professional conventions, and many are also reported in newspapers, radio, and television. Some reports of brain functioning are controversial, and it takes time to confirm or reject them. That is how scientific inquiry into brain functioning works: every study is intended to be criticized, its design and results questioned. Once a study has been confirmed by objective researchers, it becomes part of the body of knowledge we have about the brain. This is often a tedious process, but it e that the information we have about the brain is objective and accurate. By follow-ing this procedure, there is an orderly collection of knowledge in which research builds on itself.

The Brain Operates Holistically

When discussing the brain, it is important to remember that it functions as a whole. Although certain parts of the brain perform specific functions, the parts are inter-connected. Parts of the brain communicate and rely on other parts of the brain. Speaking is a good example of this holistic function. The areas of the brain used for language structure and speech planning work together with the parts that control breathing, the vocal cords, the tongue, and the lips. And the thought behind the spoken utterance drives it all. No single part of the brain is completely responsible for the utterance. Certain areas are important and even essential to producing words, but no specific area works alone.

The following discussion concerns aspects of the brain that are important to communication. Entire books can and have been written about these parts of the brain. My goal here is to review the most important parts of the brain likely to be associated with stroke-related communication disorders. Other structures will be discussed because medical professionals frequently refer to them when discussing strokes and communication disorders.

The brain has control over all higher mental functions as well as ultimate con-trol over all movement (motor) and sensory occurrences (see Figure 1.1). It is made up of billions of nerve cells; both the brain and the central nervous system are com-posed of grey and white matter. The *cortex* (Latin for "bark") is composed of grey matter and makes up the outer layers of the brain (see Figure 1.2). It is less than an inch thick, although the thickness varies depending on the area of the brain. The white matter is inside the brain. Grey and white matter get their names from the way the brain looks when it is cut open.

The brain is soft and feels like Jell-O. Both the brain and the spinal cord are sur-rounded by three membranes. Sometimes they can become infected and swollen, indicating a serious medical condition known as *meningitis*. The brain has pockets deep within the white matter that are filled with fluid and are interconnected.

The brain is divided into halves called the *right* and *left hemispheres,* which are almost identical in appearance (see Figure 1.3). However, they are not identical in function. The right hemisphere is often called the *silent hemisphere*. While it is true that this hemisphere is largely devoted to nonverbal functions, it is not silent. Some speech and language functions are located there. It is primarily involved in are called *spatial and temporal* functions. That means that, in most people, the hemisphere is involved in the planning, perception, and conceptualization of

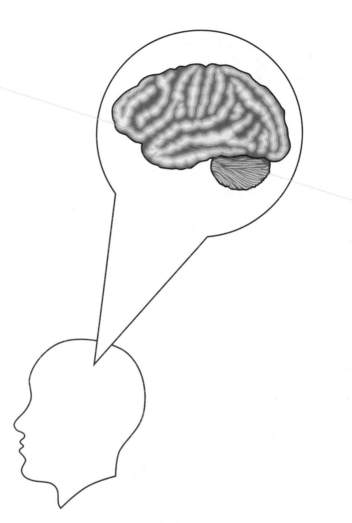

Figure 1.1   The left hemisphere of the human brain.

things related to time and space activities. A good example of this function is planning the best route to get to work. The speed of the car, anticipated travel time, and
distance covered are all considered.

The left hemisphere of the brain controls the right side of the body and vice
versa. In most people, the left hemisphere houses the speech and language functions. It is also called the *dominant hemisphere* because of the presence of language
and the fact that most people are right-handed. Left brain dominant people have a
stronger right eye, the right sides of their bodies are stronger, and they can even

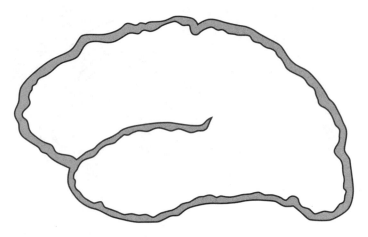

Figure 1.2   The grey matter of the human brain.

hear better with the right ear. This explains why many patients with stroke-related communication disorders have weakness or paralysis on the right sides of their bodies. The stroke occurred in the left hemisphere so the right side of the body has physical impairments. The opposite also occurs. Patients with right hemisphere strokes can have the physical limitations on the left sides of their bodies. Physical limitations and strokes will be discussed in greater detail in the section on strokes.

Left   Right

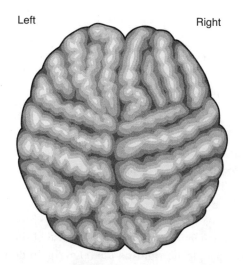

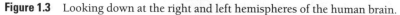

Figure 1.3   Looking down at the right and left hemispheres of the human brain.

The Special Case of Left-Handed People

Approximately 90 percent of people are right-handed. The remaining 10 percent are either left-handed or ambidextrous. *Ambidextrous* means that a person can use both the right and left hands equally well. The number of left-handed and ambidextrous people may be increasing because most teachers no longer force children to change their handedness. There may be cultural variations in the percentage of left-handers, but 10 percent is the usual figure given. Of this 10 percent of the population, most also have speech and language centers located primarily in the left hemisphere, just like right-handers. Interestingly, a small percentage of left-handed individuals have their speech and language centers located primarily in the right hemispheres of their brains. Although scientists disagree about the percentage of so-called "right language dominant" individuals, most agree that some people have language function located primarily in their right hemispheres. As a result, such a patient may have a major speech and language disorder and have physical limitations on the *left* side of the body. This is a rare occurrence, but it does happen.

The various structures of the brain are interconnected and communicate with one another. This is also true of the left and right hemispheres. A major connecting structure between the two hemispheres allows one side of the brain to know what the other side is thinking and doing. Sometimes this connecting pathway is destroyed, either by accident or by surgeons as part of a treatment. Researchers have studied these patients carefully because of what can be learned about brain function. These research projects, called *split-brain studies,* have provided much information about behavior and various aspects of language. One of the most interesting aspects of these studies is the fact that split-brain patients appear remarkably normal. For many of these patients, disabilities show up only on carefully designed tests. This tells us that, although the hemispheres communicate, they also are able to operate relatively independently.

The four lobes of the brain—the frontal, parietal, temporal, and occipital lobes—are named after the skull bones under which they are located (see Figure 1.4). When doctors discuss brain damage suffered by a patient, they often say that the stroke occurred in the frontal or temporal lobe. Doctors make this distinction because general functions have been identified with each lobe. The occipital lobe, at the back of the head, is involved primarily with visual functioning. The frontal lobe, at the front of the head, is where higher thought processes and reasoning occur. The frontal lobe is also where speech expression is located. Scientists believe that the frontal lobe is the most recently evolved in humans. The temporal and parietal lobes are concerned with understanding the speech of others and with reading.

Certain areas within the brain play important roles in communication. These roles involve memory and perception. For individuals to communicate normally,

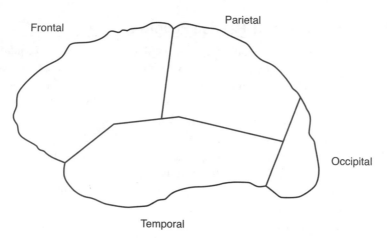

Figure 1.4   General boundaries of the lobes of the brain.

they must have intact memory both for distant events and for ongoing ones. In fact, the confusion seen in some stroke patients is directly related to memory problems. If patients could remember clearly what had gone on, they would be less confused. Because memory is so important and is involved in all aspects of human behavior, it is natural that there is no one single site for it in the brain. However, one structure—the *hippocampus* (from the Greek word for "sea horse")—is considered very important to the process of memory and learning.

What we know about the hippocampus has come from patients who have had damage to it and from the study of rats. Rats also have these structures in their brains. Scientists have purposefully damaged the hippocampus in rats and run experiments on their ability to remember how to run through mazes. It appears that damage to the hippocampus usually results in memory and learning problems. Humans with damage to this part of the brain show a variety of memory, learning, and behavioral problems. It is important to remember that no one part of the brain is completely responsible for memory, but the hippocampus is certainly an important structure.

Perception is the ability to attend to certain things and to shift attention from others. Like the functions of memory and learning, perception involves the whole brain, not just one part. Also like memory, one area of the brain is important to this ability. The *thalamus*, which gets its name from the Greek language and means "deep chamber," is located deep within the brain. Some specialists like to call the thalamus the *gatekeeper* because many of the sensations from the eyes, ears, and skin go through it. The thalamus, working with other parts of the brain, either permits or denies access to awareness from these senses.

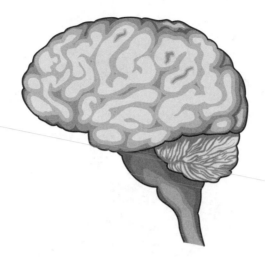

Figure 1.5   The human brainstem and cerebellum.

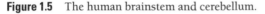

An interesting way of seeing how the thalamus works is to think about how your shoes feel on your feet. Until you allowed yourself to think about them, you had no conscious awareness. Once the gate was opened, you became aware of how they felt on your feet. Just as easily as you thought about your feet and shoes, awareness of them can be disregarded, especially when you turn your attention elsewhere. The thalamus plays an important part in this ability, not just for skin sensations but also for sight and hearing.

The brainstem is at the base of the head (see Figure 1.5). A good way of thinking about the brainstem is to imagine the spinal cord getting wider as it finally enters the brain. As a result, most of the senses coming from the body itself go through the brainstem and the impulses to move body parts go down it as well. The cerebellum is also located at the base of the head, and it is involved in the coordination of movements, which will be discussed later.

Speech and Language Centers of the Brain

Discovery of the location of the speech and language centers in the brain occurred in the mid-1800s. A French neurologist by the name of Pierre Paul Broca discovered the *expressive* speech and language center of the brain. He had a patient who had completely lost the ability to speak although the tongue was not paralyzed. After the patient died, examination of the brain showed the damage to be limited to the left hemisphere, particularly in the frontal lobe. After studying additional patients with loss of speech not due to tongue paralysis, in 1865 Broca uttered the famous

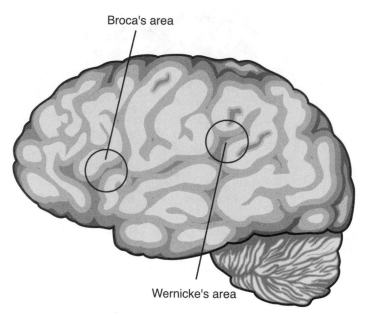

Broca's area

Wernicke's area

Figure 1.6   Approximate sites of Broca's and Wernicke's areas.

statement: "We speak with the left hemisphere." Later, Broca narrowed the area to a specific region in the left frontal lobe for most right-handed people. Over the years, doctors and scientists have come to refer to this area as *Broca's area* (see Figure 1.6). It is the primary expressive speech and language center of the brain.

Karl Wernicke was a German neurologist practicing medicine at about the same time as Broca. Using research methods similar to the ones used by Broca, he observed that there was an understanding area also located in the left hemisphere of the brain. In 1874 he presented a research paper identifying this area. Today, *Wernicke's area,* located in the temporal lobe, is an important *receptive* speech and language center. Wernicke's area is used to decode and understand the speech of others.

More than two areas of the brain are responsible for the ability to communicate. Speech and language are complicated functions; no act requires more brain power. Besides Broca's and Wernicke's areas of the brain, several other areas, when damaged, cause paralysis, weakness, or numbness of the speech muscles. An area of the brain called the *cerebellum* coordinates the production of ongoing speech; it is located in the lower part of the back of the head (see Figure 1.5). Speech requires rhythm and coordination, and this structure helps keep the output smooth and easy. And, of course, there are hundreds of nerves and muscles that must function for normal speech.

When scientists try to locate and describe areas of the brain, they engage in *brain mapping studies*. Similar to what geographers do, brain mapping studies identify an area and describe its boundaries. The goal of brain mapping is to identify a specific area of the brain with a particular function. Much of the research currently being done involves brain mapping. Broca and Wernicke were pioneers in this science. It is important to note that brain mapping is far from an exact science, especially concerning the language centers. Neither Wernicke's nor Broca's area has clear boundaries. Also, there are significant unique differences among people. The brain is as individual as fingerprints. Although certain landmarks can be identified and described, each individual has variations. Some variations are minor and relatively insignificant, but others are dramatic. A good example of a dramatic variation is that some people have speech and language centers located in the right hemisphere, not the left. With such variability, one can see why brain mapping is a difficult process and, as yet, far from precise.

Broca's and Wernicke's areas, along with other areas of the brain, perform extremely complicated functions. Speaking involves over 100 muscles and thousands of neurological impulses per second. Taking a thought and putting it into words is a complicated act. Sophisticated brain and nervous system activities are required to use the appropriate language structure; to program the tongue, lips, and soft palate muscles; and to pump air in and out of the lungs. The following general description of what is required to produce the word *Murphy* provides a glimpse into the complexity of the act.

> *Beth's brain selects the name "Murphy" from the thousands available in her vocabulary. If Beth were to say the word "Murphy" as part of a sentence, her brain would also have to select the appropriate grammar and syntax (word order). Beth has said her husband's name often in the past, and, as a result, most of the planning and production of the word are done unconsciously and in a fraction of a second. It is like typing; very little thought is given to the individual finger movements. Nonetheless, Beth's brain must first decide how much air is necessary to say the string of sounds in his name. "Murphy" has four distinct sounds: m, uhr, f, and ee. Beth's brain and nervous system determine the amount of air needed for the word and the muscles needed to take the air into her lungs. Air is compressed using the breathing muscles. Beth's lips then come together with just the correct amount of force to produce the sound m. The m sound must be made with the vibration of the vocal cords. Neurological signals are sent to Beth's vocal cords to vibrate with the necessary loudness and the appropriate pitch. A separate command is sent to the soft palate to lower, so that the m sound has the correct amount of nasalization. The next commands require Beth's lips to open gradually in production of the sound uhr. Her tongue*

also makes a slight adjustment. The speed at which the vocal cords vibrate is reduced so that her pitch drops slightly. Beth's soft palate also elevates so that the uhr *sound is not produced with too much nasalization. The production of the* f *sound requires Beth's upper teeth to touch her lower lip, and the compressed air coming from the lungs is squeezed through the opening between them. Separate neurological commands are sent to the vocal cords to stop them from vibrating, because the sound* f *is not produced with vocal cord vibration. The final* ee *sound requires the reactivation of the vocal cords and smooth, gradual adjustments of Beth's tongue and lips. Her soft palate must remain elevated on this sound. All the time this is occurring, Beth's breathing muscles must create just the correct amount of breath support, or the word will sound uneven and jerky. In addition, her brain, via the hearing mechanism, monitors the sounds. There is also feedback to the nervous system on the force, pressure, and touch of the speech muscles as they make the sounds. Beth's brain and nervous system must also plan and produce any accompanying gestures and facial expressions.*

The preceding example contains only a few of the requirements to simply say a single word. The whole act occurs in less than a second. The thinking, planning, and movements involved in speech are marvelous skills. A minor error, a slight irregularity in producing the word, would have been detected. Adjustments would have been made for serious errors in output. Scanning for errors occurs constantly. Considering the complexities of speech and language, it seems remarkable that we can speak at all and with so few mistakes.

Blood Supply to the Brain

Doctors have found that at any given time, the brain contains over 20 percent of the body's total blood supply, and it consumes over 25 percent of the oxygen. When there is a complete interruption of blood flow to the brain, consciousness is lost within 10 to 15 seconds. Permanent brain damage occurs when the blood supply is lost for more than a few minutes. This is because the brain has no backup oxygen reserves; it is completely dependent on ongoing blood supply.

Blood, rich with oxygen, is pumped into the brain from the heart through the neck. You can feel the pulsing of the blood flowing to the brain by putting your finger on the side of the windpipe a little above the voice box. Each pump of the heart causes a swelling of this artery. As the blood moves higher, the main arteries pool the blood into a common area. This is an important site because it is a place where blood from each artery combines. As a result, a person can have an interruption of blood flow below the common area in one of the arteries and yet not necessarily have significant brain damage. The reason is that the other arteries, if they are healthy, pick up the slack and keep blood flowing to the cells of the brain. Interruption to blood flow beyond the common area, within the brain, often results in brain damage because there is no way for the other arteries to compensate for the blocked one.

Before discussing strokes, it is important to explain how the arteries branch into smaller sizes. Arteries start off large but get progressively smaller as they branch out. This reduction in width continues until they are so small that they allow only individual blood cells to pass through. Brain cells use the oxygen and food in blood. The waste is deposited in the blood and returned to the heart and lungs to be replenished. This is how the brain, and other parts of the body, get the food and oxygen to function and stay alive.

Three important arteries in the brain, when plugged or broken, are often linked to communication disorders. You may hear the doctors talk about one or more of these arteries when referring to the type of stroke. One artery supplies a lot of blood to the front of the brain. Another provides blood toward the back of the brain. The middle artery is important because many significant speech and language centers get much of their blood from it.

Strokes

Stroke is defined as an interruption of blood flow to the brain. Some doctors call a stroke a CVA, or cerebral (brain) vascular (blood vessel system) accident. Sometimes, family members confuse a heart attack with a stroke. A heart attack occurs when blood flow is interrupted to the heart muscle. When an artery to the heart is plugged or bursts, part of it dies, and this is called a heart attack. Certainly, if the heart stops pumping blood for a period of time, brain cells will die, too. But this is a heart attack, not a stroke.

Doctors have identified two broad types of stroke. One type is the result of a blockage to an artery of the brain. The plug can be a blood clot or something else that stops the flow of blood. There can also be a gradual narrowing and hardening of the artery, which results from a buildup of plaque inside it. The other type of stroke occurs when the wall of the artery cannot tolerate the blood pressure. The wall is not strong enough to contain the blood and it bursts. Both types of stroke have one thing in common: They cause lack of oxygen to certain areas of the brain, resulting in the destruction of brain tissue.

According to medical researchers, the blockage type of stroke is the most common, accounting for about 75 percent of all strokes. The damage done to the brain depends on the site of the blockage in the brain and the size of the area damaged by the lack of blood. When a large plug stops the blood from flowing through one of the larger arteries, the brain damage is extensive. It is greater than if the plug were smaller and blocked only a small artery. A big plug deprives a larger area of the blood it needs.

Some plugs develop in other places of the body and lodge in the brain. For example, a blood clot may begin in an artery in the leg and eventually travel to the brain. Sometimes, blood will pool in the heart for a longer time than it should and clotting occurs. When the clot in the heart breaks loose, a shower of plugs can travel to other parts of the body, including the brain. This can be the result of a heart irregularity.

A burst type of stroke is often called a hemorrhage or *bleed*. There can be a buildup of blood below one of the membranes that surround the brain. The bleeding can affect only a small area of the brain or it can be large and result in extensive brain damage. Because of the broken artery, the blood spills out into the adjacent tissue and the area that needs the blood does not get enough. After a short period, the brain tissue is destroyed. In this way, the burst type of stroke is similar to a blockage. It is different in that a sizable amount of blood can escape and cause serious medical problems. One of the biggest problems is the pressure buildup in the brain caused by escaping blood. If the heart cannot overcome the pressure and get the required amount of blood supply to the brain cells, then brain death can occur. To combat this buildup of pressure, brain surgeons do an operation to remove the blood and release the pressure. Sometimes a tube is kept in the brain to drain the fluids.

When a wall of an artery becomes weak, it balloons outward due to the pressure exerted on it by the blood. This ballooning of an artery may precede a stroke. You may have observed the effects of a weakened wall of a bicycle tire inner tube. When the tube is filled with enough air, part of the tube, the weakest area, balloons out. This is similar to what can happen to an artery. When this occurs, the symptoms are similar to those seen in a stroke. The swollen part of the artery presses on a part of the brain, causing weakness or numbness. Speech, language, and thinking problems can also result. Surgeons can sometimes fix the balloon before it bursts if they discover it in time and can get to it, and if the ballooning is a part of the brain that can be operated on. These ballooned arteries can also exist without symptoms, and there may be no need to operate.

A person can also experience a temporary loss of blood to the brain as the result of a spasm in the blood vessel system or a blockage that clears by itself. The patient experiences a temporary loss of function because of the disruption of blood flow. Although like a stroke, the symptoms are temporary and do not leave the patient with a permanent disability.

High blood pressure is often linked to strokes. Normal blood pressure in an adult is about 120/80 units of pressure. Doctors and nurses sometimes just say that blood pressure is "120 over 80." These numbers reflect the pressure changes in the blood system during the contraction and relaxation of the heart. The top number is the pressure during the contraction phase of the heartbeat; the bottom one is the pressure during the relaxed phase. When people have high blood pressure, they are said to be *hypertensive*. Medications and lifestyle changes can help bring the numbers down.

Doctors and scientists have discovered that heredity, diet, and lifestyle patterns all contribute to the risk factors for a stroke. Heredity is an important factor. The tendency to be at risk for a stroke runs in families. Doctors often counsel patients to change their diets to decrease the risk of stroke. However, the role diet plays in the prevention of a stroke is a subject of controversy. Generally, the goal is to reduce the amount of fat in meals. Lifestyle changes involve getting more exercise and reducing stress. Once an individual has had a stroke, the doctor usually orders diet and lifestyle changes; once a person has had a stroke, there is a greater likelihood of having another.

Head trauma and certain diseases of the brain can cause communication disorders similar to those that occur in strokes. When these conditions affect the speech and language areas of the brain, they produce communication disorders. They also produce other kinds of problems typically not seen in stroke-related communication disorders. Many diseases of the brain can also result in communication disorders. One of the most severe is cancer. Cancer of the brain may cause communication disorders for two reasons. First, the tumor may be located in one or more areas necessary for normal speech and language. Second, sometimes brain surgeons must sacrifice some aspect of the ability to communicate to get to the tumor to remove it. In addition, radiation and chemotherapy to kill the cancer may affect an individual's ability to communicate.

Some of the other medical conditions that can cause a communication disorder include infections and degenerative diseases. When an infection occurs within the brain, there may be pockets containing bacteria and other products related to the infection, such as white blood cells. The brain is damaged in two ways. First, the infection destroys brain tissue at the site of the infection. Second, there is frequently an increase in the pressure within the brain. Too much pressure can destroy brain cells as well.

There is a long list of degenerative diseases that can affect the brain. Alzheimer's disease, chronic alcoholism, and Parkinson's disease are among the more common. These diseases, and others like them, can directly result in communication disorders by impairing the functioning of one or more of the speech and language areas. Indirectly, they can affect communication because of impaired memory or difficulty attending to people and things.

As you can see, the human ability to communicate is a marvelous skill. We communicate on many levels all of the time. Communication is an extremely complicated ability involving the thoughts behind the utterance, hundreds of muscles, and thousands of neurological impulses. Although specific areas are important to normal communication, the brain operates as a whole. The hemispheres, lobes, and other areas of the brain are in constant contact with one another, communicating and sharing information. A stroke occurs when blood supply to the brain is interrupted and permanent damage occurs. There are different types of strokes, and the impact on the patient's ability to communicate is dependent on the area of the brain deprived of blood and the amount of brain damage, although small areas of damage can result in major communication disorders.

It is a difficult time for family members when a loved one has suffered a stroke, perhaps especially difficult if he or she has been left with a communication disorder. There are many unknowns, especially early on. What will life be like for the patient and for loved ones? What will the patient's quality of life be like? How effective will the medical treatments and rehabilitation be? There are often many medical professionals to deal with, each with a specialty. Patients and family alike can feel overwhelmed by the medical words, diagnostic tests, and expensive treatments. Although it may sound like a cliché, information is the best antidote to fear and uncertainty. In the next chapter, we will discuss the nature of stroke-related communication disorders. Reading about them will help eliminate some of the unknowns about stroke and the communication disorders sometimes caused by them. By learning about these disorders, you and your loved one can better overcome those that *can* be overcome and learn to accept those that are permanent.

CHAPTER 2
Loss of Language

The limits of my language stand for the limits of my world.
—LUDWIG WITTGENSTEIN

Rarely do we use the word "lucky" when referring to a person who has suffered a stroke. But some people are lucky indeed. Some people who have strokes are spared problems with most day-to-day activities. Thinking, walking, dressing, and eating are still done easily. By far the luckiest of them all are the ones who can still communicate. A stroke can lead to many kinds of communication disorders. It can weaken the tongue, causing sounds to be slurred. The vocal cords can be completely or partially paralyzed. When a stroke impairs the muscles of breathing, the patient can have problems compressing air to be used for speech. A category of speech disorders includes those that disrupt the planning of muscle movements necessary to produce strings of sounds. Some patients cannot understand the speech of others. Strokes can destroy the ability to read and write. Some stroke survivors cannot remember any words; others just forget pronouns or certain verbs, although this is a rare occurrence. More often than not, two or more of the above, and a host of other problems, combine to paint a complex picture of silence and isolation for the patient and pain and frustration for the patient's loved ones.

In severe cases, a stroke can render a person unable to walk, talk, eat, dress, or even go to the bathroom. Those close to the stroke survivor also suffer. They confront major family changes in the wake of highly charged emotions. A stroke is an emotional event for the entire family. But this is not a time for despair, either for you or the patient. It is not a time to give up. There is light at the end of the tunnel.

Communication disorders resulting from stroke have been studied for decades. Much is known about them and more is being learned every day. Millions of people have had stroke-related communication disorders and gone on to lead relatively normal lives. Even patients who have suffered major communication disorders have been able to overcome many problems. As for the insurmountable problems, patients have learned to go around them. Many family members and friends have been able to adjust, too. By learning about these disorders, you and the patient can gradually adjust to the changes caused by the stroke. Caring family members, armed with knowledge and teamed with rehabilitation specialists, can make this difficult time much easier. The adjustments and changes required of everyone can be made smoothly. The first step in making the best of this difficult situation is to learn as much as possible about the communication disorders resulting from a stroke.

A few words must be said about how these disorders are presented in this book because not all professionals look at them in the same way. In the world of academics, professionals are divided into "schools of thought." This means that like-minded people think about these disorders in similar ways. We have all heard of the parable of the three blind men and the elephant. Each touches the elephant in different places—the trunk, tusk, and tail—and has a different idea of the nature of the creature. Each of the blind men perceives only a part of this big animal and thus has a unique way of looking at it. In many ways, the communication disorders resulting from stroke are like the elephant and the professionals are the blind people. The many different types of stroke-related communication disorders are viewed differently by different professionals.

Physicians are most concerned with the patient's medical condition. Naturally, they want to reduce the effects of the stroke, including the communication disorder. But their concern is not limited to the communication disorder; they must treat all of the stroke-related issues. Consequently, doctors see communication disorders as only one of many symptoms of the stroke. To the physician, the communication disorder is similar to the other symptoms of the stroke in that it needs to be evaluated, treated, and monitored. If there are therapies, drugs, surgeries, or other treatments available, the physician will want the patient to receive them. As such, the physician's view of stroke-related communication disorders focuses on medical diagnosis and treatment. The physician is responsible for the whole patient.

Researchers and other people who develop theories are mostly concerned with the brain, nerves, and muscles of speech. They collect data, usually from large groups of subjects. Frequently, their interest is in gaining more knowledge about general evaluation and treatment approaches. Sometimes, researchers engage in what is called "pure" research. Here, the goal of a study is not necessarily applied to a particular treatment. In fact, there may be no practical goal to the research. In pure research, studies are conducted just to find out something and to satisfy the scientific quest for knowledge. As a result, researchers tend to look at stroke-related communication disorders as a part of human existence that needs to be explored. They create theories to try to increase the general knowledge base about humankind.

Speech-language pathologists are concerned with therapies to help patients overcome stroke-related communication disorders. The evaluations they conduct are designed to find out what type of communication disorder exists in a particular patient. The goal is to discover the patient's individual strengths and weaknesses in the area of communication and to apply the best therapy. These therapies are taught in speech-language pathology and audiology programs in colleges and universities, and many are teaching, counseling, and behavior modification techniques borrowed from education, psychology, and other professions. Although speech-language pathologists are also concerned with the whole patient, their view of stroke-related communication disorders is primarily therapeutic: What can be done to help patients help themselves?

Other professionals who study stroke-related communication disorders also have their own perspectives. Linguists and psychologists study these disorders either directly or indirectly for a variety of reasons, and they often have unique ways of looking at strokes and the communication disorders that result from them.

As you can see, there are many professionals with unique perspectives on this complex subject. It is not surprising that there are many different schools of thought. Some schools of thought revolve around a theory or diagnostic test or are based on the writings of a leader in the profession. There is a geographical trend as well; people in some regions of the country look at these disorders in the same way. Although there are schools of thought with loyal followers, many professionals are eclectic, meaning that they do not rigidly follow a specific approach to viewing stroke-related communication disorders. They apply the school of thought most appropriate to the needs of individual patients.

This book deals with the most common stroke-related communication disorders in the most basic terms. We will not delve into extremely rare communication disorders. For one thing, there are too many to cover in a book of this size. Additionally, there is no need to get into a discussion of every school of thought as it pertains to stroke-related communication disorders. Some are complex and draw heavily on neurology. Others are primarily of interest to specialists.

The "Big Three" Communication Disorders

This book covers the three basic types of stroke-related communication disorders: amnesia (loss of memory) for words, tangled tongue, and nerve and muscle deficits. Medical professionals refer to them as *aphasia, apraxia of speech,* and *dysarthria,* respectively. Other frequently occurring symptoms of a stroke that may indirectly disrupt communication will also be discussed.

Stroke can impair a person's use and understanding of language. Although there are many forms of this disorder, the essence of it is that the patient loses the memory of words. A host of other ills, including head trauma and diseases that affect the brain, can also cause amnesia for words. *Aphasia* is the medical term for the loss of language due to brain damage.

Speech planning and sequencing are important parts of communicating normally. When an individual produces speech, all of the muscle movements must be planned and the string of sounds produced in the proper sequence. When there are problems with this ability, the tongue and other parts of the speech mechanism become tangled. *Apraxia of speech* is the medical term referring to problems with planning and sequencing speech due to brain damage.

Strokes often impair the speech nerves and muscles. When this happens, patients slur their sounds and have problems with rhythm and speed. *Dysarthria* is the medical term for these types of disorders. Actually, the term *dysarthria* represents a group of disorders that is the result of specific types of paralysis or weakness. Some patients with dysarthria also have problems chewing and swallowing.

In a medical environment, you often find professionals using medical labels that begin with the letter *a* and some words that begin with the letters *dys*. As a rule, when a term a health care professional uses begins with the letter *a*, the *a* means "without." Therefore, the word *aphasia* technically means "without language." *Apraxia* means without the ability to plan and sequence movements. *Anarthria* means that the patient has no speech because of nerve and muscle problems. When the core of the word is preceded by the letters *dys*, it means "impaired." Therefore, *dysphasia* means "impaired language." Although there is some language, what is produced is impaired. *Dyspraxia* means that there is impaired ability to plan and sequence the speech remaining after the stroke. *Dysarthric* patients can produce some speech, but the speech is impaired due to nerve and muscle deficits. Many words in medicine can be broken down into segments of separate meanings based on the core word and prefixes and suffixes. For example, the *itis* suffix usually means inflamed or swollen. The word *tonsillitis*, then, means that the tonsils are inflamed or swollen. Another example is the suffix *ectomy*, which means surgical removal. Tonsillectomy, appendectomy, and laryngectomy mean surgical removal of the tonsils, appendix, and larynx, respectively.

Amnesia for words (aphasia), tangled tongue (apraxia of speech), and nerve and muscle disorders (dysarthria) are the "big three" communication disorders associated with strokes. Although both aphasia and apraxia of speech begin with the letter *a*, many medical people do not make the "without/impaired" distinction. Therefore, the distinction will not be made in this book. It is easier to talk about these disorders using the common usage of the words. For example, when referring to a stroke patient who has lost some of his or her language functions, the traditional word *aphasic* will be used rather than the technically correct word *dysphasic*.

Aphasia: More Than a Speech Disorder

The patient with aphasia has lost all or part of language. This disorder has many aspects because human language has many aspects. Obviously, before a disorder of language can be understood, we must first explore our ability to use language normally. Only in understanding normal language can we appreciate what happens when it is lost.

Language is broader than speech. Language has to do with words, letters, gestures, numbers, and thinking; speech has to do with sounds. Speaking is just one part of language. Language includes reading and writing as well as gestures and signs. Language is made up of nouns, verbs, adjectives, prepositions, and those other parts of speech we try so hard to learn in school. Language is word order and it is grammar.

Communication is never one-sided. Like a tango, it takes two. Someone expresses an idea and another receives the information. Language is both expressive and receptive. The person speaking has someone who understands what was spoken. The writer communicates with the reader. Gestures are both expressive and receptive, too. A fist held in the air in congested traffic expresses the anger of the driver. Anyone who sees it understands the frustration. We wave "good-bye" and "hello." The expressive modes of language are speaking, writing, and gestures. The receptive modes are listening, reading, and gestures. We also send and receive information with numbers. Ten dollars, whether written or spoken, means 10 one-dollar bills to both the clerk at the store and the customer.

Hopefully, when we hear someone speak, understanding takes place. The speaker's thoughts, ideas, and feelings have been shared through language. He or she has taken an idea and put it into a form and structure shared by people who speak the same language. Because the speaker and listener are speaking the same language, the idea is communicated. For there to be communication, the sounds that make up the words must follow the rules of a common language. Vowels and consonants must be spoken correctly. The words must be put in proper order. For example, the meaning of the phrase "Dog bites man" is drastically different from "Man bites dog." Finally, for there to be communication of an idea, both speaker and listener must share a common meaning of the words. The word *comb*, whether spoken in English, Spanish, or Hopi, must refer to the same grooming tool. Any breakdown in the rules of the language can cause communication to be impaired. The words of any language are made up. Over thousands of years, groups of people gradually agreed that certain sounds, when said in a particular word, have a certain meaning. People who speak English agree that the sounds *c* and *ar*, when put together, refer to a machine with four tires, a steering wheel, hood, and engine. *Car* refers to a category of vehicles. Everyone who speaks French agrees that *Oui* means "Yes." Spanish speakers agree that *Dios* means "God." People who learn Morse code agree that the clicks or tones *dit dit dit, dah, dah, dah, dit, dit, dit* mean "SOS" or "help."

Children start to learn the meanings of words at an early age. The buildup of a vocabulary begins with words such as *Mama* and *Dada* and grows by leaps and bounds, especially during the first seven or eight years of life. By adulthood the average speaker understands more than 20,000 words but typically uses about 2,000 words in everyday speech.

Language, then, consists of sounds built into words and words built into phrases. When language is written, it consists of letters built into written words and words connected to make up sentences. Rules must be followed to build words and to string them into phrases and sentences. Language requires that the words have a shared meaning. When the rules are followed and the meaning is understood, language allows communication.

Language is also used in thinking. People think in words, too. This is called *inner speech*. In a way, inner speech can be viewed as the way people talk to themselves. We use words to solve problems, and our inner voice often serves as our conscience. Some types of thoughts are primarily verbal; they cannot be thought clearly without using words. Thinking with words (verbal thought) and other types of thought processes in aphasic persons will be discussed in Chapter 6.

Language is more than just sounds and words. Words carry meaning; they represent underlying concepts. Language has both deep and surface meanings. A good way to understand these differences is to examine sentences that have two or more meanings. On the surface, there is one meaning, but there can be a deeper one as well. The following sentences have two or more meanings:

"The man decided on the trains."
"The girl broke the window with her brother."
"The Cannibals had the Missionaries for dinner."
"She dislikes big dogs and cats."

If you think carefully about the preceding sentences, more than one meaning can be attached to the same combination of words. The meaning is dependent on the context of the statements. Language is often dependent on context.

Aphasia is not a speech disorder; it is a breakdown in language. This is an important distinction for all family members, friends, and acquaintances to understand. Your loved one with aphasia may have the muscle ability to speak normally. The ability to compress the air in the lungs for speech might be normal. The vocal cords, tongue, and lips might also be unaffected by the stroke. Because of aphasia, however, the patient's ability to communicate can still be impaired. This impairment may be so severe that the patient is left without the ability to read, write, speak, or understand the speech of others. Many professionals use the word *global* to refer to severe or complete aphasia. At first, to you and to the patient, this seems like an unusual and bizarre disorder. It is not. Aphasia has been around for centuries.

The early Egyptians suffered from aphasia. One scholar wrote about a patient with a head wound who was "speechless." The early Greeks and Romans also had words for patients who were unable to speak and write. Some writers of the past tried to locate the area of the body that caused the communication disorder, although most missed the point by quite a distance. Before the correct parts of the brain responsible for language were discovered, incorrect theories abounded. Looking back, it is amazing that so little was known about the brain. Some early theories proposed that aphasia was caused by too much fluid in the brain or because there was damage to areas deep within the white matter. In the early 1800s, it was believed that medical people could tell an individual's personality by feeling the bumps on the skull. Some thought that these lines could reveal how intelligent, verbal, or creative a person was. Of course, this theory was false. It wasn't until the mid-1800s that the specific areas of the brain responsible for aphasia were found. The way they were found and the pioneers who discovered them are discussed in Chapter 1.

Most people have had problems at some time remembering the name of a thing or an acquaintance. We are all too familiar with the embarrassment of being unable to remember the name of a particular tool or object. We are left to describe it or explain its function to an impatient clerk. Being unable to remember a person's name is also a common occurrence. Though we can remember the person's face and other details, the name escapes us. Then, minutes later when it is too late, the name pops into our head. Because we all experience these minor word-finding problems, it is easy to understand what it is like to have a very mild case of aphasia.

It is much harder for us to understand what it is like to have complete aphasia: the total loss of language. There are three reasons for this. First, we take language for granted. Thousands of times a day we read, write, speak, and understand what is spoken to us. We are constantly thinking to ourselves in inner speech. We do it so automatically, so unthinkingly, that we are unable to fathom what it would be like to have it completely taken from our lives. Second, to understand well what it is like to have complete aphasia, we would need to talk to people who have recovered from this condition. We would need to have many patients describe, in detail, what it is like to have language removed from day-to-day routines. Patients who have lost all of their language only to regain it could provide valuable insights into this disorder. Unfortunately, few, if any, patients who have suffered complete aphasia for an extended period ever have all of their language return. Many patients with severe aphasia do make good gains in their communication abilities, but they are unable to explain and describe their experience in detail.

The third reason it is difficult to understand what it is like to have complete aphasia has to do with testing. The tests that could provide insight into what it is like to have severe aphasia would require good language abilities by the person taking the test. Many of these reading and writing tests are simply beyond the ability of the severely impaired aphasic person. Even clinical interviews require the subject to understand the questions and be able to express the answers in sufficient detail. It would be wonderful to have a stethoscope that could be placed on the severe aphasic patient's head to listen to his or her thoughts, to understand the emotions, and to see the world as the patient sees it. Then we could truly understand the disability. Unfortunately, no such tool is available, and understanding what it is like to have complete aphasia is a difficult task indeed.

What remains in our attempts to understand complete aphasia are incomplete reports from partially recovered patients. These reports are certainly valuable and are perhaps the best sources of firsthand information. Much understanding has been gained from such reports, especially about the emotional and psychological aspects of aphasia. Family members and friends of patients also have provided useful information. Because they knew the person well before the stroke, they are able to give valuable insight into the changes that have occurred. Clinical observations also provide important information. Looking at what patients can and cannot do in therapy gives clinicians some understanding of patients' thoughts and emotions. We can also understand more about what it is like to have severe aphasia by listening to reports from patients with mild and moderate aphasia and generalizing from their reports to severe ones. Finally, research conducted on the brain provides more information about complete aphasia. By discovering the areas of the brain that are responsible for certain functions, researchers better understand what it is like to suffer a complete loss of language. Knowing the function of a particular area of the brain helps give insight into what has been destroyed by a stroke.

To date our understanding of what it is like to have complete aphasia, the total loss of language, is incomplete. At best we have unproven theories, superficial test results, observations, and insufficient reports from patients and family members. Taken together, these sources provide an increasing understanding of the trials and tribulations of the severely impaired aphasic person. We do know that aphasia is much more than a speech disorder. Hopefully, someday all aspects of aphasia will be known. But until that day, patients, family members, clinicians, and all who study aphasia must operate on the facts, data, and theories available. Because we have an incomplete understanding of something does not mean that we give up; we do our best with what we have.

One way of understanding what it would be like to have complete aphasia is to imagine that you suddenly have been transported to a different country with a strange, new culture, where everyone uses a language unfamiliar to you. You find yourself in a familiar situation, such as in a restaurant, classroom, or church. You look around and most of the objects are familiar. You know that a fork is for eating, a pencil is for writing, and the pew is for sitting. There are written words everywhere: on the menu, chalkboard, program. You try to read them, but the letters do not look like letters you know. Perhaps, you think, they are Japanese or Chinese letters. Some are recognizable as letters but they seem to spell nonsense words, words without vowels, words with only vowels, or words with strange combinations of consonants. Occasionally, you recognize the words but are unable to remember what they mean or you give them the wrong meaning. Attempts to communicate in writing to the server, teacher, or minister result in garbled letters and words that communicate nothing except your frustration and dismay.

To you, the speech of others is a jumbled mess. You do not recognize many sounds and when they are combined, the words are strange and foreign. More often than not, the server, teacher, or minister shouts them in a failed attempt to improve your understanding by increasing the volume. Occasionally, you recognize the word only to be confused about the meaning. This is painfully apparent when requests are made of you. You reach for the fork instead of the knife, the pen instead of the pencil, your hat instead of your coat. Longer utterances are even more confusing.

Your attempts to speak are met with failure. Sometimes you have difficulty remembering how to begin a word. Other times you begin the word only to forget how to string together the rest of the sounds correctly. The harder you try, the more errors you make. When you do form a word, the meaning is either lost or wrong. Although it is difficult to monitor your output, you can sense the errors. Then, out of the blue, a swear word or a family member's name is uttered correctly, almost perfectly. These words come best when you give them no or little forethought. Even gestures such as where to sit or stand are confusing, as are coins and counting. After several failed attempts to order, answer a question, or say "good-bye," you sense the futility of it all and simply shut up.

Aphasia Disrupts All Avenues of Communication

Aphasia is a language disorder and as such impairs more than simply the ability to speak. All avenues of language can be destroyed or impaired. Each of these avenues of communication needs to be discussed separately because there are unique aspects to each of them and a variety of problems may exist. First, the reading and writing problems resulting from aphasia will be discussed. Reading and writing problems are often called *graphic* disturbances by health care professionals. They are somewhat different from the speaking and understanding problems associated with aphasia because they are products of education. Whereas all normal children naturally learn to speak and understand the language to which they are exposed, reading and writing must be taught and learned. Children are taught to give meaning to "scribbles."

Three General Types of Reading Problems

Reading problems found in aphasia can range from minor confusion about the content of a long passage to the absolute inability to read anything. The extent of the problem is related to site and size of the brain damage. Many reading problems are associated with damage to the parietal lobe of the left hemisphere of the brain (see Chapter 1). Researchers have identified three general types of reading disturbances occurring in stroke-related communication disorders. Sometimes a stroke can cause only a reading problem while leaving other forms of communication normal.

The reading problems in aphasia are not the result of the patient being visually impaired or blind. Although it is certainly true that strokes can cause a variety of vision problems, the reading defects in aphasia are not caused by problems seeing the letters and words. Of course, some stroke patients can have both vision and aphasic reading problems.

In a common type of reading problem, patients can read some words aloud but have poor comprehension of the material. Sometimes they can comprehend the written material better during silent reading. With this type of reading problem, patients' writing is also impaired and so, too, are their other language functions. The reading comprehension problems are not just for long, complicated passages but also for simple, elementary school types of sentences and paragraphs. Generally, these comprehension problems are caused by poor attention, not remembering what the words mean, and not being able to follow the idea of the text. Some people with aphasia get stuck on a particular word and cannot go forward. Others cannot shift their attention from one idea to the next one fast enough.

The second type of reading disturbance is one in which patients cannot remember phonics. Instead of sounding out a word, patients read what they "think" the word says. Patients with this type of problem, when reading aloud, might say words that are similar in meaning to the correct ones. For example, the sentence, "He looked at his watch to see if he was late," might be read aloud as, "He looked at his clock to see if he was early." Although what is read is incorrect, there is an association between the correct word and the one spoken by the patient.

The final category of reading disturbance is rare. In these few cases, a patient cannot recognize words but retains the ability to write. This is sometimes called *pure word blindness,* though there is nothing wrong with the patient's eyes. Although the patient cannot read words, he or she can often understand them when they are spelled aloud by someone else or when they are traced on the palms or arms. Some of these patients cannot read what they have just written!

Like most communication disorders resulting from stroke, the type of reading problem is dependent on the site and size of damage in the brain. Many patients have a combination of these reading disorders. With reading problems, the nature of the disorder is also dependent on how the person was taught to read. Some people were taught the sound out method while others were taught using sight words. Many were taught to read using a combination of methods. Some people were never taught to read and others do so poorly.

Most Aphasic Individuals Write Like They Speak

As previously explained, the left hemisphere of the brain controls the right side of the body, and the right side of the brain controls the left side of the body. Many communication disorders are the result of damage to the left hemisphere of the brain. While it is true that some disorders may result from damage to the right hemisphere of the brain, most occur because of left hemisphere damage (see Chapter 1). This is the reason that many patients with stroke-related communication disorders have weakness or complete paralysis of their right arm and hand. Most people use the right hand for writing.

Right-hand weakness or paralysis is not always the source of the writing problems found in stroke-related communication disorders. If hand paralysis were the main source of the writing problem, most patients would simply put the pen or pencil in the left hand and write that way. Sure, when right-handers write with the left hand the writing is clumsy and awkward, but most people can get their thoughts on paper albeit with poor penmanship.

The writing problems resulting from stroke have to do with remembering what letters mean and how to create them on paper. Occasionally, the writing problems involve the patient writing words that do not belong in a sentence. Some patients mislabel objects and things; other patients make one or two scribbles that go on and on.

Problems with writing can include difficulty copying forms. For example, if a triangle or square is drawn on the top of a sheet of paper, a patient with severe writing problems would be unable to copy it. Copying letters, words, and sentences can also be difficult. One of the most difficult tasks is to write to dictation. When the patient is asked to write the words spoken by someone else, a major breakdown in communication often results. This may be primarily a problem with writing, but it may also be one of understanding the words of the speaker.

Simple Arithmetic Impairment in Aphasia

The problems aphasic patients have with arithmetic are not restricted to complex formulas and problems in geometry, algebra, or calculus. Most of us have problems doing complex math, especially if we have not done it for a long time. Problems doing high-level math can be likened to speaking a foreign language that you studied in high school. If you have not had an opportunity to practice it since high school, you likely will be very rusty. The same holds true for high-level mathematical problems and concepts. But the problems aphasic patients have doing math go beyond long-forgotten skills. They have difficulty doing simple and common problems. Their deficits involve day-to-day activities such as counting, knowing that two plus two equals four, and that ten minus seven equals three. Making change is one of the most practical problems. For example, many aphasic people would find it difficult to know how much change to give a customer if a purchase cost $8.95. It would be hard for many stroke patients to make the correct change for a 20-dollar bill.

Problems understanding money significantly limit a person's independence. Buying a blouse, hat, hammer, or even a hamburger requires that the patient know whether the prices are reasonable and within budget. Large purchases are even more critical. Purchasing a television, stereo system, or car involves price comparisons and math calculations. The aphasic person may be taken advantage of financially. Consumers are often warned to "let the buyer beware," and this is certainly true for the aphasic person. Of course, the severity of the math difficulties must be considered when deciding how many limits must be placed on your loved one.

There are two reasons why aphasic patients have difficulty with arithmetic. First, doing math involves speaking, understanding, reading, and writing. Whatever limitations stroke patients have with these avenues of communication will also affect their success with arithmetic. Patients who have many problems putting down their thoughts on paper will also have difficulty putting down math problems on paper. When the ability to write words is impaired, so, too, is the ability to write down numbers.

The second reason patients have problems with arithmetic after a stroke involves the fact that math, too, is a language. Philosophers and mathematicians like to call it the "universal" language. In many ways, the number eight, whether written or spoken, has meaning just like other words do. When the number eight is put in this statement, "Eight plus three equal eleven," correct grammar and syntax are necessary, just as in any other language. Placement of the number on the wrong side of the equal sign causes the statement to have a completely different meaning. When the language centers of the brain are damaged because of a stroke, the ability to do and understand math is also likely to be harmed.

The degree of disability felt by aphasic patients because of reading, writing, and arithmetic problems varies greatly depending on their living conditions. A stroke patient with these communication problems who continues to work, drive, and shop faces more communication challenges than does a patient who is confined to a skilled nursing facility. Certainly, it is good if a patient in a nursing home can read, write, and do arithmetic. However, nursing homes and other long-term care facilities supervise and protect these patients. The people who live in them are not independent and the staff help them with day-to-day activities. They provide correct change and transportation and shop for them. They help with writing and reading letters from loved ones. They dial telephone numbers and do many other things to help those who cannot read or write. Not all institutions have the staff or time for all of these activities, but many are extremely helpful.

Many individuals who have had strokes continue to lead independent lives outside nursing homes and hospitals. Assessing the problems they have with reading, writing, and arithmetic is important when making decisions about how independently they can live their lives. One of the biggest concerns has to do with driving a car. Family members must ask the question: "Since the stroke, can the patient read and know numbers well enough to drive?" Often this is a difficult question for you to answer, and it is important to work closely with the health care team in making these decisions. To see how Verne and Nancy's children dealt with issues related to driving, read Chapter 13: Profiles in Recovery and the case study on page 225.

The laws governing whether a stroke patient can drive vary among states. The stroke survivor as well as other drivers and pedestrians must be protected. After a person has had a stroke, it is usually desirable and necessary that he or she retake both the written and driving tests. Most states require that a physician also verify that the patient is competent to drive a car. If patients cannot read, write, or understand numbers well enough to pass the written test, then safety dictates that they not be allowed to drive. A speech-language pathologist or occupational therapist can target the driving tests as goals for therapy. Though driving is an important part of being independent (ask any teenager), there are other ways a stroke survivor can shop, visit, and get to work. Many communities provide transportation services for the disabled.

Use and Understanding of Gestures

Family members of the patient with severe or complete aphasia often ask why the patient cannot be taught sign language; they assume that by using the hands and fingers to communicate, the speech problem can be bypassed. At first glance, this seems like a solution to the problem. For many patients who have paralyzed speech muscles but intact language, learning sign language is an option. Unfortunately, learning and using sign language is beyond the range of many aphasic patients. Recall that aphasia is a language disturbance, not a speech problem. As such, all language is impaired, and this includes the ability to use and understand signs and other complicated gestures.

Several studies have looked at how deaf people fare when they suffer from aphasia. These studies have shown that deaf individuals who knew sign language before having the stroke often lose the ability to communicate in sign language because of aphasia. The reason for losing sign language was not weakness or paralysis of the hands or fingers; it was loss of language ability.

Sometimes, speech-language pathologists will teach hand gestures along with speech. The goal is to pair the gesture with the utterance. In some patients, doing both helps the patient to be able to remember words and to get them out. Such pairing helps many patients start a word or sentence. But the goal is not to learn the complicated sign language of the deaf; it is to use signs, gestures, and speech to maximize the ability to communicate. Another big problem with teaching sign language to aphasic patients is that not many people use and understand this form of communication. Therefore, it is not a very practical way of achieving independence.

Broca's Aphasia

As previously discussed, writing and using gestures provide different avenues by which people can express themselves. When a person has a stroke, these avenues of expression are sometimes impaired or eliminated. The writing and gesture problems can be hindering and disabling to the patient. They are part of the syndrome of aphasia. The word *syndrome* means a collection or group of symptoms that often occur together. However, most people use speech as the primary means of getting across their thoughts and feelings to other people. A stroke can impair or destroy this avenue of communication as well.

Many health care professionals use the term *Broca's aphasia* to refer to communication disorders that are primarily expressive in nature. As explained in Chapter 1, this type of communication disorder gets its name from Pierre Paul Broca, who first identified the expressive speech and language center in the brain. When a person experiences damage to this area of the brain, speech is choppy and punctuated by many pauses and fillers. Broca's aphasia is nonfluent—it is a struggled attempt to talk. Selecting the correct sounds and words is difficult, so patients have problems remembering the appropriate words for expressing thoughts, naming objects, and sharing emotions. As a rule, when patients have to produce a longer utterance, they have more difficulty dealing with grammar and syntax. The rules of grammar and word order are impaired, especially in longer utterances. The severity of Broca's aphasia can range from a mild nuisance to the complete loss of expressive communication.

Actually, there are many subtypes of expressive aphasia, and authorities use a variety of labels to refer to them. The common link among them is that stroke patients have trouble expressing themselves. The words to express the ideas are not readily available. Even when the words are found, patients have trouble getting the sounds to come out. When sounds are made, they may be the wrong ones or in the wrong order. And because the understanding areas of the brain have not necessarily been damaged because of the stroke, Broca's aphasia patients often know when they make mistakes. Like everyone else, when they make a mistake they try to correct it . . . and this, too, is often unsuccessful. Errors and attempts to correct imperfect speech result in the pauses, fillers, and struggle seen in this type of stroke-related communication disorder.

Patients with Broca's aphasia sometimes "telegraph" their ideas by leaving out some words. To understand this aspect of aphasia, it is necessary to separate words into two categories. Language contains both *function* and *content* words. Content words include nouns, verbs, and adjectives, and they carry the content of the idea. Function words, such as articles and conjunctions, are only important to the proper grammar of the statement. When people with Broca's aphasia speak, they often omit the function words and leave only the content words. As a result, only the most important words carry the thought. This is called *telegraphic speech,* because when people first began to communicate by telegram, the telegraph company charged by the word, so messages contained only the most important words to express an idea.

Attention span also influences the length of speech. If a person's attention span is limited to only four or five syllables at a time, thinking in long utterances is difficult. These patients are forced to limit their speech to shorter sentences, typically like those seen in young children with immature grammar. Because of their short attention span, they have trouble expressing longer and more complicated ideas.

Specialists disagree about what causes telegraphic speech. Some believe it is caused by damage to grammar centers of the brain because the patient has lost primarily the function words. But the grammar problems can also go deeper than just a loss of function words. In some patients, knowing the meaning and importance of the grammar may be lost. The grammatical ideas behind words such as *before* and *after* may be impaired by the stroke. Some stroke patients may not remember the meaning of the words *up, down, over,* and *under.*

Some authorities believe that the cause of telegraphic speech is a general loss in the number of total words available to the patient. We have fewer function than content words in our expressive vocabulary. As a result, a general loss of words may result in only the content ones remaining. Both theories have merit, but the latter is considered the best explanation for telegraphic speech in most stroke survivors.

Automatic Speech

An interesting aspect of Broca's aphasia is that even severely affected patients may have some normal speech. In a sea of revisions, word-finding problems, and struggled attempts to string sounds together, there are occasionally islands of near-perfect words or even phrases. These are called *automatic* speech because they happen with little or no forethought. They seem to come from out of the blue. When this speech occurs, individuals with Broca's aphasia often seem as surprised by their ease of expression as are the listeners. It is perplexing to struggle and toil one minute, only to have these words and phrases come out automatically.

The occurrence of automatic utterances in Broca's aphasia is related to the idea that some speech emerges with little or no thought. Greetings and the "How ya doing?" and "How's it going?" questions are speech said with little, if any, forethought.

Few people expect, or want, for that matter, a thoughtful reply to the passing query, "How are you doing?" It is a verbal gesture, a sort of wave with words. These are the types of words and phrases available for clear, near-perfect expression by some Broca's aphasia patients. Words and phrases related to exasperation also occur easily, such as "Oh, boy," "I'm outa here," and "Now, come on." Many Broca's aphasia patients also have more access to formally *over-learned* words and phrases. The Pledge of Allegiance, days of the week, and months of the year are examples of over-learned words and phrases that are more easily remembered and spoken by some patients. Even long recitations, such as acts from plays and poems, can be spoken by some Broca's aphasia patients. There is a high degree of variability in the amount and nature of automatic speech. Strokes can leave some patients with many automatic expressions, while others have few, if any, available for automatic recall.

Swearing is a common, automatic thing to do. When you hit your thumb with a hammer, a swear word may surface with little or no thought as an unthinking expression of pain and frustration. It is common in Broca's aphasia for some of the automatic expressions to be swear words. Family members and friends of the patient are sometimes surprised by the frequency and number of them. Although they seem to occur more often in individuals who were accustomed to using them before the stroke, some patients who rarely swore before the stroke find them readily available and at the most inopportune times.

When you are dealing with a patient who has automatic swear words, it is important to keep the proper perspective. Although the occurrence of automatic swear words may be embarrassing to you, the patient, and other listeners, they are expressions nonetheless. They are acts of communication. Certainly, they are not the most desirable choice of words and phrases, but they can and do communicate. Even if they only express the frustration of the patient, they have value and should not be discouraged. This is especially true during the first weeks after the stroke. For the patient, any word correctly spoken, even a swear word, is proof that he or she can talk. Psychologically, knowing that some words can be spoken provides motivation to participate fully in therapy. In the world of aphasia, discouraging or punishing patients' ability to talk should be avoided. Encouraging, not discouraging, speech is the goal. At the same time, swear words specifically should not be practiced or encouraged, because they may be learned at the expense of more appropriate words. Later, during therapy, the occurrences of profanity can be gradually discouraged and eliminated when patients gain more words and more control over their speech.

Following is an example of the type of speech found in patients with Broca's aphasia. Here, an elderly gentleman is describing a Bounder motor home. It has two television sets and a microwave in the kitchen, and it is equipped with both power steering and power brakes.

The totor home, plotor home is a . . . , a . . . flounder, no not flounder. Mounder, sounder, sunder. It two TV. In the . . . , in the . . . , in the . . . , bedroom, no, not bedroom. In the . . . , kitchen, a microwave stuven. It's a flounder no. Darn, I just can't seem to say "Bounder" today. Brownder, I mean flounder. It has easy wheels and stops good. Love it. Love my flounder.

In the above example of Broca's aphasia, the person has difficulty saying anything clearly and easily. He pauses to search for the correct sound, syllable, word, or phrase. When the words are remembered, the sequence and correct choice of sounds are often impaired. Note the telegraphic speech: "It two TV." This is an example of telegraphic speech expressing the idea that the Bounder motor home has two televisions. Automatic speech is also present when the patient says, "Darn, I just can't seem to say 'Bounder' today." Unfortunately, he will probably be unable to make the same utterance later. As he tries to say it again, he becomes more thoughtful and applies more purpose to it. This defeats the automatic nature of the statement.

In Broca's aphasia, comprehension of the speech of others is usually good, especially with short, concise statements and questions. When the statements become longer and more complex, for many individuals, comprehension suffers.

The communication problems seen in Broca's aphasia can be viewed as two weights on a scale. On one side of the scale are those who primarily have problems remembering words. They have difficulty finding the correct word, or any word for that matter, in their vocabulary for expressing ideas. On the other side of the scale are those who have fairly good memory of words, but when they try to say them, they have difficulty programming and sequencing the strings of sounds. A person with Broca's aphasia can fall anywhere between the two extremes.

When you listen to a family member with Broca's aphasia, it is natural to feel uncomfortable and a bit anxious. Nonfluent speech creates nervousness for both the speaker and listener. It is like listening to a person who stutters. Several studies have shown that when a person listens to a stutterer, both the listener and the person who stutters feel nervous. Interestingly, the listener may feel more anxiety than the person stuttering. This is also true in aphasia. Part of the nervousness felt by the listener is founded in a perceived need to help the speaker. The listener may also feel awkward and not know what to do. Perhaps the biggest reason for the listener's nervousness is the long pauses. People are not accustomed to tolerating long pauses during a conversation. When a pause does occur, it usually signals that the other person can pick up the conversation. It is a turn-taking cue. During conversation with a patient with Broca's aphasia, you may not know whether to speak when there are long pauses. When the patient struggles to say a word, should you help? What about eye contact? Should you look away? When it becomes obvious that your loved one will not be able to complete the idea, you may feel nervous and not know what to do.

Providing guidelines about how to react to every instance of a stroke patient's nonfluent speech is impossible. There are many variations of Broca's aphasia, and each person reacts differently to the frustrations. Your previous relationship with the individual also must be considered. Try to keep the conversations as routine as possible. The key word to remember is "relax." Don't hurry the speaker and don't let on that you feel nervous. Let the patient feel that there is all the time in the world to get his or her ideas across. As the patient struggles to remember words and how they are spoken, sit or stand quietly, making casual eye contact. Do not, by word or deed, express to the patient that speech must be hurried. Trying to remember the words or how they are said is therapeutic for the patient and a natural and healthy step on the road to recovering the best speech possible. The patient should know that you tolerate and even encourage these attempts to communicate. Through trial and error, the patient may relearn some or all of what has been lost. As the patient improves, keep in contact with the speech-language pathologist for ideas about new approaches. Your visits can be therapeutic if you are patient and get the proper guidance.

Wernicke's Aphasia

The problems aphasic individuals have understanding the speech of others are known by various names. Understanding problems seen in aphasia fall into many subtypes. Wernicke's aphasia is the most common label given to a stroke patient who has problems understanding the speech of others. This type of aphasia gets its name from Karl Wernicke, the first person to identify the primary comprehension center of the brain (see Chapter 1).

Rarely does a person with aphasia have total comprehension of what other people say. This is true for most of the subtypes of this disorder. Even in Broca's aphasia, in which the primary problem is expressing ideas, patients usually have some difficulty understanding the speech of others. Sometimes it takes detailed tests to detect these problems, but for many patients the ability to understand the speech of others is impaired.

In Wernicke's aphasia, the major problem is understanding the speech of others, and this includes simple as well as complex statements. Wernicke's aphasia patients have trouble following directions and understanding questions. Some patients have only mild problems, while others have a complete inability to understand the speech of others.

The most apparent indication that patients have trouble understanding words is when they cannot follow directions, even simple ones. For example, you might be drinking coffee with a patient in the dining room. When you ask for the cream or sugar, the patient does not respond, gives you the sugar when you asked for the cream, or doesn't give you anything.

Understanding problems are even more apparent with longer and more complex communication. Asking the patient to choose one of three television programs or to express thoughts about a financial concern are examples of questions that could "fall on deaf ears." Although the patient actually has normal hearing, there is no comprehension of the questions.

There are many reasons why an aphasic person fails to correctly follow a simple command such as to pass the sugar. A review of these reasons will help you to appreciate the nature of understanding problems.

1. The most obvious reason a patient does not follow a simple request or command may be that he or she is paralyzed. The body muscles do not work well enough to reach for the sugar and give it to you. Though the person completely understands the question, he or she cannot fulfill the request because of paralysis. Here, understanding the question is not the problem. This person may be paralyzed rather than aphasic.

2. A person may not pass the sugar on request because of a profound hearing loss or deafness. If the ears do not hear the words, the request cannot be followed. Shouting will not help. If the patient is hard-of-hearing, talking a little louder and very clearly may help. "Please, Pass, The, Sugar," with each word said clearly and the sounds made as precisely as possible, will help the ears to make sense of your speech.

3. You may not get the sugar when you requested it because the patient's attention may have been directed elsewhere. Maybe he or she was blanking out and simply not thinking about anything. Perhaps the person was looking at the line in the cafeteria and thinking about something else. Sometimes the patient attends to only the first part of the request; this is called *fading out*. Other times the person attends to only the last part of the question; this is called *slow rise time*. Both problems are apparent when you ask for several things. For example, if you ask the patient to pass you the salt, sugar, and cream, if he or she is fading out, you are likely to get only the salt because the patient has not processed the last items. If the problem is with slow rise time, you are likely to get only the cream because there was no rapid pickup in attention, and the first items were not processed.

4. A patient may not pass you the sugar due to problems recognizing all or part of the sounds in your request. The areas of the brain where sounds are recognized and processed may have been affected by the stroke. To the patient, your request may sound like this: "Kese, kath, the, tuter." Your request will go unanswered because the sounds do not make sense to the patient.

5. The patient may not give you the sugar because the words no longer have meaning or they have the wrong meaning. You end up getting the salt or the pepper instead of the sugar. The patient may understand some of the

request but cannot remember what the word *sugar* means. Perhaps he or she draws a blank, or thinks the word refers to the salt. Longer requests may be perceived as a jumbled collection of unfamiliar words.

6. Your coffee may go unsweetened because the patient has severe memory and thinking problems. Maybe the patient doesn't realize that he or she is in a cafeteria and that you are taking a few minutes to have a cup of coffee. The whole idea of what is going on escapes the patient. The sounds and words may have meaning to the patient, but there is a general confusion about everything.

Understanding problems frequently are not "pure." In other words, two or more of the preceding conditions may combine to cause a patient to be unable to understand the requests of others. Perhaps the patient is partially paralyzed, hard-of-hearing, and some sounds and words no longer make sense. A degree of distractibility might be added to these problems.

Though Wernicke's aphasia results primarily from damage to the understanding center of the brain, patients may also have problems expressing ideas. Their speech is said to be *jargon:* Either the sounds are combined incorrectly to make words or the words themselves are incorrect. Sometimes the words have the wrong meaning or no meaning at all. However, many Wernicke's aphasia patients speak in nonsense fluently and easily. If you were from a foreign country and did not understand English, the jargon speech of some Wernicke's aphasia patient would appear normal, just like that of every other English speaker.

The following example illustrates the speech pattern in a severe case of Wernicke's aphasia in an elderly woman.

> *"Liver. Please get liver. In the past, from Minnesota, we have them to get ready. That's what we call them in Minnesota. The chitters and livers are the struts and the struts are the ones. Boy, in Minnesota we have them. Once in a while, it all depends, criks and criks are all that is needed. Boy."*

This woman fluently and easily talks in nonsense, almost as though she is speaking a foreign language, one understood only by her. Her facial expressions and hand gestures punctuate the nonsense. Some of the nonsense is words combined into meaningless sentences. Other contributors to the nonsense are sounds combined into meaningless words. She produces complete sentences with what appear to be proper grammar and syntax, but they, too, have no meaning. In jargon aphasia, listeners may begin to feel that if they could just try harder, they would understand this perfectly normal sounding speech.

There is some evidence that men are more likely to have Wernicke's aphasia, whereas women tend to have Broca's aphasia. This appears to be the case, but more research on the subject is needed. If indeed this is true, research into the reasons for this difference between men and women is also needed. Although men may be more likely to have Wernicke's aphasia, many women also suffer from it.

Authorities disagree about why these patients speak jargon. One theory is that because of the damage to the understanding center of the brain, they cannot monitor their own speech. Because of brain damage, some patients have lost the meanings of words. They do not know when they make a mistake in saying a word or when they have chosen the wrong one. Another theory is that these patients are simply expressing their disordered language patterns. In effect, they have nonsense verbal thoughts and the jargon is merely an expression of them.

It can be very unsettling when a loved one talks in nonsense. Because of the strange speech, you may be confused about how to respond. If the jargon speech makes you fearful, you may tend to avoid contact. What should you do?

First, it is important to remember that the Wernicke's patient is not mentally ill or crazy. He or she has aphasia, which is a language disturbance, not an emotional or psychological one. Certainly, there is a psychological component to this and other types of aphasia, but it is not a mental illness. Second, do not avoid the patient. He or she needs to feel the bonds of family and friendship to get through this difficult time. To recover from this type of aphasia, an individual needs a lot of social interaction.

How do you respond to a nonsense statement? Many factors determine how family members should respond to jargon. It is best to discuss specific issues with the patient's doctor or speech-language pathologist. Remember that jargon is a form of expression; it may not have meaning to listeners, but it is a form of communication nonetheless. To the patient, it may be extremely meaningful. For one thing, jargon sounds like normal speech and this can be comforting to the patient. The words spoken also may be a language unique to the patient. As such, it carries all of the importance of normal language. One of the best ways of thinking about jargon is as a stage in recovery. The fact that jargon occurs is not as important as whether there is less of it tomorrow, and even less the next day.

When dealing with aphasia, it is important to realize that patients must understand what a word means before they can be expected to use it correctly. This is true of everyone. For example, if you are asked to use the word *aileron* correctly in a sentence, first you must know what the word means. Without knowing the meaning of the word, you cannot use it correctly. However, once the meaning of the word is learned, you can use it in a sentence. An aileron is the part of an airplane, at the ends of the wings, that causes the airplane to bank to one side or the other. It is a crucial element in turning the airplane. Now that you know the meaning of the word, you can use it correctly in a sentence: "The broken aileron caused the airplane to be unable to turn." Likewise, the aphasic person must know what the word means before he or she can be expected to use it correctly in speech. Speech-language clinicians say that "comprehension precedes expression."

Types of Naming Mistakes: Rhyme and Reason

All aphasia boils down to a form of amnesia, a loss of memory. Aphasia is amnesia for words. Either patients cannot express the names of people, objects, actions, or feelings, or they cannot remember what words mean when spoken. Scientists have thoroughly researched the kinds of errors aphasia patients make and have found interesting results. A relationship often exists between the way the words sound, or there is an association in their meaning. The wrong words said by the patient are often related in meaning or sound similar to the correct words.

Suppose you and the patient are in the dining room having coffee. If the patient tries to ask you for the sugar, sometimes he or she will say a word that is similar to it in meaning. She might ask for salt, pepper, honey, or cream, choosing these words because they have some association with the desired word. Salt and pepper are also found on a table, and honey is sweet, like sugar. Some coffee drinkers also add cream to coffee. These are common mistakes made by some aphasic people. The meanings are fuzzy instead of completely wrong.

These kinds of mistakes can also be embarrassing to the patient and uncomfortable for the listener. Because of the tendency to say words related in meaning, a patient might accidentally call his wife his "mother." Some patients mix up the names of their children. A woman might address her present husband by a previous husband's name. It is important to realize that these errors are not mistakes in reality; they are naming errors. The patient hasn't really confused his mother with his wife.

Because of this tendency to substitute words with similar meanings, some patients are thought to be confused and disoriented when they are not. Say you ask a patient, "Do you know where we are?" in an attempt to find out if he is disoriented. When the patient responds with the name of a city in proximity to the actual one, or gives the name of another city that is similar in size and characteristics, you might incorrectly assume he is disoriented. You fear that he doesn't even know the correct city when, in fact, the patient might be perfectly oriented but simply made a mistake in naming. The key to knowing if a patient is truly disoriented is to look at behaviors and not just answers to questions. Does the patient "act" disoriented?

Yes and No are also associated words. They are short, one-word responses to questions. As such, they, too, are sometimes mixed up by the patient. "Do you want to leave the coffee shop?" can be answered with a "Yes," when in fact the patient may want to continue the coffee break. Again, the key to knowing what the patient actually wants is to look to the patient's behaviors or to ask the question again.

Some aphasic individuals also come up with the wrong word that sounds like the desired one. When asking for sugar, the person may say "tugar" or "fugar." A request for a fork can become "pork." A request for cream may become "Please pass the steam." These errors, too, can cause embarrassment and confusion.

Besides making errors with words that are similar in meaning or that sound alike, aphasic patients sometimes try to describe what they want. "Pass the . . . , it is sweet, white, and is like salt" is a descriptive attempt to get the sugar. It is a roundabout way of communicating. These descriptions can be extremely frustrating for both the patient and the listener if the correct request cannot be understood.

Some mistakes in naming have no rhyme or reason; they seem to be random errors. For example, a patient might be requesting the sugar, only to say, "Pass the boot." "Boot" doesn't sound like "sugar," nor is there a relationship in meaning. It seems to come out of the blue. These mistakes do happen and there may be no apparent reason for the mistake. Sometimes the error can be traced to what the patient was looking at. In the case of "boot" for "sugar," the patient might have been staring at someone's feet. All of us have done something like this at one time or another.

Frequently, the aphasic patient may feel as though the word is on the tip of the tongue. Not surprisingly, this frustrating memory problem is called the *tip-of-the-tongue phenomenon*. Patients who have this problem know the word when it is provided to them but cannot recall it on their own.

Occasionally, an aphasic patient, particularly one with severe aphasia, will make up a new word. Making up new words is common in Wernicke's aphasia, but it can occur in many types of aphasia. This word will be the patient's own word for somebody or something. It might be a word like *bubble*. The patient will use the word as a greeting or to request something. Alternatively, the word might be one that doesn't make sense, such as *Tula*. The patient might request a hamburger by saying "Tula, tula." After a while, you and the patient will share the meanings of the made-up words and they can become an important part of communication. Because communication takes place, it is okay that the words have meaning only to you and the patient. After all, every language is made up of invented words.

Sometimes there is an interesting occurrence when people who speak more than one language suffer a stroke. Occasionally, one language will be less destroyed by the aphasia than another. This happens rarely, but it does occur. For example, if a person spoke both English and Spanish before the stroke, in some instances, she might be able to communicate better in Spanish than in English, or vice versa. There have been reports of cases in which one language is left almost completely intact. Several possible explanations for this occurrence have been offered. One theory is that the first learned language is the least likely to be damaged. This is true of a lot of learning: things learned first are best remembered. Another theory is that the language with most prestige will be spared by the aphasia. It is thought that because one language is more prestigious than another, the person chooses to use it. The final theory suggests that the language most used before the stroke is the one likely to be spared by the aphasia. Practice makes perfect, and because one language was used a lot, the individual learned it more thoroughly.

Awareness of Naming Mistakes and the Ability to Correct Them

All things being equal, patients who know when they make a naming mistake are better off than patients who are unaware of an error. Because they are aware of the mistake, the first step in regaining memory of the words has been taken. Before an individual can overcome a problem, he or she must be aware that a problem exists. This is true of naming problems. The patient who is aware of the mistake and can self-correct is ahead of the game because self-therapy occurs every time an error happens. When a word is said in error, the patient knows it and through trial and error can eventually say the correct one. Learning has taken place. The more the person talks, the more self-therapy occurs. These individuals have a good chance of regaining as much memory for words as possible, given the extent of the damage done to the brain.

In summary, complete aphasia is one of the most disabling communication disorders. Few disorders wreak as much havoc on the ability to communicate as complete aphasia. It virtually eliminates the patient's ability to communicate through speaking, writing, reading, gestures, and understanding the speech of others.

Even mild forms of aphasia can disrupt relationships and frustrate attempts to communicate. Knowledge about these communication disorders can help defeat fear and frustration. By learning about aphasia and other stroke-related communication disorders, you can understand the process of your loved one's rehabilitation and become an important participant in it. Check out the Resources section for a list of associations and agencies concerned with aphasia.

CHAPTER 3

Motor Speech Disorders

The greater the difficulty, the more glory in surmounting it.
—*EPICURUS*

Overwhelmed. This word is often used by family members to describe their feelings when a loved one has a stroke. In an instant, both you and the stroke survivor are confronted with a new and strange world. The business-as-usual routine before the stroke abruptly stops. You and your loved one may be separated for long periods, but hopefully, relatives and friends will give you much-needed support. The sensation of "too much, too soon" can make you want to withdraw. It *can* all be overwhelming. But you do what you know you must and continue despite your negative feelings. You and your loved ones have much to learn and many adjustments to make.

The human brain is complex and dynamic. Our knowledge of the world, memories of days gone by, and fantasies and fears of the future all reside in this three or four pounds of nerves and tissue. Constant chemical reactions and electrical discharges result in thoughts, emotions, sensations, and movements. Collectively, the goings-on in the human brain have created societies and cultures. The buildings, machines, laws, schools, religions, books, and flights into space all began in the human brain and were made possible by it. It is a marvelous and amazing creation.

Given the complex capabilities of the brain, it makes sense that damage to it results in equally complex disorders. In the world of strokes, there are few simple outcomes. Strokes can cause more than expressive and receptive language disturbances, and, as if those were not enough, there may also be speech planning, movement, and sensation disorders. The purpose of this chapter is to explore the final two categories of the big three stroke-related communication disorders: apraxia of speech and the dysarthrias. Collectively, these are the *motor speech disorders.* Aphasia, the first of the big three stroke-related communication disorders, was discussed in Chapter 2. The main difference between aphasia and the motor speech disorders is the absence of language disturbances. When a patient's communication disorder is limited to the motor speech system, language is largely preserved. Unfortunately, these disorders more often than not occur together.

For simplification purposes, the following discussion will explore apraxia of speech and the dysarthrias separately so that you can learn about them as distinct and individual problems. Thus, if more than one occurs in a stroke patient, it will not be difficult to recognize the important features.

Apraxia of Speech: A Tangled Tongue

Aphasia is a language disorder that interferes with all avenues of communication. The aphasic person may have problems speaking, writing, reading, and understanding the words of others. These difficulties can range from mild problems such as remembering a few names to the complete loss of all language functions. There are two distinct types of aphasia: Wernicke's aphasia reduces or eliminates the patient's ability to understand what is expressed by other people; Broca's aphasia patients, on the other hand, have problems expressing themselves. This often results in word recall problems and telegraphic speech.

Many Broca's aphasia patients also have major problems planning and sequencing the strings of speech sounds. They remember the words and phrases but have problems getting them out. This is the "motor" aspect of Broca's aphasia-apraxia of speech.

In apraxia of speech, the part of the brain injured is the programming part of Broca's area. Unlike Broca's aphasia, in pure apraxia of speech there are few if any language disturbances. Patients with pure apraxia of speech can remember the names of people and things, and they recognize and know words when they are spoken to them. Reading, writing, and the ability to do arithmetic are not affected. Pure apraxia of speech relatively rarely results from a stroke because more than one blood vessel supplies this area and the tracts leading to and from it. Pure apraxia of speech does happen, but not very often.

Apraxia of speech is also known as *verbal apraxia* by some health care professionals. Both labels refer to the inability to perform complex or skilled speech acts. The problem is not with the muscles or the nerves attached to them; the muscles used in speech are not paralyzed. Because apraxia of speech is a programming deficit, perhaps a comparison with a computer will illustrate the nature of the problem.

The Speech-Programming Computer

Although both the computer and the human brain take in and process information, the brain is by far a greater and more complex "machine." It is true that present-day computers have extremely large memories and rapid processing times, and, in some ways, these computers seem more powerful than the human brain. But computers do not have a knowledge of the world. Unlike people, they are not conscious nor do they have a humanlike command of language. When it comes to the programming and sequencing of speech sounds, however, a computer comparison is helpful.

Before discussing the workings of the speech-programming computer, we should know the order and priority of speech in the brain. Speech is a "secondary" ability. That is, it does not have the highest priority in the makeup of the brain. The brain knows that its primary job is to sustain life. The breathing system, voice box, tongue, lips, and teeth have this as their primary function. Breathing is necessary to supply oxygen to the body. The mouth is for chewing and swallowing. Even the vocal cords close during a swallow to protect the lungs from food and liquid. Scientists believe that humans first developed these functions to sustain life. Over millions of years, the lungs, voice box, and mouth gradually evolved to produce speech. Eventually, humans learned to use the breathing system, mouth, and voice box to make speech. As a secondary function, the compressed air coming from the lungs is shaped into speech.

To illustrate the point that speech is a secondary function, the next time you are jogging or running, note that you cannot talk when you are winded. The brain knows that the highest priority is to keep oxygen going to the cells of the body, and talking interferes with that. Only after the biological need for oxygen is satisfied are you able to talk to someone. The tongue, teeth, and lips have the primary function of chewing and swallowing food and a secondary one of producing speech. This is why paralysis or weakness of the speech muscles often occurs along with chewing, sucking, and swallowing problems.

The area of the brain that plans sounds, syllables, words, and phrases can be likened to a specialized computer, one of many in the brain. This computer is responsible for programming and sequencing speech sounds, and it is connected to other computers that process information coming from the five senses: sight, smell, taste, touch, and hearing. Much more powerful and complex computers process thoughts and ideas, while others are concerned with emotions, behaviors, and movements. Life experiences are stored in huge memory banks. Working together, these computers allow people to go about day-to-day activities. They allow simple, automatic acts such as opening a door or turning a television on and more complex ones such as balancing a checkbook or giving a speech.

The "computer" for speech programming has a direct cord coming from the language computer. When the language computer needs a sound, syllable, word, or phrase to be spoken, it is the speech-programming computer's job to plan and produce the series of complex movements. Four main lines leaving the speech-programming computer go to different parts of the body necessary for speech: the breathing system, voice box, tongue and lips, and the soft palate. Feedback lines also come back into the computer from these areas.

This particular computer turns on only to produce language you have thought about. It is not for automatic kinds of statements. For example, if you were to bite your tongue while chewing, the cry of pain and exclamation "Ouch!" would not have been programmed by this computer. "Ouch!" would result from another computer that deals with these automatic, unthinking types of speech. When you want a glass of ice water to soothe the pain of your sore tongue, however, the request, "Please pass the ice water," would require the speech-programming computer to be turned on. The speech-programming computer is for voluntary and thoughtful statements.

When the speech-programming computer gets an order to produce speech from the language computer, the first thing it needs to do is to decide how much air is going to be needed. Correctly programming the amount of air to produce speech is very important. All of the subsequent programming is based on the amount of air in the lungs. You must have the air and breathing components programmed correctly, or other parts of the speech program will break down. The computer programs breathing muscles to take air into your lungs. The most important muscle for this is the diaphragm. The diaphragm is a dome-shaped muscle that separates the lung cavity from the stomach and intestines. It receives a command from the computer to contract, causing air to rush into your lungs. The many other muscles involved in breathing also receive commands at this time. For the air to rush into your lungs, the ribs and back must be elevated. The computer must not forget to open your mouth and to separate the vocal cords to let the air pass to your lungs.

Once the air is in your lungs, the programming computer must also gradually allow it to flow out, and the gradual flow of compressed air is shaped into sounds, syllables, and words. As each sound, syllable, and word is produced, the breathing system must make many minor adjustments. These minor adjustments are necessary to account for the changes that occur in other parts of the speech tract. For example, every time you close your lips to make a sound, the breathing system must make a minor adjustment to keep the desired loudness. To accomplish this, there are lines of feedback going to the speech-programming computer from the breathing system.

The next task of the speech-programming computer is to regulate the voice. Drawing from memory banks, the computer must decide the pitch and loudness of the words you are to speak. Pitch and loudness changes are made by minor adjustments of the muscles in the voice box and by the vocal cords themselves. The speech-programming computer must see to it that your vocal cords vibrate at just the right number of times per second. In the female voice, this averages about 250 times per second. Most males have lower pitches, and their vocal cords vibrate about 130 times per second. To adjust pitch, minor movements by muscles in the voice box are timed to changes in the flow of air coming *from* the lungs. It is an extremely delicate, coordinated, and complex act. Like many other things in life, timing is everything. To demonstrate the timing and coordination that must happen between your breathing system and voice box, place your hands on your stomach while making the sound *uh*. Push on your stomach and notice the pitch and loudness changes that occur unless you make adjustments with your voice box to counteract the change in force. Your breathing system is constantly adjusting pressure, which accounts for changes in resistance in the speech tract.

Not all sounds have vocal cord vibration, and the speech-programming computer must know this. For example, the sounds s and z are produced identically by the mouth. The only difference between these two sounds is voicing. The s sound does not have vocal cord vibration while the z sound does. F and v are two other sounds between which voicing is the only difference. An interesting way to understand this difference is to plug your ears with your fingers, then start saying the s sound and gradually cause the vocal cords to vibrate. You can hear and feel the s become a z. You can do the same for f and v.

Now the creation of a word must involve your mouth. The compressed air coming from your lungs must be shaped into recognizable sounds by your tongue, lips, and teeth. The tongue is the main muscle performing this job. The English language contains 44 sounds. In connected speech, these sounds are produced by small, rapid changes in the position and shape of the tongue. Many consonants require the tongue to touch, or nearly touch, the roof of the mouth or teeth; vowels are made by minor adjustments in the height and front-to-back position of the tongue. Muscles inside the tongue cause it to change its shape. Other commands require rapid movements of the tongue from one point in the mouth to another. These muscle movements happen so rapidly that one sound glides into another. The gliding is done with such speed that few sounds are produced perfectly. Most speech occurs so fast that each sound is made just close enough together to sound normal. The faster you say the word or phrase, the further away the sound is from its ideal production. Signals are sent back to the computer indicating how close each sound is to the ideal one. These signals include both sound feedback from your ears and feeling and movement sensations.

Normal speech is produced with just the right amount of nasalization. In English three sounds require a lot of nasalization: *m*, *n*, and *ng* (as in bo*ng*). They are produced in the mouth like all of the other sounds but have one other adjustment. When these sounds are made, the soft palate drops down to allow the nose and nasal cavities to be used. If the soft palate is down on the other sounds, you get too much nasality. If the soft palate is up on the production of the three nasals, or if the nasal passages are closed, you talk as if you have a cold. The speech-programming computer regulates nasality.

The speech-programming computer is responsible for all of the above plans and movements. Whether a sound is produced alone or as one of many, the computer must plan and monitor it. But speech requires more than just the planning and monitoring of individual syllables, words, and phrases. Normal speech is a highly coordinated, rhythmic event. Words and sounds must have just the right amount of emphasis. It is not enough that speech is produced; it must be smooth and fluent. This, too, is the responsibility of the speech-programming computer.

The part of the brain that is the speech-programming computer is a remarkable machine. Taking commands from the language computer part of the brain, it is responsible for the planning, sequencing, and execution of speech. Thousands of nerve impulses drive hundreds of muscles to produce speech. Each sound, syllable, and word is checked for accuracy by constant feedback. The speech-programming computer also sets tolerance levels. Sometimes the speech act is not precise enough or an error is made. This may happen at any time, but it happens most often when speech is produced too rapidly. Then the speech-programming computer sends commands to fix the error and correct the speech.

Planning the muscle movement in speech is an extremely complicated act. When this process breaks down or is injured in a stroke, apraxia of speech results. Like most disabilities resulting from stroke, the site and size of the brain damage determines the degree of difficulty experienced by the patient. If the entire speech-programming computer is destroyed by a stroke, the patient completely loses the ability to program speech. Unable to get his or her breathing system, voice box, tongue, lips, and soft palate to produce speech, the patient becomes mute. The patient cannot talk because speech cannot be planned and organized, although some patients may have a few automatic utterances.

As mentioned earlier, the degree of disability is determined by the amount of injury to the brain. Some stroke survivors have only minor difficulties programming speech, and the apraxia of their speech is no more than a minor nuisance. It is easy to understand what it is like to have a mild case of apraxia of speech. You have probably occasionally had a minor problem saying a word or two. Most people have some difficulty producing a particular word on occasion. Words such as *aluminum, phenomena, supposedly, cinnamon, linoleum, spaghetti*, and *specifically* are occasionally said in a clumsy way. Tongue twisters, such as "red leather, yellow leather," are also difficult to say, especially when you speak rapidly. Some of the many reasons that people have problems saying sounds and syllables in certain words and in tongue twisters include (1) too many consonants occur together, (2) these particular vowels and consonants do not usually occur in this particular order, and (3) the tongue has difficulty moving fast enough from the front to the back of the mouth and vice versa. Whatever the reasons, sometimes certain words and phrases are difficult to say. However, tongue twisters and difficult words may not be true programming problems. The problems might not be directly related to the speech-programming computer, and they are certainly not a result of brain damage. Even so, these types of errors are similar to what happens with apraxia of speech. When you have trouble saying a particular word or tongue twister, it is because you do not have the control of your mouth to say them. You know what you want to say but have difficulty doing it. Apraxia of speech is also a "mouth control" problem, but many times worse. Apraxia of speech is usually most apparent in attempts to program the mouth. In some patients, the voice and even the breathing system also can be difficult to program.

The following is a typical example of mild apraxia of speech. Here, the patient is describing a picture of a police officer writing a ticket to a frustrated driver.

> "The stop, top, uh, prop has told over a very trustrated, uh, frustrated sotorist. You can see that he is angry. He is trying to splain, estain, erstain. It is futile because the crop, stop, plop, stuhcop is done with it."

Mild apraxia of speech is often limited to problems programming the tongue. The patient with a mild disorder makes sound substitutions and revisions. In the preceding example, the patient's tongue is supposed to go to the position for making the *c* sound in the word *cop*. But because of the programming error, it goes to the *s* position instead. Then the patient's speech-programming computer gets an error signal and attempts to correct it. But this, too, meets with difficulty. The revisions and substitutions occur because the patient hears the wrong sounds being said and knows that a mistake has been made. Patients with pure apraxia of speech do not have receptive language problems, although some studies suggest that some patients with apraxia of speech have problems with speech discrimination. A speech discrimination problem is present when a person cannot clearly distinguish between similar sounds, such as *t* and *d* or *s* and *sh*, when they are spoken by someone else. The listener cannot perceive the differences. The research suggests that patients with apraxia of speech may also have these problems. At this time, not enough studies have been conducted to either accept or reject this observation. The research is not conclusive.

The problems in apraxia of speech occur with consonant sounds more often than with vowels. This is not to say that some stroke survivors with apraxia of speech will not struggle and revise vowels; it simply means that consonants are more often said in error. This is not unusual. Children have more problems learning consonants than vowels. Vowels are easier to say because, unlike consonants, they do not require complicated adjustments of the tongue. Also, all vowels are voiced. This gives them more energy or loudness, making them easier to hear and, therefore, easier to learn. Scientists have looked at how frequently sounds occur in a given language. In English the *n* sound occurs more frequently than the *z* sound.

Patients with apraxia of speech have an easier time making the sounds that occur most frequently. Sounds that occur infrequently and that require more complex adjustments by the articulators are harder to say. They are more difficult to get started, too. Studies have shown that sounds at the beginning of a word are more difficult to produce than those in the middle or at the end for patients with apraxia of speech.

When you hear a loved one in the middle of an apraxic episode, it may appear that the struggle to produce speech is just random. It is not. Apraxic patients are trying to gain control of their mouths, and the errors they make are usually close to the sounds they want to produce. Research has shown that the revisions are attempts to bring the speech mechanism closer to the positions necessary to produce the correct sounds. Like many people who stutter, patients with apraxia of speech also insert the *uh* sound in the middle of a word. For example, the patient may want to say *popcorn*. He or she might end up saying "pop . . . uh . . . corn."

The family member with apraxia of speech is also likely to overshoot and undershoot the "plan of speech," which comprises all of the required motor acts in the proper sequence. You can hear this by listening to the sounds that come before and after the struggled sound. For example, if the patient says, "I want some. . .pop . . . uh . . . corn," the overshooting of the "pop" may cause the word "corn" to sound like "porn." The patient ends up saying, "I want some . . . popporn." Undershooting of the speech plan may sound like this: "I want some . . . copcorn."

When you listen to a person with apraxia of speech, it is sometimes hard not to say, "Try harder." Especially when the person struggling with speech comes close to making the correct sound, it would seem that trying harder would be the thing to do. It is not. Trying harder is often a negative thing to do in apraxia of speech because it makes the effort more thoughtful and purposeful. Recall from Chapter 2 that in Broca's aphasia, automatic utterances are easier to say than ones with forethought. By trying harder, the patient gives the word more thought and effort and thus makes the word more difficult to say. The best suggestion you can give to the apraxic patient is, "Use trial and error." The patient should understand that he or she has as much time as needed to say the word. Many relaxed attempts to say the word with minor, unforced revisions may eventually result in relearning the word's program. The plan and sequence of the sound, syllable, word, or phrase need to be relearned. Forcing speech can be of no help and, in fact, may be harmful.

In normal conversations, a pause usually indicates that one speaker has finished expressing a thought and it is now the listener's turn to begin talking. The pause is a cue to take turns during the conversation. *Fillers* are sounds, words, and short phrases a speaker sometimes utters during a pause in the conversation. They fill the pause. When you hear them in a stroke patient, it may indicate that the speaker doesn't want to be interrupted and wants more time to complete the idea or the phrase. For example, if a stroke patient is saying, "I want w, w, wa . . . , wa . . . you know, you know, w, w, w, you know, water," the filler "you know" shows that he or she does not want to be interrupted; the patient needs more time to complete the thought. Fillers often suggest that the person feels pressured and fears that the expression will be prematurely interrupted. When talking to a stroke patient who uses fillers, it is important to let him or her know that there is no need to feel pressured to speak in a hurry. Explain that you won't interrupt. You and other family members and friends will allow the patient the time necessary to talk. Once your loved one understands that he or she will not be interrupted, the fillers will occur less frequently.

Sometimes patients with apraxia of speech can whisper better than they can talk aloud. This is more apparent during the early stages of recovery from the stroke. No one knows why whispering is sometimes more successful. It may be because it avoids complex adjustments in the voice box, and the whole speech program is less complicated. Whispered speech also is done easily and with less effort. Perhaps the patient feels less self-conscious because whispered speech is quieter than voiced talking. Whatever the reason, clinical observations have shown that some patients with apraxia of speech can whisper better than they can talk aloud.

Many patients who have apraxia of speech also have oral apraxia. The patient who has oral apraxia has problems programming the speech mechanism for non-verbal movements such as licking the lips, sticking out the tongue, biting the lower lip, and puckering. These oral movements do not involve speech. Oral apraxia is like apraxia of speech in that patients can make these movements normally when they give little or no thought to them. If you tell patients with oral apraxia to lick their lips, they may have problems doing it. However, if patients feel that there is something on their lips, they can automatically lick them. The same is true for puckering, biting, and sticking out the tongue.

Some stroke patients have problems programming arm and hand movements, too. When you ask them to point to something, sometimes they do not follow the command because of programming problems. They cannot get their arms and hands to do what they want them to do. When you see this happen, you might mistakenly assume that they did not understand the question. One of the best examples of this type of problem has to do with stroke patients who smoke. If you ask them to "Show me what you do with a cigarette," patients with this problem are unlikely to be able to act. They either will not move at all or the hand with the cigarette in it will move in a random, aimless direction. When they feel the need to have a cigarette, however, they automatically grasp one and easily light and smoke it.

In summary, apraxia of speech is a programming problem. The part of the brain that commands the breathing system, voice box, tongue, lips, and soft palate has been injured or destroyed. As a result, the patient struggles and misplaces the tongue in an attempt to talk. In complete apraxia of speech, the patient is unable to program breathing, voicing, tongue placements, and the soft palate. In mild cases of the disorder, only a few words or phrases cannot be programmed. Patients can also have oral apraxia, which impairs programming for oral movements that do not involve speech. The hallmark of apraxia of speech is that many patients can perform some of these acts automatically. Patients with apraxia of speech should never be forced to hurry their attempts to speak. Hurried attempts to talk make communication even more difficult.

Dysarthria: The Paralyzed Tongue

Dysarthria is the third of the big three stroke-related communication disorders. The speech pathologies classified as dysarthria are a distinct and different type of communication disorder, and there are different types of dysarthria, which are classified based on the type of paralysis or movement problems that occur with the speech mechanism. When dysarthria happens in pure form, the stroke patient's language and speech programming abilities remain intact. The person's reading, writing, and arithmetic skills; gestures; and ability to understand the speech of others are not damaged. Memory for words and the ability to program them are also not damaged in dysarthria. Scientists consider the dysarthrias a "lower" type of disorder in the sense that they happen toward the end of the chain of neurological events that produce speech.

Whereas aphasia is a language disorder and apraxia of speech is a speech-programming deficit, the dysarthrias result in weak, slow, or ill-coordinated speech. The stroke survivor remembers words and programs them correctly. The breakdown is primarily in the nerves and/or muscles of speech. Some stroke patients have complete loss of speech muscle function because their muscles are completely paralyzed. But strokes can merely weaken speech muscles; the muscles may retain much of their strength but they are clumsy or they tremble. Although strokes usually result in paralysis or weakness only on one side of the body, sometimes both sides are affected. Likewise, problems can occur only with the breathing muscles and voice box, or the tongue and soft palate can be affected too. The nature and degree of disability depends on the area of the nervous system damaged by the stroke.

Before discussing various forms of paralysis due to a stroke, it is important to understand how muscles move body parts. When you lift or move something, you set off a complex series of muscle contractions and relaxations. For example, when you reach for the sugar to sweeten your coffee, muscles attached to your arm and shoulder contract, causing the bones to move in a mechanical way to allow your arm to move forward. All the time some muscles are contracting, others are relaxing. When a movement is completed in one direction, it is the relaxed muscles' turn to contract while the others relax. This series of contractions and relaxations results in the mechanical movements necessary to grasp and retrieve the sugar.

The only thing a muscle can do with force is contract. When you push the sugar out of your way, your hand and arm movements are caused by forceful muscle contractions. The makeup of muscles can only forcibly bring body parts closer together. Muscles do not "push"; they can only, with force, shorten the distance between their origin and the place of insertion into the body part. This is true of your speech muscles as well.

The Muscle-Regulating Computers

A good way to understand the types of dysarthria is to continue the computer comparison. Recall that the speech-programming computer is one of many in the brain. When it is damaged by a stroke, the patient has problems planning the movements that go into speech. To continue with the computer comparison, the first type of dysarthria is a "lockup" of the computer that inhibits the muscles of speech. *Inhibit* means to stop or reduce the activity of something. Actually, there are two sides to this inhibiting computer. They are in each side of the brain.

One of the most important functions of this computer is to keep the muscles of speech from automatically contracting. These speech muscles want to go tight and stiff—to contract. This is a reflex. The inhibiting computer's job is to stop the muscles from going into a tight, contracted state. Medical professionals use the term *spastic* when referring to muscles in a prolonged contracted state. When all of the speech muscles are affected by damage to this computer, the dysarthric patient talks slowly, with a harsh voice and indistinct sounds. When only a part of the computer is damaged, only the voice box, tongue, or breathing muscles might be spastic.

When the inhibiting computer is damaged by a stroke, the muscles are limited in the amount of movement they can make; their range of motion is reduced. A good way for you to understand reduced range of motion is to stand with your arms to your side. If you can lift your arm up above your head, you have good range of motion. If you can lift your arm up only to the level of your hip or your neck, however, your range of motion is limited. Although speech muscles are not as easy to visualize as arms, they, too, can have reduced range of motion. This can be caused by damage to the inhibiting computer part of the brain.

Stiff, tight, spastic muscles respond better to slow, gradual attempts to move them. For example, if a person has a spastic hand pulled tightly into a fist, pulling the fingers open rapidly causes them to contract even tighter. However, if the fingers are pulled open slowly, with even pressure, there is less resistance. This is true for the speech muscles as well. If some or all of the muscles in the voice box are spastic because of damage to the inhibiting computer, the person's voice can sound harsh or hoarse. When the person tries to force the vocal cords into vibration in a sudden, hard manner, they tend to pull even tighter and stiffer. It works better to start the vocal cords moving in an easy, gradual way.

The opposite of a spastic muscle is one that is *flaccid*. Flaccid muscles are weak and limp. When a muscle is completely flaccid, it has no strength and cannot contract. Partially flaccid muscles are also weak and limp but can be contracted with great effort. You can visualize what a flaccid muscle is like by allowing your arm to hang limp at your side. To raise it, you must use your other arm to lift it, and when you drop it, it falls, swinging back and forth.

When speech muscles are made flaccid by a stroke, they cannot contract or move by themselves. A partially flaccid muscle requires other muscles to help it do its job, so the movements are slow and sluggish. If the voice box is made flaccid by a stroke, then the patient may have a breathy voice. The vocal cords cannot close together as hard or as rapidly as before the stroke. When the soft palate is flaccid, it is difficult to raise it to block off air going to the nose. The result is too much nasality. Flaccid tongue muscles result in slow speech and indistinct consonants, particularly ones that require the tongue to be lifted, such as *t* and *l*.

The Coordinating Computer

The part of the brain responsible for coordination of movements is called the *cerebellum*. It makes for smooth transitions from one movement to another, blending and timing actions. The cerebellum decides how much movement is needed and if too much or too little force is being applied. To continue with the computer comparison, it is one of many computers taking commands from others, providing feedback, and making decisions and adjustments. The cerebellum is the coordinating computer.

When you watch a skilled athlete dribble a basketball over, under, and around opponents and then leap, spin, and score, you are witnessing the power of the coordinating computer, as well as years of practice, exercise, and conditioning. But the smooth, blended movements are, to a large degree, the result of the coordinating computer. The dribbles are done with just the right amount of force. The ball's direction is changed with a slight rotation of the wrist. Fingers and palm movements send it between the opponent's legs. The jump, timed to coincide with changing the ball from the left hand to the right hand, is done in a fraction of a second. As the hoop nears, the speed of the movements quickens, and finally, "slam dunk." If any computer in the athlete's head should take a bow and take credit for the points, it would be the coordinating computer.

Located at the base of the skull, the coordinating computer is also responsible for the dancer's, rodeo cowboy's, jet pilot's, and bicyclist's smooth movements. It tirelessly computes force and timing for ordinary people's movements, too. Moving from a sitting to a standing position, opening the refrigerator, and walking to the dining room require coordination. Without the coordinating computer, you would make jerky, bumpy movements characterized by too much or too little force.

When you are sitting at a table and reach for sugar to sweeten your coffee, a series of complex and interconnected movements is required. The impulses for these movements come from various parts of the brain. The brain sends out gross and unrefined impulses or commands that the coordinating computer refines, moderates, and coordinates. The result is a movement that is smooth, properly timed, and produced with just the right amount of force. If a malfunction occurs with the coordinating computer, you might overshoot or undershoot the sugar, clumsily hit the table with your hand, or knock a fork to the floor.

Commands are also sent to the speech muscles in gross and unrefined impulses. When the coordinating computer is on the blink, the tongue overshoots or undershoots the articulation target, and the voice is explosive, with too loud and too soft sounds. The speed of speech is slow, occasionally punctuated by a word or phrase said too fast. The listener hears jerky, ill-coordinated, choppy speech. If there is a total lockup of the coordinating computer, speech becomes a series of unrecognizable sounds. When this part of the brain is damaged by a stroke, the patient has *ataxic* dysarthria.

With ataxic dysarthria, slowing the rate of speech is often helpful because it gives the damaged computer time to be more efficient. Slowing the rate of speech is also a helpful therapy for other types of dysarthrias. As a rule, the slower patients talk, the more precise they can be. They overshoot and undershoot movements less often.

Although the average person, speaking in a relaxed environment, talks at about 150 words per minute, speaking rates vary a great deal. Some people talk rapidly while others speak slowly. Most people talk faster when they are nervous. Three elements comprise the rate of speech. The first is the number of pauses. If a person . . . has . . . a lot of . . . pauses . . . during . . . speech . . . then . . . he . . . or . . . she . . . will have a . . . slower . . . rate. The second factor is the length of the pauses. If . . . . a person has fewer pauses . . . . but they are longer . . . . , this can cause . . . . speech to be slower. The final aspect of the rate of speech is the length of the sounds. Wheeeeen a persoooon drawsssssssss out words, theeeeeeeen speeeeeech proceeds more sloooooooowly. Each of these three factors determines rate of speech. Slowing the rate of speech allows time for each sound to be made more precisely.

Other Computer Malfunctions

Facial tics and body jerks are also malfunctions that can occur because of a stroke. You have probably had these things happen while you were sleeping. You awake to a sudden hand or head movement, as though an electrical discharge jolted a body part. A stroke can cause these things to happen during waking hours and with increased frequency and severity.

You probably have also experienced a muscle tremor, perhaps in your arm, hand, or jaw. This normal tremor usually occurs when you are cold or nervous. Strokes can also cause muscle tremors. Although they are most apparent when patients hold something in their hand, some people have tremors when they are resting. When the tremors happen in the speech tract, the patient may have a quivering voice and irregularly produced sounds.

Doctors make a distinction between quick and slow unwanted movements. A facial tic or body jerk happens quickly. When the tics and jerks affect the speech mechanism, speech impairment results. Unwanted sounds are made and the normal flow of speech is interrupted. Slow, unwanted movements can blend into one another, causing sounds to be made in an exaggerated, overemphasized way. Unwanted movements, whether tremors, body jerks, or facial tics, sometimes occur because blood supply is cut off to an area of the brain that prevents such movements. The brain chemicals responsible for keeping this from occurring cannot be produced because of the stroke. When these movements occur during speech, they can result in unwanted or imprecise sounds.

These unwanted movements can happen to normal people, but in stroke patients they happen too often. They can also happen with more severity. These types of electrical surges or unwanted discharges are not common in strokes, but they do occur. When they affect the speech mechanism, the result is difficulty making clear sounds and words.

As with aphasia and apraxia of speech, the severity of dysarthria also varies. The degree of variation depends on the severity of the stroke and the motor systems that are impaired. Researchers have found that about 50 percent of the time, two or more of the dysarthrias occur together. This is called *mixed* dysarthria. Sometimes a patient will start off with one type, and gradually it will change into another. At other times, a patient will have two or more types of dysarthria occurring simultaneously.

In summary, the big three communication disorders that can result from a stroke are aphasia, apraxia of speech, and dysarthria. More often than not, two or more of them are present. Some strokes cause aphasia and apraxia of speech. Some patients have aphasia and dysarthria. It is not uncommon to find all three as the result of a stroke. Disruptions of language, impaired speech programming, and muscle paralysis can all be consequences of a stroke. These three disorders have two things in common. First, they impair or eliminate the ability to communicate. Second, they are treatable. The effects they have on communication can be minimized and, sometimes, eliminated.

CHAPTER 4

Complications

I am the master of everything I can explain.—THEODOR HAECKER

The information highway you have taken to understand strokes and the communication disorders that can result from them has led directly to the "big three" pathologies: aphasia, apraxia of speech, and dysarthria. So far the road has been direct, with few detours. But strokes do not always lead only to the big three communication disorders. Frequently, other side effects and complications of the stroke occur along with aphasia, apraxia of speech, and the dysarthrias. These complications may include impairments of perception, panic attacks, uncontrolled crying, and swallowing problems. They need to be understood so that you can deal with them properly. As you will recall, knowledge is the antidote to fear and confusion. It is also the foundation for rebuilding the relationship between you and the stroke survivor.

As discussed in the previous chapters, aphasia, apraxia of speech, and the dysarthrias are the main communication disorders that can be caused by a stroke. A stroke can result in partial or complete loss of language and compromise all avenues of expression and understanding. A stroke can also tangle the tongue by impairing or eliminating the ability to program speech acts. Paralysis or weakness of the speech mechanism can be caused by a stroke as well, and stroke patients can have trouble making sounds clearly or at all. These disorders are called the "big three" because they are the most frequently occurring communication disorders resulting from stroke. Many patients have more than one of these disorders or all three of them simultaneously. But strokes result in more than the big three communication disorders. Strokes are emotional events. Along with communication disorders, some patients have a loss of emotional control.

Exaggerated Emotions

A stroke is one of the most life-changing events that can happen to a person. Unwanted changes lurk around every corner. Being impaired or unable to talk with loved ones and having trouble walking, eating, and dressing are thrust on the patient. A stroke causes many other major and minor changes, most of them un-wanted. You would, therefore, expect the patient to experience sadness and the nat-ural response to it, crying. But some patients, because of the stroke and the injury done to the brain, have exaggerated emotions sometimes called "emotional labil-ity." They cry, often uncontrollably, at the slightest thing, and they laugh too easily at events that are marginally humorous. But because they have more to be sad about, they tend to cry more than laugh.

In the past, authorities on stroke-related communication disorders called these emotional behaviors "inappropriate." The idea was that crying, especially uncon-trolled crying, was out of the ordinary and therefore inappropriate. Nothing could be further from the truth. Crying and the feelings of sadness experienced by the pa-tient are not inappropriate. It would be inappropriate *not* to have an emotional re-sponse to the stroke. But some patients cry more than the occasion calls for. Such crying is "exaggerated": too much and too often. Stroke patients themselves report feeling as though they have lost emotional control.

The exaggerated crying seen in some patients is the result of a lowered emo-tional threshold. A *threshold* can be defined as the level at which something is set off. With some patients, this threshold has been lowered after the stroke, resulting in crying over little things or crying too much over the big ones. Some people be-lieve the lowered threshold is purely a response to brain injury. Others consider it both a consequence of injury to the brain and a psychological response. This type of exaggerated emotional response is seen more often when there has been damage to the part of the brain that is the "inhibiting computer" (see Chapter 3), support-ing the idea that such exaggerated reaction is a physical response to brain damage rather than just a psychological response. Some researchers have implied that the exaggerated crying seen in some stroke patients is just a motor act and that the tears, sad face, and sobbing are simply behaviors—actions lacking the emotion of sadness. However, it should always be remembered that a person has a stroke, not just part of a brain, so there is always a psychological component. Three general conditions can set off a bout of exaggerated crying: words and thoughts, people, and situations.

Words and thoughts trigger exaggerated emotions in some stroke patients be-cause some words are more emotional than others. The emotional response to many words can be tested by placing them on a continuum between opposite val-ues depending on how they affect and trigger emotions in the stroke patient. For example, consider the word *father* in relation to the following ranges of thoughts and feelings:

Masculine	Feminine
Bad	Good
Friendly	Aloof

Strong	Weak
Sad	Happy
Kind	Mean

Depending on the patient, the word *father* could be placed anywhere on the above ranges of ideas about the word. Many other ranges of ideas and emotions about the word can be added to the list. *Daughter, nursing home, stroke, doctor, nurse, sister,* and other words can be thought of as emotional triggers. By looking at words this way, you can see that some are more emotional than others. The words with more emotional content tend to set off bouts of exaggerated crying in some stroke patients.

The following is an example of exaggerated crying in a stroke patient caused by hearing certain words:

> *"How are you? What did you have for lunch? Are your grandchildren [crying] going to come and visit you today in the nursing home [crying]? Did you walk [crying] by yourself today? I understand that your sister [crying] called and she says she will visit you tonight."*

Visits by relatives and friends can cause exaggerated crying. Often, just having the patient's grandchildren walk into the hospital room can cause it. Pictures and videos of family gatherings are emotional triggers as well. Situations that can cause outbursts of emotion include returning to the hospital after a home pass, going into the speech or physical therapy room, returning home, or going to church.

It is important not to believe that all crying is exaggerated, inappropriate, or simply a result of brain injury. Improper or inconsiderate actions by people around the patient can also cause emotional reactions. Look for the cause of the crying when it happens and try to eliminate it. This is particularly important with patients with total aphasia because they cannot tell you why they are crying.

A goal of counseling and therapy is to gain more control over the frequency and severity of these bouts of exaggerated emotions. You and other family members can help decrease the number of bouts by avoiding topics that set them off. If your loved one is having uncontrolled bouts of exaggerated crying, try to avoid sad or emotional discussions. You should learn which words and ideas set off the crying. Of course, you cannot avoid all emotional discussions, but it may be a good idea to postpone some until the patient has more emotional control. You may need to avoid some situations, too. If the sight of a patient's motor home causes exaggerated crying, try to avoid confronting the emotional situation for the time being. Postponing visits from people who are likely to set off the crying may be a wise decision. I am not suggesting that you deprive the patient of visits by loved ones or that you stop visiting with the patient. Whenever possible, however, try to reduce the number of things that set off the crying behavior. Postpone them until the patient has gained more emotional control.

Once the patient has started a bout of exaggerated crying, you can help to reduce the length of it by shifting the topic of discussion. Once the crying begins, talk
about something more emotionally positive. Rather than let the crying run its
course, change the topic or shift the patient's attention to something more positive,
perhaps by commenting on how pretty the sunset is or how good the food tastes.
Do not be abrupt in these attempts to decrease the crying, but gradually and gently
shift attention. You should not by word, deed, or facial expression communicate to
your loved one that he or she is doing something wrong or bad. Exaggerated crying
is a natural and predictable part of having a stroke in some patients. Your goal is to
help reduce the frequency and severity of it. Read Chapter 13 and the "Three P"
therapy for minimizing or eliminating emotional lability.

Sometimes exaggerated crying does not stop or even gets worse. The crying
episodes may persist for weeks and even months after the stroke. Crying can be a
symptom of clinical depression. In such cases, the crying is part of a serious medical condition (see Chapter 7). The patient's physician should be consulted to determine the reasons for too much crying. The physician may want to prescribe
drugs to help eliminate it or recommend counseling by a psychologist. Sometimes,
physicians recommend both treatments. You must work closely with the physician
and the rehabilitation team in dealing with patients who cry.

Panic Attacks

Some stroke patients are prone to panic attacks. The medical term for stroke-related
panic attacks is *catastrophic reactions*. They can be set off by many things, but stress
is the biggest trigger. Because stress comes from many sources, if you are not careful,
you and other family members and friends can set off a panic attack accidentally.

The panic attacks seen in aphasia have been studied for decades. Observers
have reached the general conclusion that they are not just a psychological reaction.
During a panic attack, although patients experience feelings of *fear* and *anxiety* and
a sense of being bombarded by too many things, they also have physical symptoms
that can include sweating, rapid heart rate, shaking, striking out, and crying. These
episodes may range from minor attacks in which the patient appears mildly distressed to severe ones that include a loss of consciousness.

Frustration is the single greatest element in a panic attack. Frustration follows
certain laws of cause and effect. When people seek to do something and are
thwarted in the attempt, frustration arises. The opposite also occurs. When people
seek to stop something unwanted from happening and are unsuccessful, they become frustrated. Frustration arises when people don't get their way. Of course, life
is full of frustrations and most people deal with them routinely, having learned over
the years how to cope with these situations. Avoiding the sources of frustration is

one way of coping with them. Escape from frustrating predicaments is also a way of finding relief. Using psychological defenses also can be successful. Some people embrace frustrations as challenges, and others deal with frustration by becoming "thick skinned." These strategies and a host of others allow most people to suffer the pangs of frustration with a minimum of energy and negativity. Stroke and the communication disorders that result from them can change all of that.

Some patients have likened these panic attacks to feelings of claustrophobia. You probably have had similar feelings in a crowded store. The aisles are full and customers are making a lot of noise. Overhead, the clerks use the intercom to request price checks and other services. Because of the crowding, it is hard to move around and you feel bombarded by all of the stimulation. This type of environment carries the seeds of a panic attack. Frustration surrounds you. You want to get out as fast as possible. You want your environment to be quiet, calm, relaxing, or you want to find a serene place, but you cannot get your way.

For patients with stroke-related communication disorders, frustration, stress, and an inability to get their way are constant companions. Many hospital rooms are noisy. Doctors are being paged overhead; cleaning crews run noisy vacuums; doctors, nurses, and other staff members can be heard talking at the ward station. Visitors in the room can be talking too much and too loudly at the same time. A patient might be confined to bed or a wheelchair, and, even if easy escape were possible, there are few accessible places of tranquility. Even worse, attempts to talk and to understand the speech of others might be frustrating. Word-finding problems or a paralyzed or tangled tongue frustrate attempts to calm down. These and other sources of stress combine to cause the psychological and physical reactions of the panic attack. The patient's past tried and true methods of dealing with this barrage of frustration no longer work. It is understandable that some stroke patients suffer panic attacks.

The panic attacks seen in some aphasic patients are caused by more than just environmental noise and confusion. Over the years, it has been observed that many of these panic attacks occur when patients are placed in situations in which they cannot communicate successfully. Confronted with too many demands on their now limited ability to communicate, they are subjected to one failure after another. These situations threaten their perception of themselves and cause self-esteem to tumble. Feelings of inadequacy, loss of control, and failed attempts to communicate create a spiral of negative feelings, and some patients understandably panic.

Some authorities believe that aphasia patients who have panic attacks were likely before having the stroke to feign illness to get out of difficult or unpleasant tasks. For example, they would get headaches to avoid unpleasantness. Psychologically, they dealt with unpleasant situations by either getting physical ailments or pretending to have them. This pattern of coping continues after a stroke, and the result is the panic attack. This theory has not been researched carefully and at present is just an observation by a few authorities on the subject.

Only a small percentage of aphasic patients have panic attacks. However, not all panic attacks are observable nor are they recognized for what they are by the medical staff. Therefore, they may be more common than generally assumed by experts. Recent studies have shown that Broca's aphasia patients are most susceptible to having panic attacks. Some researchers who do brain mapping studies (see Chapter 1) assume that this is because damage to Broca's area of the brain destroys brain cells or chemicals that prevent panic attacks. When the stroke interrupts the workings of the brain, the patients are prone to panic attacks. A more compelling reason for the higher frequency of panic attacks in Broca's aphasia patients is the fact that this type of communication disorder is extremely frustrating. This type of aphasia is characterized by frustrated attempts to find the correct word and then struggled attempts to say it correctly. Panic attacks also happen in Wernicke's aphasia, but they are more unusual. Indifference to, or at least a casual disregard for, the communication disorder is typical of someone with Wernicke's aphasia.

You should alert other family members to the potential of panic attacks and what can be done to avoid them. Even if the patient is not prone to panic, certain principles of interaction should be followed with every patient who has a stroke-related communication disorder. First, keep noise and distraction at a minimum. Keep the patient's room as relaxing as possible. Do not allow too many visitors. Discuss with family and friends the need to be relaxed, calm, and supportive during visits with the patient. Second, try to make sure the patient succeeds more than he or she fails. Try to tailor visits and communication with the patient to reduce the level of frustration. The patient should succeed at communication more than he or she fails. Third, look for signs that the patient is going to have a panic attack: irritability, sweating, shaking, or crying. If these signs appear, immediately reduce the level of stimulation. Also, provide the patient with avenues for escape from the pressures. Ask visitors to leave the room or take your loved one elsewhere. Provide reassurance and soothing encouragement. You can calm the patient by gently stroking his or her arm or back. Other strategies for reducing anxiety and tension are discussed in Chapter 8.

Difficulty Shifting Thoughts

Strokes can sometimes cause a patient to get stuck thinking a thought repeatedly, like a car that gets stuck in one gear and cannot shift to another. You are probably familiar with similar situations, only to a much less severe extent. For example, perhaps you hear a song, jingle, or melody in the morning, and you cannot get it out of your mind. Gradually, as the day progresses the tune fades away. This is similar to what happens with some aphasic patients. They, too, can have difficulty with songs, jingles, or melodies, but their problems shifting thoughts can be more pervasive. They can get stuck on sounds, words, and ideas. Even writing can get stuck. Although they are aware that they are stuck on a particular thought, many patients have trouble shifting to another, as though their whole mental set is fixed. This tendency to get stuck on a mental set has not been identified with damage to any particular area of the brain. However, it has been noted that the more severe the brain injury, the more likely the patient is to experience this problem.

You might observe this inability to shift thoughts when you ask the patient questions. When you say, "Good morning, how are you?" the patient might answer, "Fine." Initially, the response is normal. Then, if you ask, "Do you want orange juice for breakfast?" the patient might respond with another "Fine." The tendency to be stuck on a word will become apparent when you ask, "How do you want your eggs cooked, scrambled or sunny side up?" The third response of "Fine" shows the problems shifting from one answer to another.

Clinicians see these difficulties shifting from one idea to the next during therapy sessions. Physical and occupational therapists might observe a patient who is unable to change easily from one activity to another. During a speech and language drill, the speech clinician can see such fixations in the patient's responses that require rapid or frequent shifts in mental sets, particularly in sentence completion drills. The clinician might ask the patient to answer rapidly a series of closed-end questions. When the patient is asked to complete the statement, "Knife, fork, and _____," the patient might answer correctly with "spoon." Then, because of problems shifting from one mental set to another, the patient will answer "spoon" to the next statements: "Red, white, and _____," "The United States of _____," and "Bring me a glass of _____."

Similarly, a writing fixation is the patient's inability to stop writing a particular letter or symbol. When asked to write her name, the patient might start correctly with the first few letters and then trail off into a meaningless series of scribbles vaguely resembling the last letter of the name. Some stroke patients also get stuck while drawing pictures and when copying letters and forms. This fixation on a mental set and inability to shift from one thing to another might contribute to the depression that occurs in some stroke patients. Some cannot get negative, depressing thoughts out of their minds. These and other contributors to depression are discussed in Chapter 7.

Echoed Speech

Children go through a stage of language development in which they echo what has been said to them. Parents are familiar with the child who simply answers every question with the last word spoken. Adults also echo speech. When bidding for time, a person might repeat a question: For example, when someone asks you the question, "Do you have that money you owe me?" you might repeat the question while trying to remember if you have ever borrowed money from that person. Echoed speech is a normal part of language development and adult conversations. Stroke patients also exhibit this normal type of echoed speech, but some have too much echoed speech and for different reasons.

Echoed speech in stroke patients is related to the problem of shifting mental sets. When someone says something, the patient will echo what has been spoken because the words are still being replayed in his or her head. The patient simply says what has been spoken because it is still being processed in the brain, as though the patient's thoughts are contaminated by the last thing said.

Breaking out of a fixed mental set requires mental discipline. Some patients benefit from playing games that require shifting from one idea to the next. One such game requires the patient to say the next word in a series. You might say the first day (Monday) in the days of the week. The patient then says the next day (Tuesday), after which you then say the third day (Wednesday), and so forth. The same game can be played for the months of the year, counting, and spelling. The goal is for the patient to resist the tendency to say the last thing heard. Each patient should begin at levels established by the speech-language pathologist. Before attempting these types of games with your loved one, you should discuss them with the attending speech clinician.

Perceptual Disorders

The fictional sleuth Sherlock Holmes was famous for his highly developed perceptual skills. Although both Sherlock Holmes and Dr. Watson would be present when questioning a suspect in a crime, Holmes would come away from the meeting knowing much more than Dr. Watson. Both Watson and Holmes would see the same person, but Sherlock Holmes would perceive much more. The suspect's slight accent, aftershave, red clay on his shoes, and uneven suntan would all spark meaning in the sleuth's mind. Sherlock would know where the person was born, where he vacationed, his annual salary, and his preferred mode of travel. It was "elementary" that Sherlock Holmes perceived more and better than the average detective.

Your knowledge of the world is dependent on the keenness of your senses, which permit and exclude parts of reality. Your eyes see only the visible light. Infrared and ultraviolet waves can be seen only with special aids. Your ears only hear the vibrations of the world from 20 to 20,000 cycles per second. Too few cycles per second and you feel only vibration; too many cycles per second and sound enters the realm of the ultrasonic. Your tongue can taste only bitter, salt, sweet, and sour, but their combinations bring richness to a fine meal. Running your hand over a fine cut of cloth results in feeling only the texture of it, not the feel of individual atomic particles. Your nose, too, is limited in its ability to detect odors. A drug-sniffing dog has many times the sense of smell as humans. Your senses send the information they are capable of detecting to the brain, and your perceptual abilities ignore some while recognizing and organizing others. The brain filters those that are not deemed immediately important and allows recognition of those that are significant. Perception is the ability to identify and assign meaning to the senses.

Perception is more than sights, odors, tastes, sounds, and things touched. You see with the eyes, smell with the nose, taste with the tongue, hear with the ears, and feel with the skin, but you perceive with the brain. Your brain ignores those things you want to ignore and attends to those things you find important or valuable. The use of perception is learned.

People learn to perceive those aspects of the world that are important and to filter out the rest. Every normal person is born with this ability to sense the important things and disregard those things that get in the way. A lifetime of learning refines perception. For example, if you have learned to play a band instrument, you are much better at hearing and appreciating that instrument when you hear a band play. The trombone, trumpet, or tuba is perceived with more clarity and sophistication by people who play these instruments. When a carpenter, bricklayer, or landscaper drives through a neighborhood, each perceives the homes a little differently. The carpenter is attuned to the quality of the framing, the bricklayer notices the masonry, and the landscaper focuses more closely on the placement of the shrubs. This is because each has learned the intricacies of working in these occupations; their perceptions have been heightened and refined.

It is easier to perceive variations when there is a big difference between things. When contrasts are great, it is easier to distinguish between variations. Most people can tell the difference between extremely bad carpentry, bricklaying, or landscaping and work that has been done well. It is easier for professionals to tell the difference between excellent and marginally good work. The same holds true for the symphony conductor, auto mechanic, and surgeon. They are more attuned to the subtleties in concerts, auto repairs, and surgeries.

Strokes can cause perceptual disorders, which are a distinct class of disorders. Although they frequently occur with communication disorders, they can occur alone. Because strokes can cause reading disorders and problems understanding the speech of others, vision and hearing perception disorders often occur in patients with aphasia. Perceptual disorders can cause an attention problem called *figure-ground*. The *figure* is that which you should attend to and the *ground* is the background sensations that need to be ignored. A figure-ground problem causes a person to be unable to concentrate on the figure when there is a lot of background interference. This interference can be related to any of the senses: hearing, vision, smell, taste, and touch.

People with a visual figure-ground problem have problems concentrating on something they are looking at, such as words on a page, objects on a table, or pictures on a wall. Ordinarily, people can concentrate on words, objects, or pictures and not be distracted by other things seen by the eyes. People with normal perception can focus their attention on the words on the page of a book while ignoring the table and objects sitting nearby. These visual-perceptual disorders can also occur with drawings, faces, and colors. The role of visual-perceptual disorders in the problem some aphasic patients have with reading is not completely understood. However, some patients have more of a problem reading than just remembering what the written word means. Some aphasia patients with reading problems do not recognize some letters for what they are—letters. This can be due to a visual-perceptual disorder.

A good example of figure-ground abilities related to the sense of hearing is the person who can study or read a book while the radio is turned on. Some people can direct their attention to the study materials or book and shut out the noise of the radio. They have a lot of control over their hearing attention. Other people cannot read or study with competing sounds. They cannot concentrate through background noise.

Many stroke patients who have auditory (hearing) perceptual disorders may have difficulty dealing with background noise. They may have trouble concentrating when there is competition from overhead announcements and machines and when more than one person talks simultaneously. Confusion also results from two sounds or words that are similar. Sounds such as *b* and *p, m* and *n,* and *k* and *g* are more likely to be confused because they sound similar. Words that differ only by one sound also can cause confusion. For example, *bill* and *pill, head* and *shed,* and *pen* and *Ben* are more likely to be misperceived by the stroke patient with perceptual disorders.

Some stroke patients have problems perceiving common, everyday sounds such as a car horn, a telephone ringing, or a knock on a door. Patients with this type of problem do not know what these sounds mean. When the telephone rings, a patient with this type of perceptual disorder is likely to check the door to see whether anyone has knocked on it. The meaning or significance of the sounds of children playing, a dishwasher, chickens clucking, or a fire alarm has been lost because of the stroke. Music, tunes, and rhythms may also lose their significance.

Perceptual disorders can occur with aphasia or by themselves. When these disorders occur by themselves, they are usually specific to one avenue of communication. For example, when a perceptual disorder occurs alone, a stroke patient may only have problems understanding speech, and reading, speaking, and writing are unimpaired. Another patient may only have difficulty reading, and the other avenues of communication are left intact. Perceptual disorders differ from aphasia in that the former is usually limited to one avenue of communication. Recall that aphasia cuts across all avenues of communication.

When perceptual disorders occur with aphasia, it is hard to tell them apart. Are the problems with reading due to the patient not recognizing the letters for what they are, or are they a result of not remembering the meaning of the word? Does the stroke patient have problems understanding what you say because the sounds cannot be separated, or because the word has lost its meaning? These questions go to the core of the disabilities, and they are difficult to answer even for health care professionals. Fortunately, the therapies used to treat them are general enough to cover both types of problems. Helping a patient learn to read or to understand the speech of others is general enough to cover communication problems, regardless of their source.

Loss of Half the World

Some stroke patients experience a unique and strange perceptual disorder primarily involving sight and sound. Some will not recognize one entire side of their world, unable to look past the middle of their range of vision to focus on people or things on the left or right. Some patients will not acknowledge the existence of people talking on one side of their midline. Usually in patients with aphasia, it is the right side of the body and visual field that is lost. The name of this disorder is *one-sided neglect*. The examples and discussion that follow focus on right-side neglect because it is the most likely kind to occur with aphasia.

When visual neglect occurs, it may be associated with a vision impairment. Many patients with this neglect have blindness in the right sides of both eyes. The right eye is not blind, but rather the right halves of both eyes. Some patients have visual neglect with no blindness.

Three common behaviors of a stroke patient signal the presence of visual neglect. The first may be observed when the patient is eating. When a plate is placed in the center of the stroke patient's field of vision, he or she will eat only the food on the left side of it. The food on the right side remains untouched because the patient does not acknowledge it. The food on this side of the plate goes uneaten even though the patient could turn his or her head to the far right to compensate for the blindness. The patient will not move his or her eyes across the middle of the plate to see the food.

The second behavior that signals the presence of neglect is when the patient will not look to the right side of the room, even when people are talking there. Such patients will not acknowledge your presence until you cross the middle of their field of vision and get to the left. Then they will acknowledge you. They behave as though you do not exist until you reach the left side of their world. When you are talking to them and begin walking to the right side of the room, once you cross their midline, they stop acknowledging your presence.

The third behavior occurs in women when they put on makeup. They apply lipstick, mascara, and eye shadow only to the left sides of their faces because, when they look in the mirror, they see and acknowledge only the left sides of their bodies.

Patients with visual neglect also have trouble reading. Because their eyes will not cross the middle of a page, they read only the left side. Obviously, this leads to comprehension problems. Their writing is also impaired. When they are finished writing a letter, for example, one entire side of the page is left blank.

The reasons for this visual neglect are not completely understood. Damage to specific areas of the brain seems to cause it. There may also be a psychological component. The stroke patient's hand, arm, and leg may be paralyzed on one side. The patient refuses to acknowledge that side of the world because that is where terrible things have happened. On an unconscious level, the patient does not want to look to that side because it causes negative feelings and a loss of the sense of wholeness. As the patient consciously begins to realize what has happened, he or she gradually learns to look at the disabled body parts and accept them.

The rehabilitation team offers programs to help patients with visual neglect. Some patients are placed in rooms where the television is located only on their neglected side. Occupational, physical, and speech therapists work to bring the neglected side of the patient's world back. By gradually requiring the patient to cross over and see people and objects in the neglected world, the patient can work toward a fuller and more complete life. All attempts on the part of the patient to cross over to the neglected side are supported and praised. Check out how stroke survivor Allison and husband Stephen learned to deal with blindness (homonymous hemianopsia) and visual neglect in Chapter 13: Profiles in Recovery.

Eating Problems

When a stroke causes numbness, weakness, and/or paralysis of the tongue, soft palate, and muscles in the voice box, patients have trouble chewing, sucking, and swallowing because the same muscles are used for both speaking and eating. These problems can be mild, requiring only that the patient slow down and think about eating safely, or they can be life-threatening. Choking and pneumonia can result from these eating problems. The pneumonia is a special type caused by getting food or liquid into the lungs. The bacteria in the food or liquid causes the lungs to become sick, and fluid builds up in them. This type of pneumonia is known as *aspi-*

ration pneumonia. *Aspiration* means that foods and/or liquids were taken into the lungs. Eating problems usually occur when the patient has dysarthria, but they can also happen when the patient has no communication disorder.

When the physician makes a patient "NPO," this usually suggests that the stroke has affected the muscles of eating. The doctor believes that if the patient eats, he or she could choke or get aspiration pneumonia. To eliminate this risk, the order "NPO" means the patient should not take in anything orally. You should never give an NPO patient anything to eat or drink by mouth, especially water, without consulting a physician. To provide the patient with nourishment, an intravenous drip, or IV, is sometimes placed in the patient's arm. The gradual dripping of liquids directly into the vein provides fluids and some nourishment. Sometimes a patient is given a nasogastric or "NG" tube, which goes through the nose and into the stomach, to provide nourishment.

To know what kind of swallowing problem a patient is having, it is necessary to understand a normal swallow. In a normal swallow, first the food must be chewed. The tongue, teeth, and lips chew the food into small enough pieces to be swallowed. But there is more to chewing than simply getting the pieces small enough to go down the throat. Saliva lubricates food and molds it into a small ball. When all of the food has been cleaned from the mouth and rolled into this ball, the tongue pushes it to the back of the throat. Then the ball of food drops down the throat. While this is happening, the vocal cords close, and a flap drops over the opening of the voice box and the tubes leading to the lungs. These two actions help prevent the airway from getting food in it. After passing this point, the food is gradually squeezed into the stomach by a series of muscle movements. Liquids are swallowed in nearly the same way except for the chewing stage.

The main reason some stroke patients have problems swallowing is that in humans, only one opening—the mouth—takes both food and air into the body. After food has been placed in the mouth, there are two possible places it can go—to the stomach or, accidentally, to the lungs. You have probably experienced having food go "down the wrong tube." Through coughing and throat clearing, hopefully you were able to redirect it to the correct tube. Sometimes strokes cause the muscles involved to be weak or paralyzed, and because of this, they cannot direct the food properly. The way the body protects itself from getting food in the lungs is damaged.

When the normal swallow breaks down due to a stroke, it is important to see where the difficulties lie. Is the problem because the ball of food is not moved to the back of the throat? Sometimes poor chewing results in little pieces of food being left in the mouth and not rolled into a ball. Is the problem because the drop of the ball is not timed properly for the protective reflexes? If there is a delay in this aspect of the swallow, the patient might accidentally breathe in the food or liquid. Is the problem with the swallow because the vocal cords and the bonelike flap do not completely close or they close too slowly? Sometimes the muscles in the throat cannot perform this job well enough to protect the airway. This is usually caused by weakness or paralysis of those muscles. Some patients are easily distracted or confused and they have problems swallowing because they are not careful enough. The evaluation of swallowing problems will be discussed in more detail in Chapter 11.

Liquids are harder to swallow than solid foods because they are harder to manage and control. Thin liquids, such as coffee, tea, water, and thin soups, are the hardest to manage. Sometimes a thickener is added to thin liquids to make them more manageable for a stroke patient. Often, either hot or cold foods are easier to manage than tepid foods or drinks because the patient can better sense where they are in the mouth and throat. Although ice cream is cold and thus easier for many patients to monitor, it creates a *rope* mucus. In some stroke patients with swallowing problems, ice cream should be avoided because this stringy liquid can be sucked accidentally into the lungs.

You might assume that patients have a normal swallow if they do not choke or cough. Although this appears to be a reasonable assumption, it is sometimes wrong. In patients with numbness or muscle weakness in the throat, the lack of choking and coughing can result in something called *silent aspiration*. Food and liquids are sucked into the lungs accidentally, but there is no coughing or choking—the intake is silent. It appears that these patients swallowed correctly, but food or liquid entered the lungs. Some patients with swallowing problems do choke and cough, and you can sometimes hear a gurgle in the lungs or throat. If the swallowing problem is serious enough, patients will often "spike" a temperature. Especially in weak and feeble patients, this can be a serious medical condition requiring the physician's immediate attention. Any time you suspect or wonder if your loved one is accidentally breathing food or liquids into the lungs, you should contact his or her physician.

As you see, several complications can arise when your loved one has a stroke-related communication disorder. Some patients have a lowered threshold for emotional expressions and tend to cry too easily. Stroke patients may also experience panic attacks, especially when there are too many distractions or too much pressure is placed on them. Strokes can cause patients to have trouble shifting from one thought to another. A word, thought, or action cannot be dropped from the mind and it taints the thoughts and actions that follow. Sometimes this results in repeating the last sound or word that was heard. Several perceptual disorders can cause confusion about sight, odor, taste, sound, and touch. Visual neglect also occurs, and the patient cannot or will not look to one side of his or her world. Paralysis or weakness of the speech muscles can cause sucking, chewing, and swallowing difficulties. These can be serious, even life-threatening problems, and require immediate medical attention.

Like the big three stroke-related communication disorders, these complications have happened to many people and they are treatable. At first glance, they may appear too complex and insurmountable. But, while complex, they, too, can be overcome or adjustments can be made to reduce them. The important thing to remember is that every patient has room for improvement. With proper care and strong support from family and friends, patients can and do improve. There is always room for optimism.

CHAPTER 5

Loss of Awareness

Set up as an ideal the facing of reality as honestly and as cheerfully as possible.—DR. KARL A. MENNINGER

A stroke can affect a person's perception of the world. Even when the brain injury is minor, difficulties communicating affect the way the patient views the world. There is likely to be a changed awareness of things previously taken for granted. The act of communicating normally takes on new meaning and has broader implications. Also, the patient's perception of health and wellness changes significantly. In these ways, even a minor stroke changes the way a person views the world. Severe strokes also can affect dramatically an individual's awareness, often compromising and completely changing a person's perception of "self" and the surrounding world. Strokes may cause disorientation, memory deficits, and learning problems. In one of the worst case scenarios, a stroke can leave a patient in a deep coma.

Many stroke survivors suffer no loss of awareness. However, some strokes reduce or eliminate the person's awareness of self and the world. As far as we know, a patient in a deep coma has no awareness and does not communicate. Some people survive strokes only to emerge confused and disoriented. Of course, when these people talk, their speech reflects their disorientation and confusion. Many patients have one or more of the big three communication disorders along with reduced awareness. Their communication is a mixture of aphasia, apraxia of speech, and the dysarthrias, all occurring within and contributing to the blur of confusion and disorientation.

"*I think therefore I exist.*" Put in modern terms, this ancient maxim might read, "I am conscious, therefore I have an awareness of myself and my environment." Consciousness is the same as awareness. Mental health professionals call this *orientation*. Orientation means you remember what happened in your youth, last month, yesterday, and 10 seconds ago. You have an idea of the time of day, the season, and the decade. You know who is president of the United States, and you know the names of the country and state in which you reside. You know your parents and children and the neighbor next door. Dogs and cats are familiar, as are jet vapor trails and the smell of freshly baked bread. Muffled traffic noise and certain types of music are familiar, comforting sounds. And as disturbing as it may be, humans are aware of mortality, which means "destined to die."

Humans possess a special kind of awareness that is different from the awareness of the dog, cat, or worm. It is doubtful that the dog wonders what it is like to be a cat and vice versa. A worm is unaware that it is a worm. Some authorities believe that human awareness is shaped and framed by language. For example, the Eskimos have many words to describe snow, allowing them to think more clearly and succinctly about this major part of their lives. Because they possess many words for snow, they perceive of snow differently than does someone who lives in the Caribbean. One theory asserts that humans became aware of themselves because of language. Words allowed humans to be able to think about themselves in the abstract. There are many theories about how humans developed this special type of awareness—self-awareness. Some people believe that the origin of human awareness is God-given. In the Christian Bible, the origins of awareness go back to the parable of Adam and Eve and the tree of knowledge of good and evil. Some people trace consciousness to learning; because humans can learn, they gradually became more aware of themselves and the environment. A theory that is appealing to some scientists is that awareness is a property of matter: Given enough time, consciousness will arise from matter. According to this theory, human consciousness evolved from matter over the billions of years the universe has been in existence.

When it comes to strokes and awareness, where a patient *is* is not as important as where he or she is *going*. The road to the return of awareness can be short and straight. It can also be long and never-ending. Progress can occur in leaps and bounds, just as gains can also be "three steps forward and one step back." The most important thing for you to remember is to meet your loved one wherever he or she is on the road to recovery. Assuming that or acting as if the patient is more aware than he or she really is creates a frustrating relationship for both of you. Likewise, regarding the patient as less aware than he or she actually is reduces the potential for the best recovery possible. Underestimating your loved one's position also limits your relationship and the joys and pleasures it can bring.

Coma

A patient in a coma appears to be asleep. A person in a deep coma cannot be awakened even with strong prompting and also does not respond to internal needs such as hunger. Although there are similarities between coma and sleep, they are two very separate states. The main difference is that the sleeping person can be awakened; the patient in a coma cannot. In fact, studies have shown that patients in a coma also sleep, going through several states of sleep found in normal people. Some patients in a coma do not appear to be asleep. This sometimes occurs when both sides of the brain are damaged severely. In this form of coma, the patient appears to be awake because the eyes are open, but the patient exhibits no speech, thought, or purposeful movement.

You have probably heard of people in deep comas who suddenly awakened from them. This is rare, but it has happened. Sometimes a coma is caused by pressure or another problem on the part of the brain that regulates alertness. When this problem is removed or subsides, the brain again functions normally. If there has been no other damage to the brain, a person who was in this type of coma often returns to normal levels of awareness.

As you can see, there are levels of coma. Not all patients in a coma are in a deep one. Many patients progress to more alert and less confused states. Specialists use several scales to measure levels of awareness in these patients. These scales rate how well patients talk, move, and keep their eyes open. Memory and orientation tests also help evaluate patient awareness. Sometimes patients are said to be delirious or stuporous, or that their consciousness is clouded. There have been many studies conducted to predict the patient's eventual recovery. Because of these studies, a particular patient's ultimate prognosis is now fairly accurate. The length of time in a coma and the degree to which the patient can pass these tests are good indicators of how he or she will ultimately fare.

Although strokes can cause coma and reduced levels of awareness, these conditions are most often seen in head injuries. There are two general types of head injuries: closed and open. A closed head injury is the kind frequently seen in car accidents and falls. The person's head hits the dashboard or highway, and the force of the impact damages the brain. An open head injury consists of a hole or opening into the brain. This can be caused by car accidents and falls, too, but they are caused primarily by gunshot wounds. When a bullet or shrapnel enters the brain, damage is caused by the impact and by the tearing of the brain due to the foreign object. Like strokes, head injuries often reduce blood flow to the brain. This is because some vessels burst. Coma and reduced levels of awareness can also be caused by poisons, infections, cancers, and other diseases.

Memory deficits and confusion are at the heart of problems experienced by patients who are coming out of a coma. In many of these patients, as the coma lifts, these orientation and memory problems gradually improve. Unfortunately, some patients remain at a particular level of confusion and disorientation. Some are generally confused about everything while others have more specific types of disorientation. Other stroke patients have problems of memory and disorientation but may never have been in a coma.

Disorientation

Being aware of yourself and your orientation to the world around you can be divided into four categories: time, place, person, and situation. Some stroke patients have difficulties in one or two of these areas and other patients are completely disoriented in all areas. Patients confused in all four areas are said to be disoriented "times four," meaning that the disorientation cuts across time, place, person, and situation.

The first category of orientation—orientation to time—is awareness of dates and the passage of time. It involves knowing the hour, day, month, year, and season. Disorientation to time is the most common type of confusion, probably because time is fleeting and an intangible. A patient with time disorientation may consistently report the wrong date and time. He or she might be confused about when to eat meals or when to go to bed. When asked the season, the disoriented patient might report that it is winter, when in fact it is summertime. The patient's perception of the passage of time may also be confused. If you have set aside an hour for a visit, the patient might think that the allotted time has already passed when only 10 minutes have gone by.

Disorientation to place usually occurs along with time confusion. Patients disoriented to place may not know their city, state, or even the country of residence. Some patients report that they are in a city or state they have never even visited. Other patients believe that they are at home instead of at the hospital, and it is difficult to convince them to the contrary. Other types of disorientation to place include believing that a dining room is a movie theater, a hall is a tunnel, or that the hospital room is a sleeping compartment on a train.

The third category of orientation is to person. In disorientation to person, the patient may be confused about whom he or she is and about relationships. Patients may experience confusion about their gender or about their previous occupation. In the broadest sense, patients completely disoriented to person have lost their identity. As with the other types of disorientation, the confusion can be complete or selective. Selective disorientation to person occurs when the patient knows some aspects of his or her life but is confused about others. The patient may know you and other members of the immediate family but be confused about friends and acquaintances.

The final type of disorientation is that of situation. Some authorities call this type of confusion *disorientation to predicament*. Patients disoriented to situation do not have complete awareness of their medical condition. They might report that they are in a hospital for routine tests when in fact they are having intensive rehabilitation following a stroke. Some patients with confusion about their situation believe that their problems are nonexistent or minimal. There is often an element of denial to this type of confusion. These patients believe their problems are of minor consequence, when in reality they are debilitating.

Confusion or Aphasic Naming Errors?

It is easy to diagnose disorientation in a patient who has normal powers of speech— the patient talks as though he or she is confused, making mistakes about time, place, person, and situation. The confusion is apparent to all who meet the patient. However, the patient with aphasia might be misdiagnosed as disoriented when in fact he or she is just making naming errors typical of aphasia. Recall that many aphasic patients mistakenly say words that are related in meaning: *car* for *truck, pen* for *pencil,* or *fork* for *spoon.* Some aphasic patients confuse these words because the words share similar or related meanings. These are naming errors and not indications of confusion. Though confused about the names of people and things, the aphasic patient is not likely to try to eat soup with a fork.

Understandably, it is a source of concern when a patient says, "This is my mother," when in fact the woman is his wife. The fear is that the individual does not know his wife from his mother. To know whether the error was just a naming problem or an indication of general confusion, look to the patient's behaviors. Does he or she act confused? Does he treat his wife like his mother? When a patient says she is in the wrong city, does she act confused? If the patient says the next holiday is Christmas when in fact it is Easter, do his behaviors support the error? Does the patient exhibit behavior that indicates he does not know Christmas from Easter? Unfortunately, some patients may be both aphasic and confused. If you have difficulty knowing whether the patient is confused or just making a naming error, you should take these concerns to the medical staff. Wrong assumptions can cloud your relationship with the patient.

Memory Problems

We are products of our experiences. Our memories of the past allow us perspective on the present. Our knowledge of the past is merged with our view of today. The way we deal with challenges, successes, and failures and our attitudes about the nature of life are based on our personal and collective memories. Experience is only a great teacher if we remember the lessons.

Psychologically, memory provides our lives with continuity and predictability. It is comforting to have a history. Normal memory is also the foundation on which learning occurs. Learning can be defined as the ability to profit from experience. But to profit from experiences, one must have a memory of them.

Memory problems are at the core of the confusion and disorientation seen in some stroke patients. If the patient could remember facts about time, place, person, and situation, he or she would not be disoriented. Without memory a person is bound to current events and is less aware of his or her environment. Memory problems and confusion go hand in hand.

Three processes are essential to normal memory, and the disruption of any one process can impair memory and contribute to confusion and disorientation. Discovering which of these processes is defective in the stroke patient provides valuable information about how to deal with your loved one's memory problems and disorientation. The processes are attention, storage, and recall.

Attention

All of us have had the experience of being asked a question when our minds were elsewhere. While we were daydreaming or distracted, information was presented and when we were asked to comment on it, all we could provide was an embarrassing confession of our lack of attention. "Please repeat the question," is the admission of this lack of attention. A general level of attention must be present for a patient to have unimpaired memory. For normal memory to be possible, the patient must have awareness of the environment. If a patient is in a deep coma, very little can be done to improve memory.

Selective attention is also important to memory. The patient must have the ability to attend selectively to important things and ignore others. (See the discussion in Chapter 4 on figure-ground problems.) For patients coming out of a coma, poor selective attention may be the reason for memory deficits. These patients can be bothered by too much noise and too many distractions. For example, they may have difficulty attending to conversations while the television is on because the sounds and images from the television interfere with their ability to attend selectively to visitors.

Storage

Storage of information is the second stage of memory. Human memory comprises two types of storage: short- and long-term memory. Short-term memory involves the ability to retain information for as long as you are thinking about it. Remembering a telephone number is an example of short-term storage. We have all had the experience of looking up a telephone number and saying it repeatedly. As long as we consciously attend to the numbers, we remember them. Then someone will ask a question or we run into another type of distraction and we forget the numbers. Because the telephone number was stored only in short-term memory, we must look it up again. Short-term memory requires continued rehearsing.

Authorities say that our short-term memory is "seven, plus or minus two." This means that the average person has a short-term memory of seven items, with the range of normal between five and nine. It is normal to have a short-term memory of items from five to nine. The average number is seven. It is no coincidence that telephone numbers are usually seven numbers in length. The "seven, plus or minus two" rule applies when the items are said in an evenly timed and spaced way. Some people can remember more items when they are said faster or "chunked" into categories.

Scientists believe that when information goes from short-term storage to long-term memory banks, different processes in the brain are involved. Short-term memory requires continued nerve impulses, whereas long-term memory results in actual changes in brain cell chemistry. The transition from short-term to long-term memory means that information has been internalized. When information is internalized, it is made personally relevant through association with other stored memories.

For patients coming out of a coma, storage of information can break down at the short- or long-term stages. In the midst of a lot of noise and distraction, it may be difficult for the patient to keep rehearsing important information such as the names of family members, friends, and the medical staff. Numbers, times, and schedules also may be lost to distraction and noise. Long-term storage problems often involve incidental information. When information is not made personally relevant to patients, they will have a harder time remembering it. For example, if a patient is being taught to remember the days of the week, it is better to make each day personally relevant, perhaps by saying, "Monday is the day you go outside to have lunch." If the patient likes going outside to eat, the association between Monday and going outside to lunch increases the probability of the information being stored in the long term. The information selected to be remembered should always be relevant and important. Trying to teach the patient presidents' birthdays, obscure holidays, and names of distant relatives are examples of spending time on unimportant information. As the patient comes out of a coma, he or she should be taught only the most important information that is specifically relevant to his or her situation. Superficial information should be delayed and kept as a goal for later in the rehabilitation program.

Recall

Recalling the information is the final stage of memory. Once the events and information have been attended to and stored in memory, they must be available for recall. Recall is affected by several factors, some of which cannot be controlled. Attention, general alertness, anxiety, and psychological defenses all affect the recall of events and information that were attended to and stored.

Not all stored information is available for recall, because some information is blocked from awareness. This is the idea behind subconscious memories. Certain memories, especially unpleasant ones, are sometimes blocked from a person's awareness. Although they were attended to and stored, because they are unpleasant the mind blocks them. Some mental health experts believe that these unconscious memories still affect how a person thinks, feels, and behaves. When unconscious memories negatively affect a person's life, psychotherapy may be helpful in bringing them to the surface so that they can be dealt with more rationally.

Many studies on memory have shown that people are better able to recall information when they are calm and relaxed. That is the reason hypnosis is sometimes helpful in solving crimes. Hypnosis can be used to bring about a state of suggestive relaxation. It has been shown that when witnesses to a crime are deeply relaxed, they are more capable of remembering the details and events surrounding the crime.

The recall of certain memories can be triggered by sights, smells, and sounds. We have all had the experience of a certain memory being triggered by a song from days gone by on the radio. The smell of something from our past can also trigger memories. Patients coming out of a coma can also be stimulated by the senses. Some patients talk about these triggered memories as they come up. Some patients appear to be rambling when in fact they are talking about memories as they surface. The patient undergoing therapy to improve memory should never be hurried. When you interact with the patient, be sure to project the idea that he or she has all the time in the world to recall information. Impatience on your part can cause the stroke survivor to feel hurried and tense, and tension interferes with the process of recall.

Recalling information that was attended to and stored is more difficult than recognizing the correct answer when it is provided as a series of options. For example, if a patient has problems remembering a family member's name, providing the first sound of it might be all that is necessary to recall the name. Sometimes only a cue or prompt is needed to bring the memory to mind. You should be careful to provide these cues only when you know for certain what word or memory the patient is trying to recall.

Human Memory Banks and Libraries

Whenever a person's memory breaks down, the collapse can be traced to problems with one or more of the three stages of remembering: attention, storage, and recall. These memory problems can be likened to the way books are stored and checked out from a library. Each book is an event or an item of information and the library is the person's memory. Like books in a library, each person has a vast number of individual memories.

Initially, for the library to get a new book, some employee must select it. Not all books are in every library. Some libraries are small and select ony the titles with the widest range of interest; their budgets dictate that only the most popular books are selected for the stacks. Others are specialized, such as law or medical libraries. Only books written about the legal or medical professions are chosen. Large university libraries would choose more books than would small community libraries. Employees who select the books try to choose ones that are relevant and important to the types of people who are likely to use the library.

Like a library, the human memory bank does not register and store every event in a person's life. Instead, human memory is selective. Millions of events occur each day that the individual sees, hears, touches, smells, or tastes. It would be impossible for all of these events to be placed in a person's memory bank. Only those that are attended to are selected for storage in the memory bank. Throughout life, a person learns to attend to and perceive only events that are meaningful, important, and relevant. The color, shape, and size of every bug the person sees are not carefully attended to and selected for storage. Every blast of a car's horn is not selected for storage.

Some events are more important and relevant than others, and they are immediately selected for storage. Most people will remember what they were doing when it was announced that Japan had bombed Pearl Harbor and that the United States had entered into World War II. So, too, are memories associated with President John F. Kennedy's assassination and the tragedy of September 11, 2001. These are "peak" memories, which are immediately attended to and selected for storage. So, too, are the feelings associated with them. If these memories were books, they would be best-sellers, major titles the patrons of the library would want to check out and read.

Once a book is acquired, it must be filed correctly if it is ever to be found again. Books are stored in libraries based on the category to which they belong in alphabetical order. Fiction books are placed with other novels. Periodicals and reference works are placed with similar books, magazines, and journals. Each book is assigned a number and an entry is made in a computer or card catalog. In a building full of books, the computer entry or card catalog provides a system of organization by which library patrons can find the specific book they want to read. Books are not just randomly placed in the stacks; there is a system to their placement.

The human memory bank stores events and information in a similar way. Memories are associated and follow a train of thought. Sight, sound, smell, and taste are associated in memory. Most people order and store memories in a predictable way. Events and information are often stored together with the feelings and emotions felt at the same time. Some events are stored with powerful emotions, others with little or no feeling.

Neuroscientists have conducted studies in which they touched parts of the human brain with probes having small electrical currents. The subjects of these studies were awake during the experiments. When particular areas of their brains were touched, the subjects reported seeing, hearing, touching, or smelling something. "I smell freshly baked bread" or "I see my grandmother in her driveway" were the types of reports made by these awake subjects when the probes were touched to various parts of their brains. Many subjects reported feelings associated with the memories. Not only did they smell freshly baked bread, but they also felt like the 10-year-old who was standing next to the oven.

When library patrons want to check out a book, they first go to the computer to see where it is located. The information in the computer tells patrons where the book is located. The building, floor, section, and shelf where the book is located are provided on the computer screen. Library patrons can then get the book and take it to the circulation station to be checked out.

The human memory bank is also a lot like a library when it comes to retrieving information. For an event or information to be recalled, there must be a system for access. Some things are remembered when a person consciously seeks the memory. Remembering where a car is parked in a large parking lot is an example of conscious retrieval of information. Locating your car is a process of association with rows of other cars, color codes of parking lots, and the model of the car. Other memories are stumbled on. Like browsing through a library and seeing a book of interest, some memories are incidentally recalled. Perhaps a sight, sound, or word triggers the memory. Some are recalled with no apparent association. Sometimes memories are easy to retrieve while others are stored deep within the memory bank.

Most libraries have signs that read "Please do not shelve the books." This sign tells patrons to leave the books on the tables when they are done reading them. Books can be lost in the library simply by placing them in the wrong stack or on the wrong shelf. When shelved improperly, though the book is in the library, it cannot be found. Likewise, human memory banks can contain many memories that are unavailable for recall because the brain has no retrieval method. These memories are like lost books in the library: They exist within the brain, but they are not retrievable. When books are shelved correctly in the stacks, they are easy to retrieve. A library patron can locate and retrieve a single book from thousands in a short time. Human recall is basically the same as the library system but much more efficient. Memories of what to do when confronted with a stop sign, door knob, tax bill, or poisonous snake are available in an instant. Humans are capable of retrieving millions of memories with minimal effort. You are doing it now as you recall the meanings of the words on this page. Memory is truly a remarkable process.

In human memory, there is a phenomenon known as *state dependent* learning. This means that when someone stores something in memory, the emotions he or she is feeling influence the recall. When you are happy, it is easier to recall events that happened at other times in your life when you felt on top of the world. Depressed people more readily recall sad or painful events in their lives. When a group of people goes out drinking, the alcohol affects their recall in the same way. Under the effects of the alcohol, they are more inclined to remember other times when they were drinking. State-dependent learning holds true for prescription mood-altering drugs and other substances and circumstances that affect a person's mood.

Amnesia Before and After the Stroke

Two types of memory loss can result from a stroke. The first type has to do with the loss of memory of information and events that happened before the stroke. The patient can have memory gaps about information or events that occurred before the stroke. Sometimes the blank memory encompasses all things that happened, or it can be selective and involve only certain aspects of a person's life. This type of amnesia may involve forgetting that a relative has died, that a friend has remarried, or that a business failed. It can also be for everything that happened during the past week, month, year, or even decade.

A second type of memory loss involves the inability to recall events that happened after the stroke as well as learning and remembering new information presented since the stroke. It frequently affects remembering some or all of the events that have happened since coming out of a coma. This type of amnesia can last for weeks, months, or even years. The patient experiencing this type of memory loss may not remember having the stroke even though there was no loss of consciousness. The patient's first memory might be a recent session of group therapy or a recent visit from a relative, although many sessions and visits occurred earlier.

Accurate Diagnosis of Memory Deficits

As previously discussed, it is sometimes difficult to evaluate confusion in aphasic patients. They may not know the correct time, place, or person and not appreciate their predicament. While it is true that some patients are confused, others might just be saying the wrong word when being tested because of a speech and language disorder. To separate naming problems from true confusion, it is important to observe the patient closely to see whether the patient truly acts confused. Observation is also important in determining the nature and severity of memory problems.

A patient can be given many memory tests that are important in finding out how well the patient will fare at home. These tests are often used to decide whether the patient needs to remain in a hospital or nursing home with careful supervision or whether he or she is ready to go home. Some tests have the patient memorize numbers and repeat them backward and forward. Some tests evaluate how well the patient can remember information that has been read. Other tests look at how well a patient can remember a sequence of blocks, pictures, or diagrams. Both long- and short-term memory may be assessed, and literally hundreds of memory tests can be given to stroke patients. However, one of the best tests is to have the patient's family observe how he or she does in real life. Studies have shown that formal tests often miss the mark when it comes to deciding how well a patient's memory will allow independent living. Some patients do well on the tests only to engage in dangerous activities at home, such as leaving the stove turned on. Other patients do poorly on memory tests but succeed in living at home safely with very little supervision. A patient's performance on memory tests does not always translate into an absolutely accurate picture of how he or she will fare at home.

Behavioral Problems

Behavioral problems are not common in strokes, but they do happen, especially as the coma gradually lifts. Some patients say or do things that are inappropriate, often with a sexual theme. They may play with themselves in public, make sexually provocative statements, or touch visitors in inappropriate places. Patients with behavioral problems may lose any sense of modesty and walk around unclothed. Other types of behavioral problems include acting too friendly with strangers, boasting, talking too loudly, lying, and talking on and on about irrelevant things. Some patients laugh or cry at improper times and for the wrong reasons.

Naturally, these actions can be embarrassing and unsettling for loved ones. For the spouse, the sexually provocative comments made by the patient to a stranger can feel like a slap in the face. The spouse is doing all he or she can to provide help and support and the patient appears inconsiderate or even unkind. Patients themselves often report, after they have regained awareness, being embarrassed about these things. When told that they walked through the hall of the hospital partially clothed or that they groped a stranger, they are understandably embarrassed. Some patients cannot even believe they did these things.

Although the embarrassment felt by both you and the stroke patient is a natural reaction, these behavioral problems should not be taken too seriously. In a hospital, rehabilitation center, or nursing home, these things happen frequently. Medical professionals are accustomed to such incidents and think no less of you or the patient when they occur. These behaviors are viewed as necessary and often temporary elements of the recovery process from coma or other reduced states of awareness. The patient is simply responding to his or her world differently because of brain injury and psychological needs. Of course, if the patient is physically abusive or dangerous to self or others, then medication, isolation, or a strict program of behavior modification may be deemed necessary.

As difficult as it may be at times, if the stroke patient has behavioral problems, it is still important for you and other family members to maintain emotional bonds. Maintaining the bonds of family and friendship is crucial at this time. Although it may be difficult to show love and support when a patient is behaving "badly," this is the time support is needed the most. Remember, the patient is simply reacting to the world as he or she sees it. The brain injury, emotional needs, and demands of the environment are powerful factors influencing the patient. This is not the time for the patient to have to experience feelings of abandonment by loved ones.

Improving Awareness

When a loved one is in a coma, one of the most difficult burdens for you and other family members to endure is the waiting—waiting for the patient to open his or her eyes, to grasp your hand, or to say something. You want to be able to do something, anything, that will hasten recovery. There are some things you can do that will help some patients. However, the patient must have the prerequisite levels of awareness. The main consideration is: "Can the patient profit from the experience?" It is important to know whether the patient has the attention, storage, and recall abilities to benefit from your efforts.

Some rehabilitation hospitals provide a therapy known as *coma stimulation*. Patients in a coma are read to, exercised, and given sensory stimulation. One of the goals of this therapy is to increase the patient's memory, the idea being that even patients in a coma can attend to information at some level and retain it. The belief is that this therapy increases the speed at which the patient comes out of the coma. A few studies have been done on coma stimulation, but they have produced conflicting results. Based on the research conducted to date, coma stimulation is considered an experimental therapy with little scientific support.

For patients in a deep coma, there are few direct things you can do to improve the situation. However, regularly visiting the patient, holding his hand, and providing comforting statements may provide psychological benefits to both you and the patient. It is not helpful or desirable to shake or shout at the coma patient to increase awareness. Comforting statements such as, "We love you," "Everything is okay," and "I'm with you" at least give you something to do. The comforting intent of these words also might register with the patient. Do not discuss the patient with the medical staff or other family members while in the room with the patient. Although it is unlikely that the patient understands your statements, it is possible. Besides, because the patient might detect the distressing tone of these discussions, it is a simple courtesy to leave the room to have these discussions.

For patients who are in one of the stages of coming out of a coma, there are things you and other family members can do to help the patient's levels of awareness, orientation, and memory. Before you begin to help the patient, you should discuss the situation with the medical staff. Especially for confused patients, it is important that everyone be as consistent as possible. Doing otherwise will create more confusion.

To understand the nature of the patient's confusion, you should ask three questions. First ask, "What is the theme of the disorientation?" Some patients are disoriented in a fearful manner. They have negative thoughts that cause them to be afraid. Other patients engage in commanding statements and behaviors that suggest a need to regain control over their lives. Some patients are angry and hostile and may be destructive. Emotional needs drive the actions of the confused and disoriented patient. Patients act in different ways at different times during the process of coming out of the coma. Nonetheless, you should look for the theme of the confusion at any given time. Is your loved one fearful, angry, or controlling? Knowing the patient's theme will give you guidance about how to deal with the words and actions.

The second question to ask is, "What are the environmental demands on the patient?" Everyone becomes disoriented when placed in an environment that exceeds his or her understanding. Patients can experience too much noise and too little order about meals, visitation, and sleep. There can be too many people in the dining room, too much walking in the halls, and too many announcements made over the public address system. Perhaps the beds are made by the housekeeping staff at odd or irregular hours. Your loved one may be confused because the environmental demands exceed his or her cognitive and emotional abilities.

The third question to ask is, "What is the patient talking about?" Some confused patients make unusual statements like "I am Superman." Obviously, the patient is confused, but what is meant by the statement? Does the patient actually believe that he or she is Superman? If the patient is a female, is she also confused about her gender? To understand the degree of confusion, you should look to your loved one's actions. Does he or she actually attempt to act like Superman? As reported previously, some patients produce "empty" speech, saying the first thing that comes to mind; perhaps these statements are triggered by a sight, odor, touch, or sound. When the patient remarks that he or she is Superman, was the comment triggered by a picture or the television? By listening and analyzing the patient's statements, sometimes you can discover the type and nature of the disorientation.

Once the theme of the disorientation is discovered, you can engage in some basic activities to help the patient become more alert and less disoriented. Again, before beginning these activities, discuss them with the medical staff. Family members and friends of the patient are often encouraged to be participants in a structured program of reality orientation.

Reality Orientation

Most patients who have significant memory problems and who are disoriented are put through a program called *reality orientation*. In a typical reality orientation program, all members of the rehabilitation team, family members, and friends work on getting the patient to be more aware of his or her environment and to respond appropriately to it. The team usually agrees on a treatment plan, which is then consistently applied. Everyone who comes into contact with the patient provides reality and orientation information. The patient is also given reinforcements for being more appropriate, alert, and aware. Even small indications of improved awareness are acknowledged and rewarded. The rationale behind reality orientation programs is that when all visitors provide consistent reality information, the patient is likely to become more oriented. Calendars, clocks, and family pictures are placed on walls where the patient can view them easily. Higher functioning patients work on puzzles, board games, and high-level workbooks to improve orientation and memory. Some facilities hold regularly scheduled group orientation and memory activities.

When providing reality orientation, it is important that a bridge between you and the patient be maintained or created. There is no one correct way of viewing the world; one person's perspective is neither better nor worse than another's. But productive and constructive views of the world are more likely to produce happy and well-adjusted people. The goal of reality orientation is not to make the patient conform to a particular view of life but to help him or her regain the perspectives that can lead to a productive, healthy life. Reestablishment of your loved one's healthy links to time, place, person, and current situation is the goal of reality orientation.

CHAPTER 6
Thinking Without
Language

*To understand any living thing, you must, so to say, creep within and
feel the beating of its heart.—W. MACNEILE DIXON*

What follows is a quiz of sorts, an example of a problem confronted by a patient
with global aphasia. Your answer to the question that follows the example will indicate how well you understand the thought processes in people who are deprived
of language.

*It is a cold Midwestern afternoon. The thermometer reads in the teens. Outside,
the wind is howling, blowing snow into drifts as high as a person can reach. Mr.
Robinson sits alone in the cafeteria of a large nursing home. Three years ago Mr.
Robinson had his stroke. On his chart, the speech diagnosis simply reads, "Global
Aphasia." It has been three years of life without language for Mr. Robinson. He
is confined to a wheelchair, but with careful use of his left arm and leg, he gets
around without the help of others. He comes and goes as he wants.*

*On this cold winter afternoon, Margaret, a food service worker, decides she
wants a cigarette. As is the usual custom, she must go outside to smoke so as not
to pollute the air in the nursing home. She walks by Mr. Robinson, says "Hello,"
and gives him a friendly smile on her way to the large glass doors. She doesn't
bring a coat; after all, she just wants a few drags on the cigarette before setting
up the tables for dinner. As she opens the door, a blast of cold briefly blows into
the dining room. She steps outside, carefully holding her foot so the door will
not close. As she lights the cigarette, perhaps she slips or there is gust of wind,
and the self-locking door slams closed. Now she is confronted with a long, coatless
walk to the front of the building in the freezing cold. She looks to Mr. Robinson
and knocks on the glass doors, her breath white with vapor. Shivering, she shakes
the door handle and knocks again.*

Does Mr. Robinson wheel his chair over to the door and pull down on the handle to save Margaret the long walk in the cold? Or, because Mr. Robinson has no language, does he sit oblivious to the plight of the freezing woman?

What Is Thinking?

Before we can answer any question about how a patient with global aphasia thinks about people and things, we must first define and describe *thought*. This is not an easy job. For centuries philosophers, scientists, and religious scholars have pondered the question, "What is thought?" Although some ground has been gained in understanding human thought, the topic remains controversial and subject to heated debate. However, the goal of this chapter is not to ponder the great philosophical questions about human thought but to provide a basic understanding of how normal people process information and to apply that information to the thought processes of the patient with global aphasia—one who has lost language.

A person with global aphasia has little or no language. If you have a loved one who is now globally aphasic, understanding his or her world is the key to keeping the relationship positive, constructive, and meaningful. The relationship between you and the globally aphasic person has different boundaries and features than your relationship before the stroke, but it can still be rewarding, meaningful, and sustaining. The companionship between you and the person with global aphasia can still provide satisfaction and joy. These feelings simply occur on different levels. Most important, the relationship must be based on the reality of the situation.

Perhaps the stroke caused only mild or moderate language problems. This chapter may be important to you even if your loved one has a lesser degree of aphasia because it provides information and a way of understanding how the patient with language reductions deals with the world. It will provide insight into his or her perspectives on life, and it will give you some idea of the patient's strengths and weaknesses in processing information. This chapter will also provide you with information you can use to deal with new problems and situations; this will be especially important when the patient goes home and begins life anew.

A common question asked by family members and friends of the aphasic patient, especially one with severe language reductions, is, "Does he or she understand me?" "Understand" sometimes means does he or she recognize me, remember who I am, and think of me in the same way as before the stroke. Additionally, this question is part of a larger concern by family and friends. The question reveals that they wonder about the patient's general intelligence and the nature of his or her thought processes in the aftermath of the stroke. This is a natural question as family members and friends seek common ground with the stroke patient to reestablish relationships.

Misjudging the global aphasic patient's thought process creates two types of relationship problems. First, if the patient is believed to have higher and more sophisticated thinking abilities than he or she actually has, everyone will be frustrated. The patient will be subjected frequently to tasks beyond his or her capabilities and will be confronted with failure after failure, which can be devastating to an already damaged and fragile self-esteem. Second, if the patient is assumed to be lower functioning than he or she actually is, then he or she may be treated as mentally deficient or as a child, causing feelings of inferiority and resentment in the patient. The patient may also become unnecessarily dependent.

Problem-Solving and Free-Floating Thought

For the purposes of understanding Mr. Robinson's global aphasia, thought will be divided into two categories of outcomes: problem solving and free-floating. Problem solving is a special type of thinking that, as the name implies, leads to a problem being solved or answered. Free-floating thinking is everything else. People bounce freely between these two types of thinking. One minute we are thinking in order to solve a problem; the next our thoughts are just free-floating.

Problem-solving thought is directed toward a solution or a way around an obstacle. The problem might be minor, such as deciding whether to have a cup of coffee or bottle of soda, or it might be significant, involving seeking the answer to a major question such as the choice of a career, deciding to have children, or how to answer a tax audit. Such thought might result in a new outlook on life. When you are engaged in problem-solving thinking, you have a goal in mind and you want an answer or to get a solution to something. Psychologists call this type of thinking *adaptive*. Problem-solving thought allows humans to better adapt to the world.

Free-floating thought is everything that is not problem-solving. Taking in a beautiful sunrise, appreciating a Mozart waltz, remembering an experience that happened in your youth, or anticipating grandchildren visiting for Thanksgiving are all examples of free-floating thought. There is no need to seek a solution or to answer a problem. Free-floating thought includes daydreaming. Thoughts come and go, producing nothing and solving nothing.

Units of Thought

When thinking occurs, many electrical impulses surge through the brain, so thought can be described as electrical charges that occur in the brain. These electrical charges travel along nerves and signal other reactions, and they constitute the brain waves that can be read by powerful instruments. Thought can also be described as chemical reactions that occur in the brain. These chemical reactions are necessary to the electrical impulses and for changes that permanently occur to brain cells. New thoughts are the result of new connections and chemical reactions. But describing thoughts as electrical charges and chemical reactions is of little use when trying to decide whether Mr. Robinson opened the door for the food service worker. The goings-on in the *brain* are not easily translated into what happens in a particular person's *mind*.

Rather than looking at brain cells, electrical charges, and chemical reactions occurring in the brain, it is easier to understand thought as words and images. Most thought is a combination of both. After all, when you think, electrical charges and specific chemicals do not come to mind. Thoughts are images of the past, present, and future combined with narratives or self-talk about them.

Images

Much of the thinking a person does involves images, and thinking in images can help to solve problems. For example, consider the many decisions involved in driving a car. As you go from one place to another, you process images. Which lane to be in, what exit to take, and the speed you choose to drive all lead to the solution of how to reach your destination. While driving your car, the images are all around you. You see exit signs, speedometer, and lane markers. Visually, you process the information to decide how to reach your destination. The same thing occurs when you walk through a room crowded with people and objects, mow a lawn, or get dressed in the morning. On the other hand, free-floating thought using images involves looking at a flower and appreciating its beauty, or admiring how well a house has been landscaped. Such thought is not problem-solving because there is no concern about weeding the flower bed or improving the landscaping. Nothing needs to be done.

Sometimes, the images are stored in your mind. People call this the *mind's eye*. You can solve problems in your mind's eye, without the images being present. For example, you can imagine how to wash your car although you are in a place other than your driveway. You "see" where the hose is stored and whether it will be long enough to reach the car. You "see" the bucket, soap, and washcloth, and imagine taking them to the driveway. In your mind, you start washing the top of the car, then the hood, and finally the trunk. All these images are stored in your brain, and you can plan to wash your car using them. What if the hose is too short to reach the car? In your mind, you can solve the problem by either pulling the car closer to the house or by finding a longer hose. You find the solution to the problem in your mind's eye; you can see these images with or without your eyes closed.

Many kinds of problems can be solved in the mind's eye. The best route home during rush hour, washing dishes in the kitchen sink, choosing an outfit for the day, and determining how many trips it will take to the laundry are examples of everyday, mind's eye problem solving. You can also have daydreaming experiences in the mind's eye. Daydreams about lounging on the beach for an upcoming vacation or remembering the experience from a previous trip to the ocean does not require problem solving. They are simply free-floating images stored in your mind's eye.

Words

In addition to using images, you think in words, which is called *self-talk*. Although like talking to a friend, self-talk is a discussion you have with yourself. It can be used to solve a problem, or it can be free-floating.

Self-talk obeys many of the basic rules of grammar. Nouns, verbs, and prepositions are used in the same way as when you talk to a friend. The only difference is that self-talk is often abbreviated. When people engage in self-talk, the sentences are usually incomplete or lack detail. They are shorthand statements. Self-talk does not need to be elaborate or descriptive like spoken thoughts because people do not need to describe or detail things to themselves. When talking to others, it is necessary to be more specific.

Self-talk happens faster than speaking. Although it is impossible to measure how fast a person can think in words, it has been estimated that it occurs at over 1,000 words per minute. A speaker usually speaks between 150 and 250 words per minute. This discrepancy between spoken language and self-talk accounts for problems people have when they try to attend to a sermon or a lecture. Because self-talk happens five times faster than speech, the listener has time to let thoughts wander.

Certain types of activities lend themselves to thinking in images. Carpentry, bricklaying, sewing, painting, and reading maps are examples of jobs that require the ability to think in images. Other thinking tasks are accomplished primarily with language, such as deciding whether a friend is trustworthy or if it is ethical to take a particular tax deduction. Law is based on language. However, most thinking is a combination of using images and words.

Thinking, then, may be looked on as processing images and words. In our mind, we process images and tell stories to ourselves. Thoughts also seem to follow a series of associations. One thought leads to another, which prompts a related thought, which in turn causes another. This observation has led some authorities to believe that there is no such thing as a truly original thought. According to some people, all thoughts are built on other ones; even apparently original thoughts are just continuations of associations.

Some people who have been married for a long time report that they know how their mate thinks. They usually can follow their spouse's associations or even predict them. This is why it is so important for family members and friends to be actively involved in the care of the global aphasic patient. You can be helpful in knowing what the patient wants.

Other Kinds of Thinking

Besides thinking in images and words, people also process information from the other senses. When you reach into your pocket or purse and feel around for car keys, you are processing information from touch. By feeling the different sizes and shapes of the objects, you can tell which ones are the car keys. You do not need images or words to find the correct objects.

Information coming from the senses of taste and smell does not require images or words to be processed. The taste of sour milk causes you to spit it out. No images or words are required to know that it has gone bad. The gas company puts a chemical in its product to alert people when it escapes from stoves or heaters. When you detect this odor, you do not need words or images to sense the danger. The odor signals you to leave the room.

Throughout this book, it has been emphasized that the brain operates as a whole. No single part works completely independently of another. This is especially true when it comes to thinking. Images, words, and other sensations are processed together. An odor or song can trigger a variety of images and words. The emotional status of the person also must be considered because emotions have a strong influence on thought processes.

Higher Level Thinking

Many studies have been done on what is called "higher level" thinking processes in aphasic patients. Most studies agree that global aphasic patients tend to operate on a concrete level. Aphasia can cause a person to be bound to the here and now. Many aphasic patients do not engage in abstractions as well as other people. The first researcher to discover this pattern called it a *concrete-abstract imbalance*.

A good example of this imbalance has to do with the ability to categorize. Aphasic patients have more trouble putting things in categories, such as cars, foods, and animals. Other related problems experienced by aphasic patients include understanding proverbs, explaining opposites and similarities, and knowing synonyms. Of course, you would expect these difficulties in aphasic patients because of their trouble remembering words. But the trouble also extends to nonverbal tasks such as categorizing colors and shapes. The imbalance is most apparent on the more complicated categorization problems.

Neuropsychologists sometimes give intelligence or IQ tests to aphasic patients to find out how the stroke has affected their intelligence. Most intelligence tests have two sections: verbal and performance. As you would expect, aphasic patients tend to do poorly on the verbal sections and better on the performance sections. Except for difficulty doing complicated nonverbal tasks, many aphasic patients score relatively normally on the performance section of an IQ test.

Mr. Robinson

Mr. Robinson had global aphasia because the blood supply to both the expressive and receptive centers of his brain was damaged. In Mr. Robinson's case, the stroke resulted when a plug of material lodged in a major artery that supplies both of the language centers. This occurred on the left side of his brain. As is true for most people, this was the dominant side of his brain. Although he was paralyzed on the right side of his body, he could move about freely by using his left arm and leg. The stroke did not result in damage to other parts of his brain.

Because Mr. Robinson was globally aphasic, he was unable to speak, write, read, or understand the speech of others. Speaking was impossible for Mr. Robinson because he could not remember words. He drew a blank when trying to recall the names of people and things. Even when he could remember a name or two, he could not remember how to program the speech mechanism to say them. All Mr. Robinson could say were a couple of words and a few sounds. They were best spoken when he gave little or no thought to them.

The stroke eliminated Mr. Robinson's ability to express his thoughts through writing. Although his left hand could grasp a pencil, he could not write because the words and letters were no longer available. All he could do was make random scribbles on a sheet of paper with his left hand.

Reading was also impossible for Mr. Robinson. Although he recognized letters and words, he could not remember what they meant. Occasionally, he could read a single familiar word such as his name, but longer passages were beyond his capabilities.

The speech of other people sounded like a foreign language to Mr. Robinson. Occasionally, a sound or word would make sense, but most of the time it seemed strange to him. When people would say, "Good morning," to Mr. Robinson, he would not understand whether they said, "Nice day," "Good night," "Pass the butter," or "Buy it."

Global aphasia had also eliminated Mr. Robinson's ability to do simple arithmetic. When buying a cup of coffee, he was unable to provide the correct change or know if he had been shortchanged. Words that represented numbers, money, and figures were as meaningless as directions, commands, and opinions.

Mr. Robinson's family members had attempted to teach him finger spelling and sign language to communicate. They tried to teach him to use his left hand to make the signs. The first signs taught to him were "I want a drink of water," "I want to go to the bathroom," and "Where is my wife, Mary?" After a month of showing him how to make signs and how to put them together in sentences, they were disappointed.

First, Mr. Robinson had trouble learning the signs. It was as if he was learning a foreign language. This way of using language was as foreign to Mr. Robinson as German, Spanish, or Navajo would have been. Second, it was not enough to teach Mr. Robinson the signs; they also had to teach them to the medical staff and other people who worked in the nursing home. Few of them had any previous knowledge of how to use sign language. Trying to teach Mr. Robinson sign language to bypass the aphasia was fruitless.

People with global aphasia have been deprived of language. Because of the stroke, they have an inability to process information in language. This is indeed a significant disability, but it does not render the patient mentally retarded. Global aphasia does not return the patient to the thinking level of a baby or a child. Unless the stroke has taken away more than language, their ability to use and understand images remains unchanged. Globally aphasic patients know what to do with scissors, doors, straws, and spoons. They recognize family members and friends. They, too, daydream about being home, taking trips, and visiting with friends. Only when they are confronted with complicated visual tasks do they have some problems. A friendly smile, wave, or pat on the back are just as meaningful to a globally aphasic patient as they are to you. Complicated gestures such as sign language are beyond global aphasic patients, but many common everyday gestures can be understood.

> For years, Margaret, the food service worker, had been trying to quit smoking. She knew that it was unhealthy and, besides, it cost a lot. For the last hour, she had felt that nicotine urge tugging at her. After cleaning the grill, her job was to set the tables for dinner, but there was time to squeeze in a couple of minutes for a drag or two on a cigarette.
>
> She knew and liked Mr. Robinson. He was a familiar figure in the dining room. As she walked by him on her way to the door, she knew that he wouldn't understand more than a smile and a simple, "Hello." Outside, Margaret couldn't believe how cold the wind made her feel as she tried to light the cigarette. As was her usual practice, she put her foot in the door so that it wouldn't close and lock. Unfortunately, she slipped on the ice and the door slammed closed. She felt more than a little panic knowing that it was a long walk to the front of the building.
>
> She looked at Mr. Robinson and began to shake and rattle the door. He looked around to see if there was anyone else in the room who could come to her rescue. It was up to him. It took a minute or two for him to reach the door and even more time to pull the handle down, but finally the door opened. Margaret crushed the cigarette in the snow and happily returned to the warmth of the dining room. Mr. Robinson was delighted by the "Thank you" and the friendly hug he received from the cold woman. Margaret also saw to it that Mr. Robinson received an extra cup of butterscotch pudding that evening. After all, a good deed should be rewarded.

CHAPTER 7

Depression and the Stroke Survivor

It all depends on how we look at things, and not on how they are in themselves.—CARL G. JUNG

Depression is the most common psychological reaction to stroke-related communication disorders, particularly aphasia. Not all patients experience depression, but when it happens to your loved one, you and other family members and friends will suffer as well. It is difficult to know what to say to a depressed person. In addition, family members themselves often feel depressed because of the unwanted events that have occurred in their lives. Aphasia and other communication impairments are serious disorders, as is depression, and they can have a major impact on relationships. Understanding depression can help all involved adjust to the unwanted events, and there is reason for optimism: Stroke survivors and their families can have long and rewarding relationships despite the communication disorder(s). Life continues after aphasia and related communication disorders—and it can be a meaningful and fulfilling life. Depression and anxiety often occur together. However, in this book, they are addressed separately. See Chapter 8 for a review of anxiety and the stroke survivor.

More Than Sadness

Depression and sadness are two separate states. They differ in the degree of emotional pain and are often caused by different events. Sadness is a mild and temporary negative mood swing that can occur with or without an awareness of the cause. It may be felt as a letdown following a period of high activity, or it may occur for no apparent reason, just a feeling of sadness that occurs spontaneously. Often, a tincture of time, rest, and a good meal are all that is necessary for sadness to fade.

Depression, on the other hand, is a prolonged bout of negative emotions. Severe depression is associated with negative thoughts that can sometimes be self-destructive. Depression usually disrupts sleeping and eating patterns. Many depressed individuals lack concern for other people and may avoid family and friends. They lose interest in activities they previously enjoyed and may withdraw completely. Some depressed people are excited and nervous (agitated) and at times irritable and angry. Their actions may be attempts to regain control over their lives.

Crying and the Nature of Depression

Of all the symptoms of depression, crying is the most obvious. Depressed individuals cry for no apparent reason or cry too much or too often over little things. This is not to say that crying must be present for the patient to be experiencing depression; some depressed individuals never cry.

People with stroke-related communication disorders pose special problems in diagnosing depression. Some stroke survivors have exaggerated emotions and they cry or laugh too easily. Certainly, the stroke patient may be sad and the crying is an expression of that sadness, but as discussed in Chapter 4, the crying is exaggerated. It is too much, too often, as though the patient has a lowered threshold for emotional expression. You should not make the assumption that because a patient cries a lot, necessarily he or she is depressed. The diagnosis of depression in the stroke patient should be made by a health care professional. Sometimes it is difficult even for a specialist to diagnose depression because the patient may have both exaggerated emotions and depression.

Doctors do not know all of the causes of depression, especially for people who have had strokes. There are two generally accepted schools of thought regarding patients having significant or prolonged bouts of depression following a stroke. One theory of depression holds that it results from the brain injury and/or a chemical imbalance. In this view, the communication disordered patient is believed to be depressed because of physical and/or chemical changes that have occurred in the brain. This school of thought is known as the *organic* theory.

There has been much research into the organic theory in recent years, and some doctors believe that this theory of depression is the only plausible one. Studies have looked closely at the size and location of the brain damage in stroke patients. It appears that damage to the left side of the brain is more likely to cause depression than is damage to the right. Damage to the right tends to cause indifference and even a false sense of well-being. One study found that when the brain damage occurs in the front part of the left side of the brain, there is a greater likelihood of the patient becoming depressed. Larger areas of damage to the brain do not necessarily cause more depression. In fact, a recent study found that the larger the lesion, or area damaged, the less likely the patient was to suffer from depression. Studies have also shown that depression caused by strokes differs in men and women. It was found that women had more strokes in the front part of the brain, thus making them more likely to be depressed.

The second theory of depression in stroke patients, especially those with complete aphasia, involves social isolation and adjustment to loss. This theory, known as the *grief model,* argues that people who have lost the ability to communicate become socially isolated and experience a sense of loss about what has happened to them. Depression is a predictable stage in adjusting to the losses. Some authorities call this *reactive depression* and see it as a normal and necessary part of adjustment to stroke and significant communication disorders (see Chapter 10). Supporting this model are several studies showing that the emotional problems seen in aphasic persons are almost identical to those seen in persons who do not have brain damage.

The organic theory of depression looks at what has happened within the aphasic patient's brain, whereas the grief model looks at the effects of the stroke, particularly aphasia, on the patient's adjustment to unwanted changes. Most likely, both theories account for depression in different patients. It also is likely that many patients, especially those with severe communication disorders, experience both types of depression.

The medical management of depression, particularly clinical depression, usually involves prescriptions of medication as well as some form of counseling. Family participation in the treatment of depression is important. Because clinical depression is a serious medical condition, patients must follow the doctor's directions carefully and completely. The attending physician should be notified if there are any significant changes in the patient's mood, eating habits, and tolerance of medications. Any indication that the patient is suicidal should be reported immediately. The suggestions and recommendations reported in this chapter are not formal treatments for depression, they are common-sense things you can do to help your loved one. They should be provided along with the knowledge, coordination, and supervision of the attending physician.

The very presence of a communication disorder can be depressing. Being impaired and unable to express oneself or to understand the speech of others is undoubtedly cause for lowered spirits. Many patients feel isolated and lonely. Although many can communicate on a basic nonverbal level, some do not have the higher levels of speech and understanding necessary for many types of social interaction. As a result, patients find themselves in a situation in which important communication with family members and friends is no longer part of life. Lack of the ability to communicate can be sorely felt in family matters, financial aspects of life, and work-related activities.

Stroke survivors can suddenly find themselves shut out of child-rearing decisions, activities involving adult children, and issues related to grandchildren because the communication disorder(s) allows little or no discussion about these issues. Many patients with stroke-related communication disorders simply can no longer take part in decisions about child-rearing, recreation activities, major family purchases, or other important aspects of family life. Because of the understanding problems, there is always a realistic fear that the aphasic patient only partially understands the information. For patients with strong family bonds before the stroke, the inability to talk with and about children and life in general is a depressing condition.

Dealing with financial aspects of life is beyond the capabilities of the aphasic individual because of impaired communication abilities and also because of problems doing simple arithmetic, as discussed in Chapter 2. Many aphasic patients cannot comprehend complex numbers and formulas, and they may not be able to do simple arithmetic. Even shopping may be impossible. Many aphasic patients cannot provide correct change because they do not remember monetary values. The inability to engage in these activities of daily life can further create a sense of dependency and isolation and decrease the stroke survivor's self-esteem.

Communication about job and work activities may also suddenly be absent in the life of the stroke survivor and contribute to isolation and depression. Many retired individuals have maintained contact with previous colleagues and discuss past job events and participate in work-related social activities. Many retired people still revel in their past occupational successes. This type of communication provides a sense of continuity and transition into the retirement years. Co-workers who visit the patient in the hospital or home feel awkward and anxious and wonder what to talk about. Both co-workers and the stroke survivor can be deprived of the pleasure and benefit of work-related conversation. Of course, some stroke survivors were not retired. Consequently, they are at an even more serious disadvantage when it comes to discussing and understanding issues related to work.

Insight into what it is like to be unable to communicate can be learned from stroke survivors who have recovered much of the ability to talk. Reports from recovered patients suggest that they missed not just the "important" discussions; they also sorely missed the day-to-day verbal interactions with family, friends, and acquaintances. "What was the football score?" "Did you hear about Mary's new job?" "You ought to see my new tool set," or "Did you watch that TV show last night?" are the kinds of comfortable and predictable conversations that can be lost due to a stroke. Unfortunately, for the stroke survivor with a communication disorder, there is little comforting small talk and too many uncomfortable, painful silences.

Many authorities in psychology recognize the importance of strong family bonds in preventing or overcoming depression. It is in this area that the stroke survivor with a communication disorder sometimes feels the most social isolation and loneliness. Maintaining a strong intimate relationship with a spouse may be especially difficult. New obstacles arise because of the communication disorders. Certainly, however, physical contact is available, and intimacy can be fostered nonverbally. Holding the patient's hand, an affectionate grasp of the shoulder, or a pat on the back can express volumes nonverbally. Many couples are also able to maintain or regain sexual relations. It is important to remember that intimacy is more than just nonverbal communication. Intimacy also involves verbal expressions of love, acceptance, appreciation, and support. Mature, intimate communication crosses many boundaries and satisfies many needs. Painful isolation and loneliness result when the stroke patient and his or her spouse or loved one can no longer share these experiences. Unless care is taken, stroke related communication disorders can be devastating to an intimate relationship.

Feelings of Guilt and Worthlessness

Guilt and feelings of worthlessness are major manifestations of depression despite the irrationality of these feelings. All patients can struggle with feelings of guilt and worthlessness, but the aphasic patient is most at risk due to the loss of language. Because inner speech, the silent statements said to ourselves, may also have been affected by the stroke (see Chapter 6), the aphasic stroke survivor can be left without the psychological tools to work through negativity. Coming to terms with many of life's changes requires language. Without it the aphasic person is unable to say, "It's time to focus on the positive," or "There are still many things I can do that will give life meaning." Language is one tool used to adjust to changing life events, and aphasia can remove that tool.

As discussed in Chapter 4, some stroke patients have a thought, or perform a physical act (such as writing), that lasts longer than normal. Getting stuck on an idea is a common disorder associated with aphasia. As reported previously, patients with this condition are much like individuals who cannot get a song or verse out of their minds. It just keeps repeating again and again in their minds. This complication can increase depression by saturating the patient with negativity.

Clearly, strokes and the "big three" communication disorders that can result from them can be extremely negative, but even more so for patients who get stuck in negative thinking patterns. For example, the negative thought, "I'll never be a good husband again," can replay repeatedly in the patient's mind. Thoughts, and the accompanying feelings of worthlessness, guilt, isolation, and fear, can circle round and round in the aphasic patient's mind because of stroke-induced problems shifting from one idea to the next. The tendency for these negative thoughts to repeat again and again in the mind can intensify the depressive reaction. It is also possible that these depressive thoughts actually *cause* the depression. Having problems shifting from one mental set to another is also a barrier to counseling. Successful counseling requires flexibility of thoughts and attitudes, and the stroke patient may be unable to shift negative thinking patterns.

Sometimes you may feel that there is little you can do to help your loved one who is in the grip of depression. You feel overwhelmed trying to deal with the patient's extreme negative emotions. Most of us also have a natural tendency to avoid someone who is depressed; in a psychological sense, depression seems to be contagious. Being around a depressed person tends to make us feel sad because it brings our own depressing thoughts to the surface. It is also natural for you to want to cheer up the depressed aphasic patient by acting in an upbeat, happy manner. Family and friends sometimes tend to avoid the patient completely or to avoid negative issues by projecting a false happy manner. Both tendencies should be avoided.

You should try to project, both verbally and nonverbally, that the bonds of love and friendship are still intact despite the communication barrier. Particularly during the early stages of recovery from the stroke, the patient should be secure in the knowledge that family bonds and friendships are greater than the communication disorder and depression and that these relationships will continue through it all. One way of projecting these ideas to the patient is to visit him or her regularly in the hospital. During these visits, simply sitting quietly at the bedside can be encouraging. Holding the patient's hand or a friendly pat on the back can express volumes of positive support. It is not necessary to engage in long conversations with the patient. In fact, for patients with severe communication disorders, lengthy discussions can confuse, sadden, and annoy the patient, ultimately deepening the depression.

In all interactions with the patient, you should concentrate on the positive aspects of recovery and the eventual resumption of life. If the patient has the tendency to get stuck on an idea, it is even more important to focus on the positive, especially early on. Statements you make can be a source of continued thoughts that will remain with the patient long after you leave. Although it may be difficult to achieve, you should find a way to be positive and constructive without being too optimistic and upbeat. These attempts need not be verbal; a smile accompanied by a thumbs-up gesture can express the strength of your love and friendship and can set the tone for a positive approach to the challenges ahead.

Self-Esteem

Researchers have recognized for decades that when a person suffers a stroke, he or she will probably experience a major reduction in self-esteem. One aspect of a person's self-concept, self-esteem comprises the good feelings and positive appraisal a person has about himself or herself. These feelings can be shattered when a stroke occurs. The person knows that his or her wholeness, or integrity, has been compromised. Simply put, the stroke survivor now knows that he or she is impaired: "I am not the capable person I used to be." In many activities, the person feels inferior and inadequate. We call this an inferiority *complex* because the condition involves the whole personality and transcends all relationships. The stroke patient's self-esteem sometimes is battered even more when he or she is confronted with the childlike tasks of relearning speech.

Certain qualifications must be made to the statement that stroke affects self-concept, especially the person's self-esteem. First, for patients to fall into this category, they must have an awareness of what has happened. Obviously, patients in a coma are not aware of what has happened. Second, there is some disagreement among researchers about whether reduced self-esteem is the result of a physical or chemical change resulting from the brain damage or whether it is purely a psychological reaction. Third, some types of brain damage mask the expected negative emotions. Some brain-injured persons experience *euphoria,* which is the opposite emotional reaction to the expected depression. The euphoria observed in some stroke patients results from oxygen deprivation. When the brain is deprived of oxygen, the patient can experience a heightened sense of emotional well-being. The person feels "high." For example, pilots are taught that if they start to feel euphoric at high altitudes, they need to don oxygen masks because the air is too thin and they aren't getting enough oxygen. Because of poor blood flow and the reduction of oxygen being supplied to the brain cells, a stroke can sometimes cause those same feelings of heightened well-being due to oxygen deprivation.

Not all authorities believe that all euphoria is the result of oxygen deprivation and brain damage. Some patients report that they experienced a heightened sense of emotional well-being because they ignored negative thoughts. This is a psychological protective mechanism known as *denial.* The patient simply does not acknowledge that something bad has happened. This results in keeping all bad or negative thoughts from intruding so that only the positive ones, and the good feelings associated with them, remain.

The Patient's Self-Concept: Images and Definitions

Self-concept and self-esteem are complicated topics. They become even more complicated when discussed in relation to aphasia and other communication disorders. Everyone experiences fluctuations in self-esteem. A person's self-concept changes with successes, failures, and even because of the aging process. Stroke patients have these normal psychological reactions, too. But stroke patients also have self-esteem problems that can be directly related to the stroke-related communication disorder(s). The foundation of a person's self-concept is body image. Body image is the way a person views himself or herself physically in day-to-day activities. If an individual sees himself as impaired, distorted, or abnormal in body functions, these perceptions contaminate normal feelings of adequacy and self-esteem.

Feelings of adequacy and self-esteem are developed at an early age. A young person's early appraisal of self is based on comments from others. Statements made about how the person looks and acts become the basis of self-esteem. Fortunately, most youngsters are considered cute and lovable, and statements made by parents, friends, and even strangers serve as the foundation for the development of body image. Body image plays an important role in depression. Reductions in self-esteem and feelings of inadequacy have at their core a negative body image.

Not only do we have images of ourselves, but we also use language to define aspects of our behavior and personality. Concepts such as intelligence, maturity, and honesty can only be clearly conceptualized with words. These self-concept words are not visible; one cannot draw or point to *honesty*. These are abstract ideas people have about their personalities, verbal descriptions rather than images. Therefore, when a stroke eliminates a person's language, it can greatly affect his or her verbal concept of self.

Self-concept is a combination of images and definitions. We see ourselves in our mind's eye and define aspects of our personality. Of course, everyone's self-concept and self-esteem fluctuate. The process of aging is a major cause of this fluctuation in self-concept. Over time, we gradually adjust the image we have of ourselves, and we begin to use different adjectives to describe personality traits. Aging and other life changes cause us to define ourselves differently. Some verbal descriptions are lost, while others are gained.

People have varying degrees of tolerance for these changes. For example, some individuals can tolerate a relatively large weight gain and feel few negative emotions. The change in body image is tolerable. For others even a minor weight gain can cause extreme distress. There is no better example of this phenomenon than the person with *anorexia nervosa:* intentional self-starvation. Although this is a complex disorder with many facets to it, at the core of the starvation is a disturbed body image. The person constantly sees himself or herself as fat.

Stroke and the accompanying physical limitations can be devastating to the patient's self-concept. And to make adjustment more difficult, this disorder comes on rapidly, with little time to prepare for it. In an instant, a man or woman who was managing home, business, work, and family affairs finds himself or herself confined to a hospital bed or nursing home. Frequently, there is paralysis on one side of the body, which makes even the smallest activities difficult or impossible. With some patients, the face is paralyzed, and there may be drooling. These impairments can affect the person's image of self, and self-esteem plunges. What is more important, because aphasia eliminates or reduces language, self-esteem vocabulary also can be

lost. The patient has no words, no language, to deal with this great sense of negativity. Not surprisingly, depression is the most common psychological reaction in
aphasia. It has been estimated that up to 50 percent of aphasics experience a clinically significant episode of depression that lasts six months or longer.

In some individuals, depression can lift on its own, and the depression seen in
stroke-related communication disorders is no exception. Given enough time, many
depressed individuals gradually improve in outlook and mood. This may be related
to acceptance of the losses, as discussed in Chapter 10. Some authorities on depression believe that the brain sometimes gradually corrects the imbalance of chemicals
that caused the depression. It is also possible that depression lifts because of the actions and support of family and friends. Bonds of family and friendship can improve
the depressed individual's spirit and perspective

Improving Body Image

The old adage, "Clothes make the man," suggests the importance of being well-
dressed and well-groomed. We are all aware of the psychological lift a new
wardrobe can have. With the stroke patient, special attention should be given to
clothing and grooming. This is particularly important because these things are often neglected in hospitals and nursing homes. As discussed previously, body image
is central to self-esteem, so care should be taken to see that the patient is well-
groomed and dressed carefully. Most importantly, the same type of clothing that the
patient wore before the stroke should be provided in the hospital or nursing home
as much as possible. If the person liked to dress casually in jogging clothes, or as a
cowboy or a motorcyclist, these types of clothing should be made available. The
type of clothing chosen by an individual is a form of self-expression, and it may be
one of the few modes of expression still available to a stroke survivor with a communication disorder. It is a form of nonverbal communication (see Chapter 9). You
should ensure that your loved one is always made presentable prior to going out
into public. The patient's hair should be combed, teeth brushed, and face washed
before being transported to and from therapies and procedures. For female patients,
makeup should also be made available, and, if necessary, they should be provided
with assistance in applying it. Busy staff members can fail to do these things for a
patient, so family members and friends may need to assist the stroke survivor with
grooming.

As discussed previously, a person's self-concept can benefit from uplifting remarks made by family and friends. Especially during the first few weeks after the
stroke, patients may not have the working vocabulary to maintain verbal self-
esteem. They cannot find comfort from the usual ego-boosting self-statements.
With many patients, language loss reduces or eliminates the self-esteem vocabulary.

Because of the aphasia, patients may be impaired or unable to think these types of thoughts: "I'm okay," "It's going to be all right," "I'm still a good person," and "Everyone appreciates how hard I'm working." For aphasic patients, it may be impossible to utter these statements to others, much less to themselves.

It is especially important that the speech and language therapy being provided to the patient also focus on these types of words and statements. Clinical time spent on the language of self-esteem is as important as words and phrases for expressing needs and wants. Time spent on self-esteem terminology may create more motivation in the depressed patient and ultimately increase the benefits of therapy.

Sincere nurturing statements by you and other family members can boost the patient's self-esteem. Some counseling approaches call this *ego stroking,* and it can play a significant role in helping reduce the length and severity of depression. Positive, constructive statements by family and friends help to elevate the patient's mood. It is important, however, that they be based on realistic, positive observations, sincere statements of appreciation, love, compassion, and empathy.

Although it is seldom accurate to compare stroke survivors to children, some parallels can be drawn about self-esteem. If a child is constantly addressed with negative labels, he or she will learn to identify with them, and the child may adopt those personality traits. Most parents recognize the importance of using terms of endearment and positive labels to teach children to have confidence. This is also a good strategy to employ for aphasic patients. Depressed aphasic patients may be reacquiring and restructuring their identities, and the power of labels can work to their advantage when used by thoughtful, caring family members and friends. You should avoid negative labels and feel free to use an abundance of positive ones. Words such as *smart, strong, good, intelligent, kind, successful,* and *likeable* should be used whenever appropriate to label an act or to address the patient. Just as aphasic patients are relearning words to describe their environment, they are also acquiring labels to define and describe themselves.

The Value of Praise

Confidence is an essential part of relearning speech and language abilities. We are all familiar with the feelings of fear and nervousness when we have to give a public speech. In a study asking people in the United States to list their fears, it was found that speaking in front of a group was number one on the "most feared list"—higher than fear of heights, spiders, snakes, and even death.

The reason for this extreme fear is that when we speak to a large audience, we worry that one or more people will reject us. Members of the audience may leave the room, talk among themselves, or laugh. We also know that as the size of the audience increases, the chances are also increased that one or more people will not like the presentation. And most people view rejection of the speech as total rejection, which can lead to an overwhelming level of nervousness. However, many people soon learn that the audience genuinely likes what is being said, and this gives them the confidence to continue. This increase in confidence contributes to a more effective delivery, which the audience likes even more. After several successful experiences, public speaking can become enjoyable. Because of the audience's positive response, the speaker has improved confidence enough to risk rejection.

When a person suffers a stroke and has aphasia, apraxia of speech, or dysarthria, the act of attempting any speech at all can become as negative as addressing a large audience. The reason for the extreme anxiety is the realistic fear that attempting speech may result in embarrassing word substitutions, struggled speech, and distortions of sounds. Not only can these problems cause the listener to feel embarrassed and awkward, but they also can make the speaker feel mentally impaired or even out of control. When this happens again and again, the patient can fall into deeper depression, making optimal recovery of communication skills less likely.

You can reduce the patient's lack of confidence by praising every attempt to communicate. You can do this by maintaining eye contact and nodding in a positive and accepting manner when the patient expresses himself or herself. The "OK" gesture can usually be understood even by the aphasic person with severe understanding problems. Similarly, applause or a pat on the shoulder can communicate to the person that he or she can attempt speech without risking rejection. For the depressed patient, this encouragement and support can be helpful in maintaining the motivation to participate fully in the therapies.

As part of making speech a rewarding and positive experience, you should avoid continuous testing of the patient. Continuous testing is a common mistake made by well-intentioned family members. It is natural to want to test the abilities of the patient, particularly soon after the onset of the disorder. Family and friends want to know how well the patient can understand what they are saying. They might say, "Do you know who this is?" or "Can you recognize Uncle Nick?" Unfortunately, some people believe that testing the patient is the same as therapy. However, constant testing does not help the patient overcome the disorder, and it can be extremely negative psychologically. From the patient's perspective, it drives home the depressive aspects of the disability by showing what he or she cannot do. Family and friends need to communicate that they understand the nature of the deficits and accept what has happened. The goal is to create a positive and accepting environment.

Allow a Wide Range of Emotional Expression

Speech clinicians try to keep the patient on a "level of success" by arranging activities so that the patient experiences more success than failure. It is not always easy to keep the patient succeeding at most tasks. Therapy must not be too complicated, frustrating the patient, but neither should it be too simple. Activities that are too easy may communicate that no one understands the patient. These rules are important for family members and friends to remember, too. In all activities with the patient, everyone should match their communication to those of the patient's abilities. From short visits in the hospital to lengthy home passes, you should walk the fine line of not frustrating the patient yet challenging his or her attempts to communicate.

Frustration is a natural yet unwanted aspect of stroke-related communication disorders. Frustration usually leads to feelings of anger. We are all familiar with the frustration associated with traffic jams. Tempers flare when people cannot move in congested traffic. When a goal is obstructed, it is natural for frustration to occur. Similarly, when patients cannot attain the goal of communication, they are likely to get frustrated and angry. One principle of psychology suggests that if an individual chronically directs anger inward, depression occurs. Frustration leads to anger, and anger, when it is directed inward, can lead to depression.

Stroke survivors are very likely to direct their anger inward because they often cannot express it in socially acceptable ways. To reduce the psychological effects of frustration associated with these disorders, patients should not only be allowed to express anger, but they also should be encouraged to do so. As long as the expression of anger is not destructive to the patient, facility, or others, it should be encouraged.

Label the Disorders

One approach to treating depression uses the individual's rational thinking skills to combat the irrational and negative emotions. Words are the tools of thought, but some depressed aphasic patients may not have the words available to express complex thoughts and feelings associated with the difficult changes they are undergoing.

The communication disorders associated with stroke may be perceived as strange and extraordinary. Many patients may not know of anyone who has ever experienced them. Some aphasic patients simply wake up in a hospital without the command of language. They are unable to ask questions about the disorder, and they are deprived of information because they cannot understand explanations.

Once a disease or disorder is given a name or label, the individual knows that he or she is not the only one who has ever had it, and the disorder becomes less frightening and bizarre. The name does not need to be a technical medical term. Although some patients can understand and readily use the word *aphasia*, other terms for the same disorder include *amnesia for words* and *naming problems*. The important thing to remember is that these labels should be used consistently; everyone should call the disorder by the same name. Once a name is given, the mystery is removed, at least to some extent. Then the patient can use the label to help him or her adjust to the circumstances.

Time Structuring

Some depressed patients experience overwhelming lethargy. The "joie de vivre" or "joy of life" is lost. Some patients have a tendency to get caught up in a listless routine, creating a cycle in which depression causes depressive behaviors and vice versa. For these individuals, the cycle needs to be gradually and systematically broken. This can be done by time structuring.

Time structuring is the scheduling of activities on an hourly, daily, and weekly basis. It provides the patient with the ability to predict events. For the patient in a deep depression, an attempt should be made to completely structure daily activities. Meals and visitations should be at the same time each day. So should visits to the solarium and coffee shop and television viewing times. Predictability of events can give the patient a needed sense of security. Although it may be difficult to get the severely depressed patient to follow the schedule, you should provide strong encouragement and support for complying.

The schedule should be created with the assistance of the patient as much as possible because it is important that he or she be included in the decisions of when and what to schedule. The schedule should be placed in a prominent place in the patient's room. Pleasurable activities should be scheduled at regular intervals to break up the therapy and exercise routines. Times for the patient to be alone should be scheduled to provide an opportunity to grieve over the losses that have occurred (see Chapter 10). Gradually, as the depression lessens, more free time can be provided, giving the patient more control. This transition should be monitored carefully to see that the patient does not use the free time to return to lethargy and listlessness. Even patients who are agitated and depressed may benefit from time structuring, although it may be a challenge to keep them on the schedule.

Counseling

Counseling can be an effective treatment for depressed patients as long as they have the expressive language abilities and verbal comprehension to participate. Consequently, only mildly to moderately involved patients can profit from the "talking" cure. It is important that the psychotherapist, counselor, or neuropsychologist working with the patient understand the nature of the disorder(s). The counselor should understand the frustration, anxiety, struggle, and word-finding problems found in aphasia so that appropriate psychological inferences are made. One study found that when these guidelines are not followed, counseling can worsen the depression.

Many approaches to counseling can be used effectively to treat the depressed person. Each person is different psychologically, and the choice of a psychotherapist, counselor, or neuropsychologist should be based on individual factors. The patient's preexisting personality should be considered when choosing the appropriate professional. Some patients respond to a direct approach in which specific philosophies, recommendations, and ideas are strongly suggested. Other patients respond more to a nondirect approach in which the counselor indirectly guides the process of exploration and self-discovery. Both types of counseling for depression have been found to be successful, as has a combined approach. Sometimes, just having a concerned listener is beneficial. Venting emotions and concerns has therapeutic value.

Positive and Constructive Attitudes

Bookstores and libraries stock an abundance of self-help books addressing depression. A common theme among these books is that a person's attitude and mental set can play an important role in reducing the severity of depression. Humans are creatures of habit, and a negative, pessimistic, self-depreciating attitude can become a habitual part of a person's thinking patterns. These books try to provide ways of understanding those negative thought patterns and offer suggestions for correcting them. As discussed previously, a fundamental part of habitual thinking patterns is the inner speech or self-statements we make to ourselves.

Several counseling approaches consider the parts of a person's personality and how they interact with one another. Many approaches recognize that there is a critical, controlling, regulating component of the personality that is responsible for morals and for regulating urges. They also recognize a vulnerable, innocent aspect of the personality. This "inner child," as it is sometimes called, requires immediate gratification and absolute love. It is a part of the personality developed at a young age.

A third part of an individual's personality is rational, thoughtful, objective, and relatively unemotional. This is the aspect of the personality called on to bring order and harmony to the whole person when the other aspects are at odds with one another. For example, in counseling an angry person is taught to look at the source of the anger. The goal is to use the mature, aware, and rational components to regulate the angry messages sent and received by the other elements of the personality. These negative messages frequently are internal monologues that have been in the angry person's mind since the initial cause of the anger. The assumption is that the angry person can change these negative feelings by changing the pattern of the internal monologues. The goal here is to understand the source of the anger and identify the initial experience that might have been responsible for it.

It is not difficult to understand where the negative, depressing thoughts come from in the stroke patient, who often experiences job limitations, social isolation, physical infirmities, and a multitude of negative disruptions to family relationships. Depressing feelings can be triggered and then maintained if patients allow themselves to engage in patterned and repeated negative thoughts. It may be difficult to break away from negativity, especially feelings of guilt.

The guilt that often accompanies depression stems from the patient believing that he or she did something wrong and deserves the communication disorder; it is a rightful punishment. The patient can habitually allow the critical, controlling aspect of the personality to create negative inner speech statements that cause feelings of negativity. Some negative inner messages are absolutely false. For example, some strokes just happen; they are not the result of lack of exercise, poor eating habits, or other lifestyle factors. The patient could have done nothing to prevent the stroke. Guilt and depressing thoughts are sometimes irrational. In the words of one counseling approach, guilt is a series of "irrational thoughts by a rational person."

Although there may be some truth to some patients' guilty thoughts, the element of truth is exaggerated and brutal. Perhaps the stroke victim smoked, did not take medication for high blood pressure, or was overweight. These lifestyle behaviors can actually contribute to a stroke. However, ruminating about them is unproductive and self-destructive. The nurturing, self-forgiving aspect of the personality should be activated to permit the patient to overcome these feelings of negativity. Forgiveness can be found in activation of the nurturing part of the personality. In both cases, the rational, objective aspects of the personality should permit, encourage, or cause the dynamics of the personality to change. Thinking should move from the negative to the positive. Patients can accomplish this by exercising some rational control over their internal monologues. People do have some control over their habits of thinking.

You can help the patient prevent negative thought patterns by adopting and projecting a positive attitude and sparing the patient exposure to depressing ones. Although you should permit the patient wide latitude to express his or her feelings, you should actively work to decrease negative patterns of thoughts. When the patient expresses them, you should emphasize that he or she is engaging in unproductive thoughts, either exaggerated or completely inappropriate given the reality of the situation. Certainly, they are honest feelings and thoughts, but they serve no constructive purpose. Given the objective, logical realities of the situation, they are irrational. The goal is to understand the source of these thoughts and feelings and to try to reduce them. The patient will find it difficult to maintain negative, depressive thoughts in an environment of rational, positive, and constructive ones.

Positive Environments

There is a strong relationship between patients' environment and their depression. Everyone has difficulty maintaining a positive mood when subjected to a depressing environment. Unfortunately, some stroke patients may not be able to communicate the need to change the depressing environment. This is where you and other family members can play an important role in helping the depressed patient. You can use your powers of speech to convince the staff of the medical facility to change a depressing environment. This can be one of the most positive steps that family and friends can take to help combat depression in their loved one.

Depression has also been linked to lack of sunshine. Known as *seasonal affective disorder,* a lack of full spectrum light and sunshine causes some individuals to experience depression. Many stroke survivors are confined to the indoors with little opportunity to spend time in the sunshine. This lack of natural light can cause depression in some patients and deepen it in others. Family and friends of the patient should communicate to the nursing staff that regular visits to solariums and sunny rooms are an important activity for the depressed patient.

Photographs of loved ones should be available to the depressed patient. Having them within view can remind the patient of people who care. Pictures of pets, cars, hobbies, and property can also be comforting. Besides cheering the depressed patient, these pictures can be a source of drills and activities used by the speech clinician. They are particularly effective because they are relevant to the patient and can motivate him or her to relearn the names of people, animals, and objects that are dear to the patient.

Other environmental changes can be used to help improve the depressed patient's mood. These must be tailored to the person's previous interests. The rule of thumb is that those things enjoyed before the stroke are the ones most likely to be missed. If listening to a certain type of music was a frequent activity before the stroke, the music should be provided to the patient at home or in the medical care facility. Portable stereos with earphones are available for patients who are not in private rooms. Care should be taken to provide the kind of music that the patient previously enjoyed. When possible, upbeat and cheerful music should be chosen.

A change in room color also can improve mood. It has been found that red and other bright colors can elevate a person's mood, whereas blue and darker shades can have a depressing effect. If a choice is available, a light, bright room color should be selected. However, if the patient is depressed and agitated, a green-colored room might have a calming effect.

Religious pictures, paintings, and symbols should be made available if appropriate, just as regular visits from religious leaders can be a source of strength and guidance for some patients. Reading from the Bible or other religious texts also may help the depressed patient, although it is unlikely that patients with complete aphasia will understand all of the words. These activities should be provided only if they were a part of the patient's routine before the stroke. All visitors should be cautioned to be positive in their discussions with the patient.

Antidepressant Medications

The patient's physician may prescribe one of the many antidepressant medications available to combat severe or prolonged clinical depression. Most physicians rely primarily on reports from family, friends, and the medical staff to decide when these medications are necessary. Sometimes the patient's family members are disappointed to find out that it takes a few days to several weeks for some antidepressants to begin to combat depression. There is a common misunderstanding that antidepressants make the patient feel high or euphoric. Rather, antidepressants tend to reduce the severity of the negative feelings rather than eliminate them. Euphoria or "highness" should be viewed as a possible, undesirable side effect of a medication and reported to the physician immediately.

The physician will prescribe the medication most appropriate for the patient. Although all drugs have side effects, newer antidepressants generally have very few. Some patients who are depressed are *bipolar* in their symptoms, alternating between the extremes of depression and mania. These patients need careful monitoring by a psychiatrist. Family members and friends should follow the doctor's orders carefully and completely in the administration of medications. You should never stop, increase, or reduce the patient's medications without first discussing the change with and getting approval from the physician.

Depression is an emotional reaction that can be severe, and it occurs frequently in patients with aphasia and related disorders. Both the patient and family members may be affected by the depression because of the limitations and unwanted changes that have occurred in their lives. Depression can also result from the stroke-related brain injury and chemical changes. Severe communication disorders, especially aphasia, can disrupt the patient's ability to adjust psychologically and disrupt the dynamics of family relationships. You may be able to help reduce your loved one's depression by engaging in the common-sense activities suggested in this chapter.

CHAPTER 8

Anxiety and the Stroke Survivor

It is well to remind ourselves that anxiety signifies a conflict, and so long as a conflict is going on, a constructive solution is possible.
—ROLLO MAY

Anxiety has been called the feeling of impending doom. For many people, it is an unpleasant yet common sensation in this "age of anxiety." Worry, stress, tension, and fear are common reactions to the trials and tribulations of modern life. For some stroke patients, anxiety becomes a constant and unwanted companion, permeating their lives. The communication disorders resulting from strokes often trigger anxiety, and they can also be barriers to reducing and coping with these unpleasant feelings. To make matters worse, anxiety and depression often occur together in stroke patients. (See previous chapter for a review of depression.) The purpose of this chapter is to look at some common sources of anxiety for the stroke patient and to explore ways of reducing them. There are several things family members and friends can do to help eliminate or reduce anxiety in the stroke patient and ultimately to help your loved one achieve a better quality of life. Understanding anxiety and its source is the first step in helping the stroke survivor reduce it.

Some sources of anxiety for the stroke patient are easy to identify.

"Will I ever be able to go home and resume a normal life?"
"Am I likely to have another stroke?"
"Does my family understand me?"
"Is this 'brush with death' over?"
"Will I ever be able to go back to work?"
"Will I ever be able to take care of myself?"
"How much will all of this cost me?"
"Will I be a burden on my family?"

"Because I have had brain damage, can I ever trust my thinking again?"

"Will I ever be able to talk normally?"

"How will I cope with this?"

Other sources of anxiety for the patient are not as apparent as the ones listed above. Sometimes a stroke results in damage to areas of the brain that produce the chemicals necessary for feelings of security and relaxation. Because of the chemical imbalance, the patient feels insecure, fearful, and tense. Although your loved one may also be anxious because of the circumstances surrounding the stroke, the chemical imbalance may be the primary cause of the anxious feelings.

The words *fear* and *tension* are sometimes listed as synonyms for *anxiety*. They are not identical, however. All three terms are similar in that they produce unpleasant feelings, but they differ psychologically. Fear is a response to an external threat. For example, you become fearful when confronted with an angry, barking dog. The dog is the external threat. Anxiety often results from an internal conflict. You feel anxiety when you want to do something considered immoral or when you wonder about your motives for doing something. Tension refers to the muscles of the body. Increased muscle tension is often a response to both fear and anxiety.

Fight or Flight Response

When confronted with a situation perceived as threatening, a person can deal with it in two ways: run away or stay and fight. This two-pronged reaction to a threatening situation is called the *fight or flight response*, and it can be traced back to early human evolution. In primitive times, the threat may have been a large animal looking for food. In preparing to flee the dangerous situation or to stay and fight, several bodily reactions occurred. To prepare for running or fighting, the heart rate increased and breathing was deepened and speeded up. To prepare for the physical activity of fighting or fleeing the threatening animal, digestion also slowed and muscle tension increased.

Today, the flight or fight response is not very adaptive. Few of the fearful situations people confront require the physical preparations to fight or flee the threat. Of course, some threats may require a person to run away or physically to protect himself or herself. For example, the pedestrian who crosses the road in busy traffic may actually have to flee to the other side to avoid being hit by a car. Here, the threat is physical and requires a comparable response. Similarly, a person being mugged may physically have to protect himself or herself. Although it is safer simply to give the criminal the valuables, the physical preparations to fight the mugger may have to be mobilized. Fortunately, however, most present-day threats that occur on a daily basis do not require running away or physically fighting. Modern threats are often abstract.

Some psychologists separate the physical reactions that occur in fearful situations from those arising from anxiety-provoking thoughts. There are minor differences in the reactions that occur when the threats come from outside versus those within a person's mind. However, the common theme is that the person wants to escape from the threat or decides to confront it.

Again, although people today are still confronted with threats, most are not as apparent or direct as the ones faced by primitive humans. Today, people still risk losing their homes, reductions in lifestyle, or even starvation, but these threats are usually indirect and not immediate. Many of today's major threats involve losing a job, being passed up for promotion or being demoted, failing in a business, or being taken advantage of. The threat of rejection is always present, as is the risk of losing a loved one to someone else or to death. Many threatening situations arise in the workplace. In modern life, however, physically fleeing or fighting often is not appropriate, successful, or adaptive behavior. Even so, when people today are confronted with abstract and disguised threats, they still have the physical reactions developed in prehistoric times. With higher levels of fear, anxiety, and increased muscular tension, their bodies still prepare to fight the aggressor or to flee from the situation.

Anxiety is generally divided into two categories: situational and free-floating. When anxiety is associated with a specific cause, it is said to be *situation dependent*. Feeling anxious because your job is in jeopardy or because you have run up too many expenses on your credit card are examples of situational anxiety. When a person has a general sense of uneasiness and anxiety that cannot be traced to a particular circumstance, he or she is said to have *free-floating* anxiety. Free-floating anxiety is the sort of general nervousness and tension that occurs for no identifiable reason. The person just feels uneasy.

Anxiety Levels: The Good, the Bad, and the Ugly

As a concerned family member, you should realize that all anxiety seen in your loved one is not necessarily bad. Although anxiety is an unpleasant feeling, it can motivate patients to work harder to recover their speech and language abilities. Manageable levels of anxiety also help patients learn by increasing their attention and concentration.

Anxiety can be a good motivator. When people feel anxious, it can motivate them to do something to reduce the negative emotion. When anxiety is channeled correctly, the need to reduce it can cause the person to do positive things. For a good example of doing the right thing to reduce anxiety, consider what a student does prior to taking a test. Fear of failing the examination creates anxiety. To rid himself or herself of the negative feelings of anxiety, the student reads and studies the materials that are likely to be on the exam. Because the person knows that studying increases the likelihood of getting a good grade on the exam, anxiety drops and the student feels better. Because anxiety tends to increase the closer a person is to the source, the student studies more and more as exam time approaches. Because of anxiety, by the time the test date arrives, the student has studied and is likely to do well on the test. In this example, anxiety has been good. It has motivated the person to study to reduce the anxiety.

Anxiety is a negative force when the anxious feelings are so pervasive that it is difficult or impossible to concentrate. Continuing with the example of the anxious student who must take a test, too much anxiety can reduce learning. The anxiety and negative feelings still prompt the student to study, but because the anxiety is so great, he or she cannot focus. When reading the material, the student becomes distracted and restless and finds it hard to concentrate. The student focuses on the feelings of anxiety rather than on the book and lecture notes. Fear of failing the exam can be so intense that it causes poor study habits. The student might also do things to escape from the negative feelings such as talking with other people, going to a movie, or eating junk food. Some students find temporary relief from the anxiety by sleeping long hours or using alcohol. Extreme levels of anxiety cause the student to have poor concentration and difficulty seeing the whole picture. This type of anxiety is not productive.

Extreme levels of anxiety carry the seeds of terror and panic. As the test date approaches, the student who has extremely high levels of anxiety cannot focus, concentrate, or learn, as though there is a clouding over the student's mind. The feelings of anxiety are so great that the student seeks immediate relief. Learning the material is impossible because the student cannot remember new information. This extremely high level of anxiety may rear its ugly head when the student actually sits down to take the test. Because of the unmanageable level of anxiety, he or she cannot remember anything previously studied or learned. Even reading the test questions is fraught with poor comprehension. The student misreads some questions and jumps to false conclusions on others, erasing constantly because of false starts. For the student with unbearable levels of anxiety, immediate relief becomes the main goal and doing well on the test becomes secondary.

Manageable levels of anxiety can be productive when channeled properly. Anxiety about getting cancer can cause a person to stop smoking cigarettes. Anxiety over getting a traffic ticket can cause a person to drive safely. Positive behaviors such as jogging and dieting can be prompted by fear of having a stroke. The ability to learn and remember information is enhanced by productive levels of anxiety.

However, high levels of anxiety are unproductive for learning new information. Excessive anxiety has negative effects on concentration and memory. People with too much anxiety have problems "seeing the forest for the trees." They cannot grasp the whole picture and focus too much on details. High anxiety levels can result in constricted thinking. People experiencing unproductive anxiety often channel it into thoughts of escape or ways of avoiding the threat. These extreme levels of anxiety often can be counterproductive because the objective is to get immediate relief. Rather than being more alert and aware of the environment, the person is in a panic state and just reacts to the anxiety. Memory often fails, as does concentration, and the person suffering from counterproductive anxiety is driven to find immediate relief.

Anxiety and the Stroke Patient

A manageable level of anxiety can be good for some stroke patients. When the anxiety is channeled into appropriate activities to overcome the effects of the stroke, it can drive the patient to make maximum gains, motivating him or her to try harder at speech, occupational, and physical therapy. Like a student who must study for a test, the stroke patient responds to manageable levels of anxiety by thinking more clearly and attending better. Certainly, not all patients need anxiety to be motivated. Some stroke survivors are constitutionally disposed to do their best to overcome their disabilities. A lifetime habit of always doing their best causes many patients to work hard to overcome the stroke-related disabilities. For many patients, however, low manageable levels of anxiety serve as a motivator to overcome the disabilities caused by the stroke.

High levels of anxiety will have detrimental effects on overcoming stroke-related disabilities. If anxiety levels are high enough to be extremely unpleasant, they can harm the recovery process. Too much anxiety can cause the patient to avoid confronting the disabilities or to escape even thinking about them. In addition, too much stress and anxiety have been linked to depression. Too much anxiety can cause the patient to be unable to attend to therapy activities. Memory will also suffer. This is especially true for patients whose memory problems primarily affect the recall process (see Chapter 5). Too much tension and anxiety are detrimental to remembering information previously attended to and stored.

Extreme levels of anxiety in the stroke patient can even completely interrupt the recovery process and lead to panic attacks (see Chapter 4). Patients experiencing terror sensations or panic attacks at the thought of having another stroke need immediate relief from the anxiety. Their physician should be notified so that appropriate medical treatments can be arranged. Treatment may include medication, psychotherapy, or a combination of the two.

There are many real sources of negative anxiety for the communicatively disabled patient. Each person reacts differently to a stroke, and general assumptions about how the patient will respond should be avoided. However, certain sources of stress and anxiety are common in stroke patients. Fear of dependency is one of the most prominent sources of anxiety. Few people want to be at the mercy of others for the execution of day-to-day activities. Anxiety can also result from the patient's perception of dramatic negative changes in job performance and the ability to recreate. Disruption of family life is also a major source of anxiety. For patients with major stroke-related communication impairments, discovering the sources of anxiety can be a challenge. Because they may not be able to tell you why they are having high levels of anxiety, you need to look to the likely sources.

Decisions, Decisions, Decisions

Most people experience anxiety when confronted with conflict situations. A conflict occurs when a person is confronted with two or more choices, and a decision must be made. The decision may be minor and of little significance, or it can involve a major change in lifestyle. When people are placed in decision-making situations, anxiety usually results. It can range from a barely perceptible increase in tension to an overwhelming feeling of distress. For some patients prone to anxiety levels that are already too high, the conflicts can be the "straw that breaks the camel's back." Conflicts can cause panic attacks and stand in the way of optimal recovery from the stroke. What is most important, extremely high levels of anxiety cause stress, distress, and needless suffering. In these cases, the conflicts should be understood and reduced as soon as possible. Psychologists recognize four types of conflicts.

Approach–Approach Conflicts

Approach–approach conflicts generate the least amount of anxiety. Although a decision must be made, the person is confronted with two or more equally desirable and attractive options. The approach–approach conflict exists when a child in a candy store has only enough money to buy one item—so many choices and only enough money for one piece of candy. Ultimately, the child will walk away from the candy store happy, but meanwhile, the need to choose generates anxiety. Anxiety levels reach their highest when the clerk finally asks the question, "Can I help you?" Of course, approach–approach conflicts can be more significant than choosing between two candy bars. Anxiety can be generated when a person must choose between two equally desirable job opportunities or destinations for a vacation. Perhaps the most difficult approach–approach conflict to resolve is when a person must choose between two equally attractive potential mates. Choosing one eliminates having the other.

Obviously, a person caught in an approach–approach conflict eventually will choose the most desirable alternative. The path to the final decision involves thinking and rethinking the attributes of each option. As the desire for one alternative begins to get stronger, even more powerful feelings to obtain it develop. Through a snowballing effect, the closer the person gets to the goal, the drive to get it becomes even stronger. Finally, the conflict is resolved when the choice is made.

For the stroke survivor, approach–approach conflicts can range from what dessert to order for dinner to which child to visit on an overnight pass. In the morning, the stroke patient may be confronted with the approach–approach conflict of which shirt or blouse to wear. Scheduling therapies can generate approach–approach conflicts. At night the stroke survivor might be confronted with choosing between two equally desirable television programs.

Although approach–approach conflicts generate anxiety, they are usually easily resolved and the outcome is positive. After all, the person gets to choose between two good options. However, for the anxiety-prone patient, even choosing between two or more good options can add to already high levels of anxiety. Approach–approach conflicts should be reduced for the anxiety-prone patient or for the patient currently experiencing excessively high levels of anxiety.

Avoidance–Avoidance Conflicts

Unfortunately, not all choices people make involve choosing between two or more equally desirable options. Sometimes they involve choosing between the "lesser of evils." When people are confronted with making a choice between two or more undesirable options, they are said to be having an avoidance–avoidance conflict. An avoidance–avoidance conflict is the opposite of the approach–approach situation. Avoidance–avoidance conflicts occur when the person is "trapped." Most people, when confronted with making a choice from among bad alternatives, would simply avoid the decision. Doing nothing seems better than choosing any of the bad options. Many avoidance–avoidance decisions occur because the person is required to make a decision. A dramatic example of the avoidance–avoidance trap is the convict on death row who must choose the type of execution. Some states provide condemned convicts with the choice of execution method. For example, they can choose between hanging and the electric chair or between lethal injection and the firing squad. Obviously, the convict wants to choose neither, but he or she is in a trap situation. A choice must be made. For most people, the traps can be financial, social, or even psychological. There is no good choice, but a decision must be made.

Avoidance–avoidance conflicts are present when people have to choose between paying bills or going bankrupt. In the voting booth, citizens sometimes have to choose between two equally unqualified candidates. Larger and more significant avoidance–avoidance decisions occur when people have to choose between two undesirable but necessary jobs or when they must move to equally unattractive cities.

In approach–approach conflicts, as the decision maker gets closer to the desired object, a stronger desire to approach it develops. In avoidance–avoidance conflicts, as the person gets closer to choosing the undesirable alternatives, a stronger desire to avoid the situation develops. The closer a person is to choosing the lesser of two evils, the more he or she is inclined to avoid both.

Avoidance–avoidance conflicts lurk around every corner for many stroke survivors. Remaining in a noisy and uncomfortable hospital room or going to painful physical therapy are examples of avoidance–avoidance conflicts. Choosing between two equally undesirable foods from the menu can create a conflict and result in anxiety. Sometimes, out of boredom, a patient may have to choose between two equally unentertaining television programs. Many medical treatments create avoidance–avoidance situations. Which is less negative, taking necessary medications that prevent seizures or suffering the side effects of being drowsy and lethargic?

All avoidance–avoidance conflicts generate anxiety as a by-product of decision making. For many patients, these decisions are made with a minimum of anxiety and negative emotions. For the anxiety prone patient, however, avoidance–avoidance decisions can contribute to already unbearable levels of stress and tension. Family members and health care providers should do everything possible to reduce the number of these unpleasant decisions. For the ones that are inevitable, you should help the patient explore the options and support him or her in reaching a decision with the least amount of tension and anxiety.

Simple Approach–Avoidance Conflicts

When a person is confronted with pursuing a single goal that has both desirable and undesirable elements to it, an approach–avoidance conflict occurs. Whatever choice the person makes will have both good and bad consequences. Psychologists call it a "simple" approach–avoidance conflict because there is only one goal. The conflict is resolved when either the desirable aspect of the goal becomes stronger or the undesirable one weakens. A person can become trapped in an approach–avoidance conflict when both the approach and avoidance levels are equal. The person cannot act because there is no tipping of the scale either in the direction of the approach tendency or the avoidance inclination.

The need to go to the dentist is an example of a simple approach–avoidance conflict. The approach aspect of this conflict occurs when the person remembers that regular checkups are necessary for good dental care. It is important to have regular checkups to discover the early stages of cavities. The patient "approaches" taking good care of his or her teeth because it is the right thing to do. The approach tendency is countered by an avoidance inclination: the memory that dental visits can sometimes be painful. This type of conflict is usually resolved when either the approach or avoidance drive weakens. For example, a toothache can rapidly decrease the avoidance drive and prompt the person to make an appointment to see the dentist.

For some stroke patients, even simple approach–avoidance conflicts result in indecision and anxiety. This is most apparent in social interaction. Most stroke patients will be drawn to engage in social interaction for the same reasons everyone else is: Social contact can be rewarding, pleasant, and enjoyable. But because of their communication disorders, stroke patients may be put off at the idea of socialization. They will avoid it because of the embarrassment associated with flawed speech. If the drive to socialize is equally as strong as the embarrassment, then the stroke patient can be caught in an approach–avoidance trap. Here, the patient cannot make a decision. Conflicts and their associated anxiety levels involving socialization may need to be avoided, especially with patients who are prone to anxiety attacks.

For the stroke patient, socialization approach–avoidance conflicts can involve decisions about whether to eat in the dining room or simply to have the dinner tray brought to his or her room. The choice of going to group or individual therapy can create a socialization approach–avoidance conflict. Family visits, day passes, and recreational activities can be sources of anxiety for the stroke patient. The need to socialize can conflict with the potential for embarrassment due to the communication disorder.

Double Approach–Avoidance Conflicts

Most of the conflicts people experience on a day-to-day basis are of the double approach–avoidance variety. Just as people are complex, so are many of the decisions they need to make. According to psychologists, a double approach–avoidance conflict occurs when a person is simultaneously driven to approach and to avoid two different goals. Each goal has both positives and negatives, so the person has both approach and avoidance feelings about acting and remaining inactive. To act or not to act, that is the question.

A good example of the double approach–avoidance conflict is a person contemplating retirement. Retirement has both positive and negative aspects to it, as does continuing to work for a few more years. Retirement is approached because it means fewer work-related headaches. No more punching time clocks or lengthy commutes. It is avoided because the prospective retiree may be making a good salary with status, power, and prestige. To give all of that up is a sacrifice. Taking on the life of a retiree also has pros and cons associated with it. Having more free time to do the things dreamed about is certainly desirable, but being less productive and dealing with idle time can be a negative. Choosing to retire or not to retire can be fraught with anxiety, especially when a person isn't sure whether he or she really wants to quit work.

Some people with communication disorders feel anxious when they must choose either to talk or to remain silent. Speaking and silence are double goals in

this conflict, and for some anxiety-prone stroke patients, they are the main sources
of anxiety. The theory that silence and speaking are two goals, both of which have
good and bad components, has also been used to explain the feelings of some people who stutter. Some proponents of this theory have proposed that this double
approach–avoidance conflict is what causes stuttering in the first place. Whether or
not this theory has merit as a *cause* of stuttering, it can be useful in describing some
of the feelings experienced by many stroke patients when they must choose between silence and speaking. Of course, this comparison is true only in stroke patients who are aware of their communication defects. Understanding the double
approach–avoidance conflict can help you and other family members relate to the
patient's predicament. Knowing the nature of these conflicts can guide you as you
try to reduce them and be supportive and encouraging.

In the double approach–avoidance conflict of speaking and silence, both goals
have good and bad components. The patient approaches speaking because of all of
the benefits of communication. Speech provides a way for a person to get things and
express emotions. Through speaking, the stroke patient can prove that he or she is
still vital and alive. Psychologically, speech represents potency and normality. But
speech is also a negative when one has a stroke-related communication disorder.

Psychologically, the negative aspects of speaking come both from within and outside the patient. The internal negativity felt by the patient has to do with *speech impo-
tency. Impotence* here refers to the patient's inability to make his or her speech
mechanisms do what is required to talk. Because of the stroke, the patient cannot perform the normal and natural function of speech as well as he or she did before the
stroke. Understandably, these feelings of being out of control can be deeply threatening. Particularly during the early days of the stroke, the patient with aphasia, apraxia
of speech, and/or dysarthria is confronted with new and strange inabilities to communicate. The impotence felt because of aphasia can include word-finding problems,
echoing other people's speech, or getting stuck on an idea or word. Patients with
apraxia of speech have trouble controlling their speech mechanism. They feel impo-
tent when they know what they want to say but cannot say it. Because of paralyzed or
weak speech muscles, the patient with dysarthria has trouble making sounds clearly
and succinctly. For patients who are completely aware of their defective speech, these
disorders can prompt feelings of impotence and negativity.

Listener reactions may also be a negative aspect of speaking for some patients
with stroke-related communication disorders. Like everyone else, these individuals
can sense their listeners' confusion and embarrassment. For listeners, at least initially, it is hard to keep a neutral face when confronted with echoed speech, slurred
sounds, or automatically uttered swear words. Because aware patients with stroke-
related communication disorders can see these reactions in the listener, it is understandable that the reactions contribute to the negativity of speaking.

So the goal of speaking has both positive and negative elements. The aware patient is simultaneously drawn to and repulsed by the act of speaking, which is a true conflict that occurs on either a conscious or subconscious level. For the anxiety-prone patient, the conflicting feelings of approach–avoidance to speaking contribute to stress levels that already may be unmanageable.

As if the conflict to speak were not enough, anxiety also surrounds the alternative: remaining silent. For the stroke patient, silence can be a refuge from embarrassment and failure. Only until the patient opens his or her mouth to speak do the word-finding problems, struggled attempts to program utterances, or slurred speech rear their ugly heads. Silence allows the patient to avoid confronting the disability. The silent patient appears "normal" except for physical limitations that may have been caused by the stroke. Besides appearing normal, the silent stroke patient is at ease. In silence there is no struggle, no feeling of impotence, no frustration. In these respects, silence is a safe haven and therefore is approached by the stroke survivor with a communication disorder.

But silence is avoided as well. Because of silence, stroke survivors may appear more impaired than they actually are. In silence there are no requests, demands, statements of facts, or questions. A silent person projects a tacit approval of everything said and done. Some psychiatrists believe that silence in dreams represents death. Because of the lack of vitality in silence, many stroke survivors avoid it.

Therefore, in a double approach–avoidance conflict, the stroke survivor encounters two goals: speaking and silence, both of which have positive and negative attributes. The conflict is very real, and the amount of anxiety felt depends on the patient's awareness and the severity of the disorders. Most important, the double approach–avoidance conflict generates even more stress and distress in the anxiety-prone patient. Conflicts that occur directly or indirectly because of a stroke can generate unbearable anxiety or contribute to existing levels. Some of these conflicts are integral parts of having a stroke and cannot be avoided. Conflicts with speaking or remaining silent and undergoing treatments or refusing them are difficult, if not impossible, to ignore. For many stroke survivors, these are as much a part of the communication disorder as the word-finding problems or the slurred speech. But many conflicts can be avoided, postponed, or ignored. It is up to you, other family members, and the health care team to protect the patient from unnecessary conflict situations. This is especially true if your loved one is anxiety-prone.

Coping with Anxiety

How does one protect oneself from negativity?

Are some strategies more mature, adaptive, and desirable than others?

Are stroke survivors different from the rest of us in using these defenses?

The preceding questions are important for family members and friends of the stroke survivor to answer. By understanding the ways in which stroke survivors try to protect themselves against external threats, you can help the patient cope more effectively. You can help your loved one deal with some of the unpleasantness associated with the stroke and the communication disorders that have resulted from it.

Avoidance

Avoidance of an anxious or fearful situation is one of the most common defenses used by children and adults alike. People use avoidance to protect themselves from situations they deem threatening, fearful, or anxiety provoking. When it comes to an unnecessary confrontation, often "a battle not fought is a battle won." Avoidance provides relief from threats to self-esteem. This defense is also available to stroke patients with even the most severe of communication disorders.

> *Mrs. Kathryn Landon was scheduled for group therapy every day from 1:30 P.M. to 3:00 P.M. On Monday she could not be found by the aide responsible for transporting her to the group therapy room. She was found in the solarium only after a long search. On Tuesday Mrs. Landon was in the shower. Wednesday, Mrs. Landon was unable to attend group therapy because of a terrible headache. Thursday, Mrs. Landon was late to group because of the time she spent trying to express a complicated instruction to a nurse. On Friday Mrs. Landon flatly refused to go to group therapy by pushing the aide away every time she tried to unlock the wheels of her wheelchair.*

For a variety of reasons, Mrs. Landon found group therapy an unpleasant experience. Perhaps it was because group therapy required her to confront her speech and language disorder. Maybe seeing the other stroke survivors made her realize how profoundly she had been affected, because she identified with them. It is possible that Mrs. Landon was never a social person and found group therapy or any group activity unpleasant. Whatever the reasons for Mrs. Landon's negativity, she used avoidance to protect herself from the experience. It is a basic method of coping with unpleasantness.

Actually, there are two aspects of avoidance and Mrs. Landon used both of them. The first aspect is postponement. Mrs. Landon was able to delay going to group by getting in the shower minutes before the scheduled group therapy time or by being in the solarium and not telling anyone. Because of these delaying tactics, she was able to postpone the group sessions. The second aspect of avoidance is refusal. On Friday Mrs. Landon simply refused to allow her wheelchair's wheels to be unlocked. She clearly communicated her refusal by pushing away all attempts by the aide to unlock the chair.

Health care professionals and family members sometimes must force a patient into confronting negativity, such as demanding therapies, painful treatments, or confinement to a nursing home. Indeed, some unpleasant and negative aspects of having had a stroke must be confronted and endured. But stroke patients with communication disorders need special consideration. Because many of them cannot verbally express their desire to avoid a situation, you should look to their actions to discern their wishes. Encourage and support the patient for confronting negativity. In a positive atmosphere, gradually and gently nudge the patient closer to the thing he or she considers negative and unpleasant. Brutally confronting a patient with a negative situation is not the best method of dealing with avoidance. Understanding and compassion are required when helping a stroke patient overcome negativity.

Escape

Sometimes, avoidance of potentially threatening situations is impractical or impossible. As children most of us used escape when we left our frightening rooms and sought sanctuary in our parents' bed. We escaped from the impending doom, stalking us from the dark confines of the closet. Whereas avoidance prevents the unpleasant situation, escape provides immediate and effective relief from it. Both avoidance and escape are common in unsatisfying relationships.

> La Verne Warner was a successful businessman prior to having his second stroke. He was accustomed to high levels of business stress. The most recent stroke resulted in expressive aphasia (Broca's aphasia), and his ability to remember and say words was lost. During the past few weeks, he had begun to make gains in recalling words and getting them out. One of the activities in therapy was "rapid recall" of the names of people and objects in pictures. As the clinician presented each picture, Mr. Warner was to say the name as fast as he could. Mr. Warner thought, planned, and struggled to remember the names and to say them. After about 10 minutes into the rapid recall drill, he indicated an immediate need to go to the bathroom. An aide was called, and the remainder of the therapy time was spent transferring him to and from the bathroom.

Obviously, a person is not necessarily using the escape defense every time he or she requests to go to the bathroom. In Mr. Warner's case, however, the excuse of going to the bathroom was an escape from the stress and demands of the rapid recall exercise. Mr. Warner was no stranger to stress, and as a businessman he had met urgent deadlines. But the urgency of the rapid recall activity and the aphasia combined to reduce his ability to cope with the demands. He simply used escape to remove himself from the demanding therapy. Escape brought him immediate and complete relief from the anxiety.

Escape is often used when postponement or refusal is unsuccessful. Many patients with stroke-related communication disorders cannot verbalize the need to escape, but they can show it by nonverbal means. Another type of escape behavior used by stroke patients includes devoting attention to another activity. The goal is to divert attention away from the stressful activity and to concentrate on one less anxiety provoking. Sometimes stroke patients, with or without the assistance of their families, check themselves out of a hospital or rehabilitation center without the approval of their doctors. This is a radical form of escape behavior and can have serious medical consequences, but it does provide the patient with immediate psychological relief.

You and other family members should be alert to the escape needs of your loved one. If you see indications that he or she needs to escape from a stressful situation, help him or her find relief. Either remove the source of stress or provide an easy way out of the situation. The patient's wish to escape usually should be honored. Providing the patient with control over the timing of breaks and timeouts is also helpful in defusing anxiety.

Ego Restriction

Sigmund Freud's daughter, Anna, first identified the defense of ego restriction. In ego restriction, the person abandons an activity because of fear that he or she will fail at it. According to Anna Freud, this defense is found in people with severe reductions in self-esteem who have deep-rooted feelings of inferiority. The possibility of failure and the resulting threats to self-esteem are too much for patients to bear, and they abandon easily attainable goals. Ego restriction differs from inhibition. When a person is inhibited about doing something, he or she may still be drawn to it. In ego restriction, the person has no drive to do it; he or she is happy to give it up.

Many aphasic patients have generally reduced levels of self-esteem and experience feelings of inadequacy. These negative feelings about the person's "self" have been called *ego reductions*. Not all patients have them but many do. For many patients, the knowledge that they had a stroke and resulting brain damage makes them question their abilities. They wonder whether they are as mentally capable as they were before the stroke. Because of these feelings of inferiority, some stroke patients are likely candidates for ego restriction.

Candace Decker ran a successful family bakery before having her stroke. The stroke resulted in aphasia, and speaking, writing, reading, and understanding the speech of others were impaired. She also had problems doing simple arithmetic. After undergoing intensive rehabilitation, she improved considerably.

She returned home and was able to communicate almost as well as before the stroke. Her ability to do math also returned. During Ms. Decker's stint in rehabilitation, her son and daughter ran the bakery. After a year, Ms. Decker was working in the bakery preparing breads, pies, and pastries, but she would never work in the front of the store. She refused all requests to meet with customers, to take orders, and to make change.

Not all restrictions placed on a stroke patient are unhealthy. Some stroke patients in reality can never return to the practice of law, medicine, education, or sales. Because of the stroke and the resulting communication disorders, they are unable to return to careers that involved high levels of communication competence. Patients who understand this and turn their attention to less verbal and more appropriate careers simply are making healthy and logical changes in their lifestyles. Indeed, it would be an indication of an adjustment problem if a patient blindly pursued an unreasonable career choice following a stroke.

However, Ms. Decker's refusal to engage in public interaction was a self-imposed and unnecessary restriction. Her communication and math abilities were almost as good as before she had the stroke and certainly did not preclude her from seeing customers. She refused to work with customers because the potential for failure was so threatening that it was not worth the risk. As a businesswoman, she realized the importance of selling her products and accepting the correct amount of money, but she restricted her involvement unnecessarily at this end of the business because of feelings of inferiority.

What can be done to help your loved one who unnecessarily limits important activities because of feelings of inferiority and inadequacy? Perhaps the patient tried an activity and experienced failure. Rather than continuing and trying to improve, he or she abandoned the activity and refuses to pursue anything related to it. What should you do?

Patients who use ego restriction to unnecessarily limit their functioning require special consideration and support from everyone, especially from family members. Their self-esteem needs to be rebuilt. The objective is to prove to the stroke survivor that success is a realistic outcome and the potential risk of failure is low or survivable. These patients must be made to realize that occasionally failure is expected and that it is normal to make errors. Everyone makes mistakes. Your loved one should be provided the opportunity to succeed at minor tasks until a basis for more success and confidence is established. The stroke survivor's ego boundaries should then gradually extend to activities in which success is not guaranteed. Most important, the patient should learn to separate his or her self-worth from success and failure.

Defense Mechanisms

We all use defense mechanisms, coping styles, to protect ourselves from negative thoughts. We use them all of the time because defense mechanisms protect and insulate us from anxiety. These defenses are at the foundation of psychology and psychiatry and go by many names. Some are mature and desirable, and others are immature, radical, or both. Radical defenses are often last-ditch efforts to defend the psyche against unpleasantness.

Patients who have complete aphasia may be unable to use defense mechanisms as well as they did before the stroke. The reason for this is that some defenses are verbal, while others can be used without the use of language. For example, a common defense people use is called *rationalization*. Literally, the word means "making rational." When a person rationalizes, he or she is selectively aware of acceptable motivations for doing something and ignores the unacceptable motivation. Rationalization may take this form: "I didn't try hard in therapy today because they were late getting me to the outpatient clinic, and, besides, I don't think these drills help me talk better." By rationalizing, the patient justifies or makes excuses for doing poorly in therapy. It protects the ego and helps to maintain self-esteem. In reality there could have been many reasons for not doing well in therapy. Some are more acceptable than others to the patient. The patient who rationalizes thinks only about the acceptable reasons.

Patients with language disorders may be too impaired to use rationalization, which is a verbal defense employed either aloud to other people or with internal speech (self-talk), which was discussed in Chapter 6. For patients who cannot recall words or have problems making sentences, using the verbal defense of rationalization may be difficult or impossible. Intact language is a prerequisite to use the verbal defense of rationalization effectively.

Other defenses are nonverbal. Denial is an example of a nonverbal psychological defense. When a person does not perceive an unpleasant situation, he or she is "in denial." The person sees or hears what he or she wants to see or hear. Denial is a radical defense and is often the first stage in accepting an unwanted event. "I don't believe it" is a statement often uttered by people in denial. They deny that something bad has happened until the shock wears off and they can mobilize more appropriate defenses. Words are not necessary to use this defense. Denial occurs at the perceptual level and is simply the blotting out of bad news.

Although a patient with complete aphasia can use denial, rationalization may be beyond his or her abilities. The many other defense mechanisms can be divided into those that are verbal or nonverbal. What is important here is that you should understand that for patients with aphasia, the tried and true past ways of coping may also be impaired because of the stroke. If your loved one has trouble adjusting to the unwanted changes caused by the stroke, he or she may need specialized counseling, which can be provided by a psychologist.

Calming the Seas

What can a family member do to help a loved one reduce high levels of anxiety? Understanding that not all anxiety is bad is important. As discussed previously, low, manageable levels of anxiety can motivate a patient and improve learning. For patients with high levels of anxiety, you need to understand the flight or fight response, conflicts, and some of the more common defenses. But there are specific things you can do to help the patient relax and feel more comfortable. These are common-sense suggestions that can help reduce the patient's anxiety and stress and help to calm the individual. One of the most important things is for you to remain relaxed. You should try to project a calm, easygoing attitude when you visit your loved one. Try not to be hurried in your speech or actions. It is much easier for the patient to be relaxed when others around him or her are relaxed. Stressed-out people tend to cause everyone else to be tense and anxious, too. When you talk to your loved one, use soft, quiet speech and a relaxed manner.

It is not a coincidence that people describe moods using color words: "He's in a blue mood," "She is so angry she is seeing red," "The man was yellow in his cowardly action." Some studies have shown that colors not only are descriptive of moods but they also can cause or contribute to them. The colors stark white and red have been linked to increased uneasiness in people. This increase in tension and anxiety may be related to the glare given off by these colors. When rooms are painted red, they tend to increase anxiety and tension levels, whereas blue has a soothing effect. You may not have control of the patient's room color, but if you do, choose a soothing one such as blue or related shades. For the anxiety-prone patient, a blue room can contribute to a relaxing environment.

Listening to certain types of music can also be calming for the anxiety-prone patient. As the old adage says, "Music soothes the savage beast." Certain types of music can reduce anxiety levels, but care must be taken when deciding which types to play. It is important that the music be both relaxing and the type enjoyed by the patient before the stroke. Surprisingly, what some people consider relaxing can have the opposite effect on others. Obviously, if the patient can talk and understand the speech of others, you should simply ask him or her what type of music to obtain. Otherwise, trial and error and close observation of the patient are ways of selecting music that will help the anxious patient relax.

You should try to create a sense of security for the patient. Security is achieved, in part, when a person knows what to expect from day to day or even hour to hour. Try to arrange visits at regular times and suggest that other family members do the same. For patients who are anxiety prone, it can be distressing when people drop in unannounced. Also, keep the contents of the room in regular places and avoid re-arranging the furniture. Even little changes can add to already unbearable levels of anxiety for some patients.

Members of the rehabilitation team may attempt to treat, directly or indirectly, the stress, tension, and anxiety in certain patients. The patient's physician may pre-scribe one of the many anti-anxiety drugs presently available. As a rule, physicians try to keep the anti-anxiety drugs at a minimum because many can be habit form-ing. And, as with many medications, complications and side effects must be consid-ered. Many physicians prescribe anti-anxiety medications and recommend counseling as part of the treatment approach. Of course, for patients with severe communication disorders, counseling may be beyond their benefit. For a patient to benefit from counseling, he or she must have good communication abilities.

Other direct ways the rehabilitation team may want to treat the anxiety-prone patient include systematic desensitization, relaxation training, and biofeedback. One or all of these therapies may be used depending on the type of anxiety and abil-ity of the patient to benefit from them.

In *systematic desensitization,* the anxiety-prone person is gradually taught to re-place anxiety and other negative emotions with calm and relaxed feelings. System-atic desensitization involves gradual exposure to the thing that causes fear and anxiety and association of relaxed and calm feelings with this anxiety source. The idea is that the new calm feelings counter the originally negative ones. This type of treatment, which is usually done by a psychologist, can be used to calm a patient about surgery, needles, X-rays, and other medical procedures. Most parents know about systematic desensitization and use it with their children. For example, when a child is fearful about taking a bath, parents know that by creating a relaxed, calm environment, they can gradually get the child into the bathtub.

Many tense people who simply do not know how to relax can benefit from *relaxation training.* A variety of relaxation methods can be taught to anxiety-prone patients. Of course, their mental and language abilities must allow them to under-stand the instructions. Anxiety reduction can be achieved by encouraging patients to concentrate on positive images or ideas when they are tense. These are thoughts the patient finds relaxing and calming, and they are discovered during therapy with a psychologist. When a patient is confronted with an anxiety-provoking situation, he or she is encouraged to go to the "calm" place in his or her mind. This calm place might be a relaxing image from the past such as sitting under a tree or a fantasy of floating on a big, fluffy cloud. Concentrating on religious symbols can also be relax-ing and comforting.

Extreme muscle tension is addressed by teaching the patient alternatively to tense or relax specific muscle groups and gradually doing this to all of the major muscles. By tensing and relaxing certain muscles, particularly those that tighten up in stressful situations, the stroke survivor can learn when muscles are too tense. Most important, he or she can learn to relax the tense muscle groups by "permitting" a sense of relaxation to flood the muscles.

The final direct method of teaching a patient to relax is called *biofeedback*. A biofeedback instrument monitors the tension level of the body and provides feedback about it. These instruments can read a variety of physical reactions, including muscle tension, breathing, sweating, and blood pressure. The patient attached to a biofeedback device can hear noises that increase in loudness or pitch as tension levels increase. By hearing these tones, the patient can learn to bring down the tension levels and achieve a better level of relaxation. Portable biofeedback devices are available that patients can carry around with them to monitor tension levels

In summary, some patients who have one or more of the big three stroke-related communication disorders also are prone to high levels of anxiety. Too much anxiety can hinder learning and be detrimental to the rehabilitation process. The many causes of anxiety range from a chemical imbalance in the brain to distress caused by conflicts. You and other family members can help the anxiety-prone patient relax. Working with the medical team, you can help the stroke survivor achieve manageable levels of anxiety and a more relaxed approach to challenges presented by the stroke.

CHAPTER 9

Maintaining Relationships

Loneliness and the feeling of being unwanted are the most terrible poverty.—*MOTHER TERESA OF CALCUTTA*

Maintaining a relationship with your loved one may be easy if the stroke caused only a mild communication disorder. The relationship between you and the stroke survivor can continue along the same path much as before. The patient's mild word-finding problems or difficulty getting a few words to come out easily and clearly should be no real barrier to your relationship. This is a blessing because the bonds of love and friendship can still be expressed verbally during this difficult time. But it is a different story if the stroke caused a major reduction or complete loss of your loved one's ability to communicate. Communication is a bridge connecting people, and a major speech and language disorder can have a serious impact on relationships. If communication can be considered a bridge between people, then a communication disorder would be considered a fence. Your job is to tear down the fence and to begin rebuilding the bridge. In this chapter, we will explore some tools and skills needed for that important job.

Bridging Troubled Waters

Carl Rogers, a famous counselor and therapist, recognized that the underlying attitude between people can have a dramatic impact on the quality of communication between them. Based on this observation, he developed a counseling approach that uses positive communication as a basis for counseling. Called the *client-centered* approach, its fundamental belief is that, for communication to be productive and meaningful, the parties must show "unconditional positive regard" for each other. This belief is an uncomplicated idea and more of a philosophy of interaction than a counseling tool. But one does not need to be a counselor or a psychotherapist to apply this approach to communication. You and other family members and friends can use it as the foundation of the communication bridges to be built.

Simply put, *unconditional positive regard* means, "I have nothing but positive opinions about you, and you cannot say or do anything to change that." By projecting this conviction to the stroke survivor, you provide a foundation for communication that includes trust and excludes fear of rejection. The patient feels free to attempt speech without the fear of suffering the pangs of rejection and embarrassment. For the stroke survivor, the courage and self-esteem necessary for expression are fostered by knowing that loved ones have positive regard for him or her and that nothing can change that.

One of the most important aspects of unconditional positive regard is that you separate the patient's speech and behavior from negative judgments. This attitude can be summarized by this statement, "I may not like or approve of some of the things you say or do, but unconditionally, I have a positive opinion of you, and that will not change." This philosophy is comforting for the patient troubled by slurred sounds, word-finding problems, automatic swear words, and a host of imperfect and often embarrassing utterances. Knowing that he or she has your unconditional positive regard can provide your loved one with a secure foundation to engage in the trial and error necessary to recover as much speech and language as possible.

The Stroke Survivor's Perspective

For satisfying communication to occur, the parties involved must understand each other's perspectives. Sharing information, ideas, emotions, and philosophies requires that each party appreciate the other's perspective and is vital when discussing emotional issues. Understanding where your communication partner is "coming from" is fundamental to rewarding and satisfying communication. Appreciating another's perspective is also known as *empathy*. Without it, communication becomes just the exchange of facts and information, lacking the richness of truly connecting with another person.

Strokes and the communication disorders that can result from them often cause changes in perspectives. Little things, especially those related to communication, naturally become more important. For stroke patients with major disabilities, the whole idea of social interaction can change. The disabilities caused by the stroke, the brain damage itself, and the patient's previous personality can combine to change perspectives about family relationships and life in general. These changes can be frightening at first for both you and the patient. They can cause insecurities about how to continue your relationship with the stroke survivor. Change is inevitable following a stroke, but one fact can help guide you during this transition: Most stroke survivors do not experience major personality changes. In fact, your loved one may well exhibit characteristics even more like those he or she displayed before the stroke.

Research has shown that when people suffer brain damage, their previous personality traits tend to be exaggerated. The brain-injured person tends to display more of what he or she was before the stroke. Dependent individuals tend to become more dependent on others; those who were easygoing tend to be even more relaxed and mellow. A person who was sensitive to criticism before the stroke becomes more so, and the perfectionist becomes even more obsessed with perfection. While it is true that some patients undergo major changes in their personalities because of brain damage, most simply have an exaggeration of previous traits. Most likely the stroke has not dramatically changed your loved one's personality, and this is important to know when you reach out to him or her. The stroke survivor is basically the same person as he or she was before the stroke.

Nonverbal Communication

The clothes people wear, the tone of their voices, facial expressions, body positioning, and how close or far apart they stand from one another are all forms of nonverbal communication. Being late or early to a meeting, a friendly touch on the shoulder, or a soft-spoken voice also communicate something. Like it or not, nonverbal communication occurs on many levels all of the time. Although a patient may be mute, he or she is "shouting" nonverbally to anyone and everyone. So are you and everyone else who meets the patient.

To illustrate the power of nonverbal communication, following are two scenes of a doctor and a stroke patient meeting during the doctor's rounds. In each scene, both patient and doctor exchange the same words; only the nonverbal communication changes.

Scene I:

A doctor opens the door to the patient's room and walks in, trailed by a nurse and an aide. The doctor says with a flat tone, "Good morning, Mrs. Fisher, you're looking well." Mrs. Fisher, in an anxious, weak whisper, responds by saying, "Thank you." The doctor looks around for a chair but does not find one, so he sits at the foot of the bed. He reviews the patient's chart. He then says matter-of-factly to no one in particular, "Mrs. Fisher is stable now. We should begin with physical, occupational, and speech therapies." He stands, pulls a pen from his white lab coat, and hurriedly makes notes. As he walks out, he turns to the nurse and says, "She passed the swallowing tests. Start her on a pureed diet for now." He then walks out, with the nurse and aide trailing, to the next of many patients.

Scene I: Instant Replay

By entering Mrs. Fisher's room without knocking on the door, the doctor expressed his insensitivity to the fact that this was Mrs. Fisher's room, not just another hospital entrance. By not allowing her time to prepare herself for the unexpected visit, he also communicated that he was unconcerned about the patient's privacy. The flat tone devoid of expression also communicated that Mrs. Fisher was just one of many patients he had to see that day. By sitting at the foot of the bed without permission, he gave the impression that either Mrs. Fisher was unable to give permission or that her wishes were unimportant. The good news that the patient was stable was spoken without any indication that the doctor was happy about it. Statements made about passing the swallowing test and a pureed diet were also made without feeling. On leaving the room, he did not hold the door for the nurse or the aide, nor did he bid the patient goodbye. To the patient and anyone who witnessed this encounter, the impression given was that of a somewhat arrogant doctor who lacked social graces and was insensitive. Mrs. Fisher was left with the impression that she was just another name on a chart, another job to be done that day.

Scene II:

A doctor, dressed comfortably in a sport coat and tie, knocks on the patient's door. After a brief delay, he opens it, smiles, and says "Good morning, Mrs. Fisher." He walks closer to the patient and says, "You're looking well" while reaching for her hand and still wearing the broad smile. "Thank you" is Mrs. Fisher's reply, accompanied by an attempt to return the smile. While a nurse and aide enter the room, the doctor looks around for a chair. Seeing that none is available, he gestures to Mrs. Fisher for permission to sit at the foot of her bed. She graciously allows him to do so by moving her leg to make room on the narrow bed. The doctor looks to both the nurse and aide and says: "Mrs. Fisher is stable now. We should begin with physical, occupational, and speech therapies." He indicates his pleasure at the statement by patting Mrs. Fisher gently and giving the "thumbs up" gesture. While gesturing to Mrs. Fisher that time is short and he must leave, he makes a few notes on the chart and starts to walk out of the room. Then, with obvious pleasure in his voice, he turns and announces: "She passed the swallowing tests." With a low tone, he says, "Start her on a pureed diet." Then, with an upbeat voice and the return of the broad smile, he turns to Mrs. Fisher and says, "For now." He opens the door for both the nurse and aide and waves "Good-bye" as he leaves Mrs. Fisher's room.

Scene II: Instant Replay

By knocking on the door and waiting a few seconds, the doctor showed that he was aware of two facts. First, although rounds are generally conducted in the mornings, they happen at irregular times. The knock on the door and the brief wait expressed his sensitivity to the fact that the visit was unannounced. Second, the knock and brief delay allowed Mrs. Fisher the opportunity to prepare herself. The doctor recognized that she might be partially clothed or uncovered and needed a brief time to prepare herself for the visit. Holding the patient's hand and smiling while saying that she "looked well" expressed his personal concern and involvement in Mrs. Fisher's care. Asking for permission to sit at the foot of the bed also expressed his understanding of space and privacy needs. The "thumbs up" gesture, along with the statement about the stroke stabilizing, expressed his personal involvement and happiness about Mrs. Fisher's improved medical condition. Most patients can understand this gesture, even those with complete aphasia. The doctor's tone of voice expressed to the patient that he understood that pureed food may not look or taste good, but fortunately, it will be a temporary diet. Mrs. Fisher understood that the doctor would try to get her "real" food as soon as possible. By holding the door for both the nurse and aide, he also communicated respect for them. The most important fact communicated by this doctor was that he knows he is treating a person and not "just" a stroke patient.

Personal Space

Most people have had the experience of getting on a crowded elevator and feeling uncomfortable as the door closes. The elevator riders stare at the changing floor indicator while silence reigns. They feel uncomfortable because their "personal space" is being violated.

Personal space can be described as a bubble of privacy. For most Americans, it extends about four feet all around them. This distance varies from person to person and culture to culture. Studies have shown that women and children tend to interact with others at a closer range and feel less discomfort when the space is small. Not surprisingly, people stand closer to friends than to enemies or strangers. More distance is maintained for authority figures, people of higher status, and individuals from different racial groups. One study showed that people tend to stand further apart from the disabled. Of course, the degree of attraction one person feels for another overrides these rules, and the opening up of personal space is the first step in fostering an intimate and personal relationship.

For stroke survivors with physical limitations, violation of their personal space happens all of the time. Because of paralysis or weakness, many patients must rely on others to help them get in and out of bed, get dressed, or go from a chair to the bathroom. They require assistance to do these things, and it is often necessary that their personal space be violated. But stroke survivors feel like everyone else about people entering their personal space. They can feel awkward, uncomfortable, and uneasy. Stroke survivors with major communication impairments can be unable to protest verbally or resist this invasion. Or, like most people when their personal space boundaries are violated, the patient may not be aware of the source of his or her discomfort.

When you must enter the person's intimate space, take care to read his or her nonverbal messages. Look at the patient's facial expressions and body movements for clues about how he or she is tolerating this close contact. Although it is likely that the patient welcomes the help, especially from family members, you should understand the intimate nature of what you are doing. When you must enter the patient's personal space, do it gradually and indicate that you appreciate the intimate nature of what you are doing. After a time, the patient may no longer feel as uncomfortable.

Personal Territory

We all know that animals are territorial. Dogs, cats, and wild animals mark their territories and defend them, sometimes viciously. People also have this instinct. Territorialism is the most common reason countries go to war. First-class seating, doctor's lounges, private parking areas, and executive dining rooms are all indications of human territorial needs. People often display the boundaries of their homes with rock markings or by shrubs, although they do not serve as barriers. A student will leave a coat on a table in a library to mark his or her territory. "No trespassing" signs and wedding rings are symbols of territorialism. It is often easy to tell when a person feels that someone is violating his or her territory—he or she stands with hands on hips, feet apart, and elbows extended. The nonverbal message is, "This is my territory." Whereas personal space surrounds a person wherever he or she goes, territory is a fixed location.

Patients in hospitals and nursing homes experience frequent violation of their need to stake out and keep a territory of their own. Although patients continue to feel the need for a defined territory, they are rarely able to claim an absolute area of the facility. After all, the hospital or nursing home and most of the furnishings belong to someone else. After a time, however, patients confined to hospitals or nursing homes stake out certain areas—a part of the hall, lounge, or dining room—as their own exclusive areas. Unfortunately, and usually inadvertently, nurses, aides, and others often violate these territorial claims. Verbal patients can protest the violations, but patients who are communicatively disabled may not have the ability to express their displeasure. For example, if a verbal patient in a nursing home has claim to an area of the dining room and prefers to eat alone, he or she can tactfully express such preferences. The patient with a communication disorder may be unable to explain the nature of the violation. Nonverbal indications of anger, frustration, or sadness may go unheeded or misinterpreted. The staff may not see these behaviors as related to an incident of territorial violation.

You and other family members should recognize the stroke survivor's need to make territorial claims. Communicatively disordered people are no different from the rest of us when it comes to privacy and territory needs, so care should be taken to consider them. A good start is to ask courteously, or in some way obtain permission, to join the patient in his or her designated area. This clearly sets a tone of respect and consideration for the patient's territorial needs.

Touching

People need physical contact. Researchers have found that monkeys deprived of touch at birth have abnormal social patterns compared to those of other monkeys. Children deprived of touch become apathetic and listless and sometimes also do bizarre things. Some researchers even believe that children deprived of touch will die because of this lack of nurturing, even if they are given food and water.

Because touching is such a powerful form of communication, there is much variability in how, when, and where it is acceptable. The most important consideration is *where* a person is touched; an innocent but misplaced touch can be misinterpreted. Studies have shown that women tend to be less inhibited about social touching, as are people in some European countries. In North America, the first contact with a stranger is usually preceded by a handshake, and much is communicated by the strength of the grasp. Both parties make an immediate impression based on this handshake.

The largest organ of the human body, skin provides one of the most effective means of communicating. Touching is a powerful way of communicating with speech- and language-disordered patients. It can express understanding, affection, and sympathy, and there is every reason to believe that most stroke survivors, even those with major communication disorders, can appreciate it. Unless the stroke has numbed the skin, even the patient with complete aphasia can understand and appreciate this form of communication. Of course, you should exercise caution if your loved one felt uncomfortable when people touched him or her even before the stroke. For some people, touching is an unwanted intrusion into their personal space.

One caution should be exercised with some stroke patients. Strokes sometimes cause an increased sensitivity to touch. Some patients have described this as feeling as though their arm has "gone to sleep," with the unpleasant "pins and needles" sensation associated with it. Because of this, what ordinarily would be a pleasant touch on the arm or back can become irritating or painful.

Body Language

Facial expression, eye contact, gestures, and the way a person stands or sits communicates nonverbal messages. You and your loved one send these nonverbal messages all of the time. A person's facial expression usually provides information about whether he or she is happy, sad, afraid, surprised, disgusted, or angry. The eyes and mouth are the most important areas in expressing these emotions. For some stroke survivors, paralysis or weakness of the facial muscles can impair this form of communication or cause it to be misinterpreted.

Gestures are good indicators of the speaker and listener's anxiety levels. Some people and some cultures naturally use gestures more frequently. According to some studies, women tend to use more gestures than men. Certain gestures are universal in their implications, and others are specific to a culture. Hand wringing, for example, usually shows higher than normal levels of discomfort, and finger drumming suggests boredom or impatience.

Authorities on speech communication have identified two types of gestures: descriptive and reinforcing. A *descriptive* gesture helps the speaker describe what is being said. For example, some communicatively disordered people use elaborate gestures when trying to talk, as though they are using their hands and arms to draw or describe what they are tying so hard to say. A *reinforcing* gesture emphasizes what is being said. A fist slammed onto a table is a gesture reinforcing the strong emotion of the speaker.

A person's posture—the way a person carries himself or herself—is also a form of nonverbal communication, providing information about self-concept and mood, among other things. Unless the person is feeble and suffering from weak body muscles, a hanging head and stooped shoulders are good indicators of sadness and poor self-esteem. Counselors are taught to sit with their arms and legs arranged in an expansive and open fashion because a "closed body" can be an expression of a negative attitude about what is being said.

A person's voice, the clothing and jewelry someone wears, and whether a person is frequently early or late to meetings also communicate on the nonverbal level. The pitch, loudness, and quality of a person's voice send information about masculinity and femininity. Men with lower pitches and women with higher ones are considered more masculine and feminine, respectively. Loud talkers are considered more assertive than those who speak softly. If there is a conflict between the speaker's tone of voice and what the words mean, the listener usually believes the tone of voice. For example, a father might say to his daughter, "Oh, you don't need to do any homework tonight!" If the words are said sarcastically, his daughter will understand that the true meaning of the statement is that she should do homework.

You should be careful in interpreting your loved one's nonverbal voice messages, especially if he or she has dysarthria. Because of the communication disorder, he or she may have a changed voice quality, loudness, and/or pitch. Be alert to the possibility that you can misinterpret nonverbal communication based on these cues.

The clothing and jewelry people wear accentuate the roles they want to project. A cowboy hat, designer jeans, expensive suit, or tightfitting sweater are extensions of a person's identity. Clothing provides physical and also psychological protection Many patients complain about hospital clothing. Not only does it often expose the patient, but he or she is also deprived of clothing and accessories that provide psychological expression. Although it is sometimes necessary for the patient to wear hospital gowns, regular and comfortable clothing should be made available whenever possible. This appears to be a minor consideration, but the patient without communication abilities can express something about his or her personality by the clothing, jewelry, and other accessories worn.

When a person is late to appointments all of the time, other people sometimes think of him or her as being disorganized or inconsiderate. Being too early to meetings also expresses information about a person's eagerness. However, these generalities are sometimes not appropriate for stroke survivors. Certain types of brain injury can cause a patient who was otherwise prompt and time conscious to lose this ability. Some strokes can cause the person to have problems accurately judging the passage of time.

One of the philosophies of treatment for stroke-related communication disorders is to encourage any and all communication. No matter whether the stroke survivor speaks haltingly or normally, all that matters is that communication takes place. Often, nonverbal communication is as important, if not more so, than the speech of your loved one. You and other family members should be alert to your loved one's nonverbal communication and be aware that you are also communicating in that way. Remember, because of nonverbal communication, "you cannot not communicate."

Family Dynamics

It goes without saying that a stroke can dramatically and permanently change a family. This is especially true when the stroke causes a major communication disorder. Strokes often make it necessary for family roles to change, and actual reversals in expectations often result. In most families, roles are shared, and they change over time and in response to circumstances. However, many family members assume a particular set of jobs and responsibilities that define their relationship to others in the family. For example, the "provider" of the family may lose that role following a stroke and become dependent on other members of the family. The "helper" can become the one to be "helped." The stroke survivor may no longer bring home a paycheck, monitor investments and balance checkbooks, make repairs of household appliances, and keep cars and the lawn mower going. Role reversals occur because someone else in the family must take charge and do them. In many families, there is someone "ready, willing, and able" to "rise to the occasion" and take over. In other families, the transition is more difficult. Strokes often change roles in and expectations about business, cooking, driving, cleaning house, washing clothes, shopping, paying taxes, and gardening, to name a few. Today's families are more broadly defined and unique, and there is virtually no limit to the role changes that may have to be made because of a stroke.

Role reversals also happen in the emotional and social areas. Strokes may change or cause reversals about who in the family is the nurturer, communicator, leader, socializer, or mediator of family problems. Families operate on many levels and in many dimensions, but certain members assume specific emotional and social roles, and a stroke can change all of that, too. In some families, other family members may readily embrace these changes, but in others a void may be left. If it is true that "all the world is a stage," then a stroke can dramatically change the script.

Give and Take

Good long-term relationships operate on many planes and levels, but they have one thing in common: They satisfy, more or less, the needs of the parties involved. Although no relationship can completely satisfy a particular individual, to no small extent the strength and endurance of a relationship is determined by the needs it meets. Each person in a relationship brings to it a myriad of needs that are as unique and varied as the people themselves. People enter into relationships for love, for companionship, and/or to rear children. Sexual, financial, and security needs draw people together, as does the need to escape loneliness. Although the parties in a relationship do not fundamentally change because one of them has a stroke, the complexion of the relationship can be altered dramatically. This is especially true if the stroke causes a major communication barrier between you and your loved one. After all, communication is the glue that holds relationships together. Communication is the bond that permits relationships to grow, change, and adapt to new circumstances. When the parties in a relationship stop communicating, the relationship suffers, and the loss of communication can be the beginning of the end.

A stroke with a resulting communication barrier need not be the end of your relationship. Even if your loved one is rendered unable to speak, read, write, or to understand what you say to him or her, the two of you can continue to engage in rewarding and satisfying communication. No matter how severe a speech and language pathology, there is always the potential for satisfying and intimate communication between you and your loved one. You simply will need to be more creative about it. Avoid slipping into poor or unmeaningful communication. The degree of disability the person has because of a stroke is largely dependent on how many limits you and other members of the family put on him or her.

Communication and Money

As a rule and as much as possible, you should try to bring the stroke survivor into discussions and decisions about household finances. Gear the discussion and decision-making levels to those that were typical of your relationship before the stroke. If, for example, you typically balanced the checkbook and paid bills, you should not set these up as the stroke survivor's new responsibilities. However, if before the stroke your loved one was actively involved in setting budgets, setting aside money for saving, or making monthly car payments, you should allow him or her to continue to be involved with these activities. Because of the stroke, he or she may not be able to participate fully in these discussions and decisions, but continued inclusion in them is an important part of family dynamics and communication. Recall that many patients with significant language impairments have problems expressing, manipulating, and understanding monetary values.

As a result, you should adjust the discussion and decision-making levels to fit any problems the patient may have with arithmetic and monetary values.

Pam and Ken Feld had been married for 52 years. During that time, Pam had been primarily responsible for financial matters. Not only did she take care of long-range financial planning, but she also took care of the monthly car and house payments, wrote checks for car and home insurance, paid credit cards, and got "walking around cash" from the bank machine. Her stroke resulted in aphasia, which severely limited her ability to speak and to understand the speech of others. It also reduced her ability to do arithmetic and to understand the value of money, such as how many quarters in a dollar or how many "fives" a person can get for a 20-dollar bill. Since Pam's stroke, Ken has assumed many financial responsibilities previously done by his wife. Although he was not accustomed to the new responsibilities, he sought help from his son and daughter and soon was able to do what was required. Because Ken realized how important it was to keep Pam actively involved in the family finances, he makes a special effort to involve her. For example, when he pays monthly bills at the dining room table, he encourages Pam to sit with him at the table. As he pays the bills, balances the checkbook, and sets aside spending money, he confers with his wife. Although the stroke has eliminated much of her ability to understand the details of the family finances, he manages to explain what he is doing and occasionally asks for her opinion or advice. Ken is careful not to frustrate or confuse her. He understands the importance of keeping Pam involved in the family finances, and he communicates to her that he still values her participation in these matters. The stroke has not changed the fact that he respects and values her as a vital member of the family.

Of course, many stroke survivors can continue to handle financial responsibilities as well as they did before the stroke. Other stroke patients may have only minor limitations doing these jobs. The only adjustment in the routine may be to have the figures checked for accuracy. What is important is that you and other family members understand that communication about money matters should continue at an appropriate level. A stroke should not be the end of this aspect of family dynamics and communication.

Communication and Social Activities

The stroke survivor, even one with a severe communication disorder, should be encouraged to continue to participate in social activities. Once again, these activities should usually be the same as those the patient enjoyed before the stroke. Not only will continuing to participate in these activities contribute to a better quality of life, but they also will provide speech and language stimulation and practice, which can be therapeutic for many patients.

Some social activities will be physically impossible for the stroke survivor. Direct participation in golf or dancing may be beyond the stroke survivor's abilities because of physical limitations. Speech and language disorders may eliminate singing in a barbershop quartet or a church choir. However, even these activities can be participated in at a different level. Many stroke survivors can ride in golf carts even though they do not actually golf and enjoy the festivity of a dance although they cannot actually get on the dance floor. Stroke survivors can still attend choir practice as limited participants or observers and have the uplifting experience of socializing and interacting with fellow churchgoers.

Ed Blakely and Marilyn Hickman loved to play cards. In the condo, a close-knit group of bridge players had formed who met three times a week in one of the card rooms of the condo's recreation center. Because Marilyn's condo was next to Ed's, on "card night" she would knock on his door and together they would go to the game, both bringing their share of snacks. When Ed had a stroke and was in a rehabilitation center for two months, his empty chair at the game was a reminder to all of the seriousness of his illness. After Ed returned from the rehabilitation center, Marilyn would still knock on Ed's door, only now she assumed responsibility for the snacks and would push his wheelchair to the card room. Although Ed's stroke had left him unable to understand and participate in the card game, he was seated at the table where he could watch the activities and share in the socialization. Although Ed could no longer play bridge, the members continued to treat him as one of the group. They valued having him at the game, not as a participant but as an observer.

By encouraging Ed to continue to attend card night, Marilyn and his other friends expressed their continued friendship. Card night was still something he could look forward to. Rather than staying in his room, isolated and lonely, he was brought into the social activity at a level that was appropriate, given the limitations caused by the stroke. It was important that his friends understood his limitations and did not try to force him into playing bridge; they did not require him to confront failure. By allowing and encouraging Ed to be in the card room and to continue to be part of the group, they expressed their friendship and acceptance of him.

Communication and Family Routines

For the stroke survivor, being able to continue with daily chores and participate in family routines is a crucial part of maintaining a sense of continuity. After a person has a stroke, it is important to gradually ease him or her back into typical family routines. These daily chores and family routines should be geared to the realities of what the individual can and cannot do. This is particularly true of people who have suffered major speech and language impairments, because there is a tendency to exclude them from activities that involve communication. You should remember that although the patient may not understand all of what is said or be able to express himself or herself completely, he or she can often participate at some level in daily chores and routines. Although participation levels may not be the same as before the stroke, participation is nonetheless possible. It is sad to see a stroke survivor relegated to a corner of the house or in front of the television while the rest of the family goes about their daily routines. When your loved one is unnecessarily excluded from family activities, his or her communication disorder becomes a true handicap.

Thanksgiving was always one of Judy Hunter's favorite holidays. Her large family converged at her house every Thanksgiving for the feast she prepared. She would often start the preparation days in advance, and the result was a meal fit for a king. Her children and grandchildren would bring necessary soups, salads, sauces, and silverware, but the feast was clearly Judy's creation. Her reward for all of the time, work, and energy that went into the meal was the pleasure she received watching her family enjoy the feast.

There would have been fewer thanks to give this Thanksgiving had Judy's family done too much for her after her stroke. But Judy's children were careful to bring her back into the tradition. Although she could no longer continue to do many things because of the paralysis and communication disorder, she was still active in the food preparation. She helped mash the potatoes, prepare the side dishes, and set the table. She decided where people sat and even when the meal was served. Although it took a little longer and certain accommodations had to be made, Thanksgiving was still Judy's event because her children and grandchildren recognized the importance of not excluding her from this tradition.

Being impaired or unable to communicate should not exclude a person from family traditions or even daily routines and chores. Everyone wants to be appreciated and to contribute, and stroke survivors are no different. Activities may take more time and involve some inconveniences, but you should make every attempt to bring the stroke survivor back into the family milieu. It goes without saying that you should respect your loved one's wishes in these matters and never force him or her to do things he or she does not want to do.

Intimate Communication

After your loved one comes home from the hospital or rehabilitation center, you may feel some awkwardness in resuming the intimacies of your relationship. This is especially true if the stroke has resulted in paralysis or weakness. Barriers to communication caused by the stroke may add to the awkwardness. Knowing whether, when, and how to resume the intimate aspects of your relationship can be difficult for both you and your loved one. Two principles can help guide you through this awkward time.

First and foremost, remember that this part of your relationship need not die because of the stroke, no matter how serious or debilitating it was. Even if you and your loved one cannot continue to relate at the level you were accustomed to before the stroke, intimacies can still be shared. In fact, because of the verbal communication barriers, it is more important than ever to relate to each other on an intimate level. If you shared the same bed before the stroke, try to arrange it so you can continue to sleep together. The companionship and physical contact can provide needed emotional support for both of you. The stroke survivor may be self-conscious about weak or paralyzed body parts, so try to communicate your acceptance of him or her as a "total" person. By word and deed, let your loved one know that the intimate feelings you had for him or her before the stroke have not changed.

Second, if you do have problems with sexual relations after the stroke, do not be bashful about discussing them with your doctor. Doctors are trained to deal with these stroke-related problems, too. Instructions, counseling, and medication are available to help you reestablish this aspect of your relationship.

One of the most important responsibilities of the stroke survivor's family and friends is to guard against unnecessary reductions in the patient's quality of life. Strokes and the communication disorders that result from them need not result in loneliness and isolation for either you or the patient. Try not to be intimidated by the stroke and communication disorder. Remember, the fact that your loved one has had a severe stroke and is severely disabled in communication is not the end of your relationship. This is a time to rebuild bridges and to tear down fences.

CHAPTER 10

Accepting Unwanted Change

I not only bow to the inevitable; I am fortified by it.
—THORNTON WILDER

In the aftermath of a stroke, there comes a time when you and your loved ones must shift your focus from overcoming disabilities to accepting them. Unfortunately, some individuals never recover what the stroke has taken from them and many others only partially recover what was lost. No matter how hard you try, and despite the time and energy you, your loved one, and the rehabilitation professionals put in, strokes often leave in their wake a multitude of permanent unwanted changes. These unwanted changes happen to both you and your loved one, and they all have one thing in common: loss. The purpose of this chapter is to discuss some of the ways in which people accept unwanted change and to provide perspective on the adjustments that must be made. With this in mind, it should be comforting to know that most stroke survivors and their loved ones are able to make these adjustments. They go on with their lives, accepting the unwanted changes brought about by the stroke.

As has been the theme throughout this book, it is important to learn as much as possible about the direct and indirect aspects of having a stroke. Only through knowledge and understanding can the stroke survivor, you, and other members of your family deal with all of the aspects of the stroke. Knowledge and understanding will help you learn to accept the changes that prove to be permanent. The goal here is not to wallow in the negative aspects of the stroke, nor to cause unwanted sadness by discussing what has been lost, but to learn as much as possible about the dimensions of life that can be affected by a stroke and to understand the psychology of adjustment to these unwanted changes. In addition, there are certain things you and other family members and friends should and should not do to help the patient (and each other) reach the stage of acceptance of what the stroke has wrought. In acceptance, people feel neither good nor bad about what was lost; they simply accept what has happened as part of a greater picture, a larger context.

As humans we are no strangers to loss. It permeates our existence. Loss is a significant part of all aspects of living, and it begins early. For example, a baby learns to cope with the loss of intimacy from the mother because of weaning. The security and warmth of being held during feedings is gone. When older, that same child may have to give up the role of "baby of the family" when a brother or sister is born. Young men and women give up freedom and independence when they accept the responsibilities of marriage and children. Too often the middle years are associated with the loss of dreams and aspirations. To the aged, loss is a frequent companion with few new treasures to replace the ones lost. All growth requires change, and that transition often involves losing something of value. But without change, life becomes stagnant. Loss is a natural consequence of life, and so is grief, the human reaction to being permanently separated from someone or something of value.

Dimensions of Loss

Strokes and stroke-related communication disorders can result in three dimensions of loss. A stroke survivor experiences loss (1) because he or she is psychologically (and sometimes physically) separated from loved ones, (2) because the stroke has taken away some of his or her abilities, and/or (3) because valued objects can no longer be used. Your loved one will feel the brunt of the unwanted changes that have happened in these three areas.

Stroke survivors are like everyone else; they experience feelings of loss over the unwanted changes caused by the stroke. The stroke survivor's family and friends also feel a sense of loss about what the stroke has taken from their relationship with the loved one and the necessary changes that must be made in their lives.

Psychological Separation

The first category of loss is called *loss of person*. In strokes, and especially with patients who have suffered severe communication disorders, loss of person is a psychological separation that occurs because meaningful and satisfying communication no longer takes place; you and your loved one feel distant and separated due to a lack of communication. This sense of separation may be felt even when both of you are in the same room. Although your loved one has not actually been lost in a physical sense, such as through death or divorce, meaningful communication has been lost. Given the circumstance, it is natural for you and the stroke survivor to feel that something important has been taken from your relationship.

The role of communication in a relationship cannot be overstated. Psychologists have long known that many of the ills married couples experience stem from a lack of communication. Marital communication problems usually result from one partner's refusal to communicate significantly with the other person. With the stroke survivor and his or her family, however, the issue is not a lack of desire or willingness to communicate. The communication barrier is caused by the stroke and the resulting damage to the speech and language centers of the brain. This psychological separation is often compounded by actual physical separation when the stroke survivor is placed in a hospital, nursing home, or other medical care facility.

With respect to maintaining a strong relationship, the communication disorders resulting from strokes are two-edged swords. Not only does a major communication disorder cause an inability to communicate normally, but it also causes stress, anxiety, and negative emotions for both the patient and his or her family and friends. During this time of many unwanted changes, when you and your loved one most need to discuss issues, share feelings and ideas, and give one another verbal support, the ability to communicate has been taken from the relationship.

> *Cheryl and Blair had been married for six years. Both had lost their first mates to cancer a few years earlier. Their married life had been stimulating and exciting. Both were avid readers and kept up with current events. Both were active in the same political party. In fact, that was how they met, at a political fund-raising event. Although they did not agree on every issue, their lives were full of exciting political discussions. Since Cheryl had the stroke, however, life had changed considerably. Instead of lively political discussions at the table, dinner was a silent affair. After the meal, both would sit in the living room watching television; communication was limited to the basics. Cheryl's stroke had also eliminated her ability to read and understand newspapers, and she could only partially understand news reports on television. Whenever Blair would bring up a political subject, Cheryl would try to discuss the issues but because of the communication deficit, there was no closure. Blair would no longer argue a political point because he worried about her feeling rejected. After a while, they did not discuss political or current events.*

Much of the social structure and communication that had initially drawn Cheryl and Blair to each other was taken from them because of the stroke and the resulting communication disorder. Discussions about politics and current events became unsatisfying for both of them. Although the stroke did not require Cheryl to live apart from Blair in a nursing home or extended care facility, they experienced a psychological separation. The loss of the ability to communicate about current events and political issues had taken away an important part of their relationship. In addition, because of Cheryl's stroke, they were unable to talk meaningfully about other issues and concerns. On several occasions, they tried to discuss the nature of their relationship and the changes that had occurred, but this also was impossible and unsatisfying. Cheryl and Blair were still very much in love, but the stroke had taken from their relationship much of the excitement and intensity they had valued. Blair felt separated from the intelligent and exciting woman he had been so attracted to in the first place. The sense of loss was no less for Cheryl. At some level, Cheryl was aware of what had been taken from them, and she felt a sense of loss for the relationship.

Loss of Objects

The second category of loss is when one is separated from a valued possession. The most obvious object in this category is a person's home. People who lose their homes to natural disasters and other events can be expected to grieve over that loss. The material possessions that people devote a large part of their lives to acquiring can create a significant void when they are taken. The value the person places on an object determines the impact its loss will have on him or her. The objects people value are as varied as their interests, such as cars, computers, sewing machines, recreational vehicles, and kitchens designed to prepare gourmet meals can be lost to a stroke. They are lost when the stroke survivor can no longer use or enjoy them.

The objects lost can have both real and symbolic value. The real value of an object is lost because the person can no longer use it and enjoy the accompanying feelings of gratification. The real pleasure in driving an antique vehicle or taking a trip in a motor home can be lost to a stroke. The relaxation and joy of gardening, sewing, or preparing gourmet meals also can be lost in a "real" sense. An object's symbolic value is as individual as people. For example, as well as a way of relaxing, being able to garden may have the symbolic value of leisure or independence. In a larger sense, people can also feel a sense of loss over intangibles such as innocence, religion, beliefs, and attitudes.

> *Norman and Ruby Blakely had a comfortable retirement. Throughout the years, they had acquired a large portfolio of stocks and bonds. Although both were retired teachers with good retirement programs, Norman continued to invest and actively manage his supplemental retirement accounts, mutual funds, and individual stocks. After the youngest of their children had left for college, Norman had converted her bedroom into an office where he would spend most of his free time trading via computer and telephone. He carefully researched each stock fund and individual company before buying and selling. Each transaction was monitored on his state-of-the-art computer. His office was full of research materials, financial magazines, and company reports. When Norman had his stroke, it caused him to have global aphasia*

and paralysis on his right side. Because the converted office was on the second floor of their house, he was unable to get upstairs easily. At first, after returning from the rehabilitation center, Ruby would help him up to his office, but this was a difficult and time-consuming task. Once in his office, he would try to work on the computer or read a fund prospectus, but neither made sense to him. As time passed, he no longer asked to go to his office and he stopped actively managing his supplemental retirement accounts, mutual funds, and individual stocks. Ultimately, Ruby had to turn everything over to a financial planner.

The stroke took Norman's ability to manage their stock and bond portfolio. Because of the trouble getting to his office, it took his office, too. Although not everyone would consider this a serious change, it was a major loss for Norman. His office and stock portfolio had both real and symbolic value. The real value lay in the money and assets he had acquired, which had resulted in a higher standard of living in retirement than Ruby or he could have expected as teachers. His office and stock portfolio also had symbolic value. To Norman, they were symbolic of his vitality as an investor and a tribute to his resourcefulness. They were a major part of his self-concept.

Loss of Self

Loss of self is the final and most significant loss that many stroke survivors must deal with. It is a broad dimension and can involve changes in the individual's health, body function, and sense of worth, self-concept, and attractiveness. Loss of self can also include functions the individual *perceives* as lost that in reality may not have been taken from him or her.

The list of what can be taken physically, psychologically, and mentally from the patient because of a stroke is long. In severe strokes, the patient may not be able to walk, use the toilet without assistance, or transfer from bed to wheelchair without help. It is not uncommon for some patients to lose the ability to chew, swallow, and, therefore, eat normally. Loss of physical sensation, usually on the right side of the person's body, also occurs. Blindness, visual field cuts, and hearing problems occur. A stroke can also take high-level reasoning skills, orientation, and memory. Sadly, some strokes are fatal and take the most valued possession of all—life itself.

A significant reduction in or the complete inability to communicate is one of the most serious losses many stroke survivors experience. Loss of language and motor speech abilities can be all-encompassing, including inabilities to read, write, and do simple arithmetic. Many stroke survivors also have problems finding the words to express themselves and understanding the speech of others. Motor speech disorders often result in a loss of the ability to make sounds easily and clearly.

These tangible losses are certainly grievous events. But just as the loss of objects is both real and symbolic, so is the loss of self. The effects of these losses on the patient's self-esteem should never be underestimated. For example, to the paralyzed patient, the loss of the symbolic ability to "stand on one's own two feet" may be more difficult to adjust to than the physical restrictions on mobility. Similarly, to speak, read, and understand what is spoken or written also carries symbolic importance. To speak is to be potent and vital. To be deprived of this ability reduces an individual to near-primitive levels of existence. Even emotion is reduced to nonverbal expression and may be misinterpreted by listeners. Because of the loss of ability to communicate, the patient's needs and desires sometimes go unmet. Thoughts cannot be declared, particularly abstract and complicated ones. In patients with irreversible and severe communication disorders, the real and symbolic aspects of the loss of self can combine to create a deep sense of bereavement.

Alejandro Perez took pride in his high school and college football career. As a freshman in high school, he was moved up to junior varsity after the first three games. Starting in his junior year, he played varsity football, and his school ultimately took the state championship. Even the local newspaper called him one of the finest receivers ever produced by his small town. Though no major college recruited him, a small private school had given him a full-ride football scholarship, and he played for them with distinction. After college, he volunteered as a "pee wee" coach and played football with his friends and family every chance he got. He never lost the joy of stretching to grasp a well-thrown football and running for the touchdown. On Alejandro's sixty-third birthday, a stroke leveled the playing field forever. A stroke reduced this fit, athletic man to a wheelchair, unable to speak or to understand the speech of others. The pain he felt because of his condition was worst when on weekends family and friends would play touch football while he watched through the dining room window.

Alejandro did not need to be an athlete to experience this great sense of loss. Confinement to a wheelchair, being unable to move about freely, and difficulty doing even the most basic of tasks such as going to the toilet unassisted or eating without assistance would be a great loss to anyone. It was especially painful for Alejandro because of his natural athletic abilities and the joys they had brought. The physical loss was exacerbated for Alejandro by his inability to communicate. Because of the aphasia, he was unable to talk and reminisce about his past football victories.

The Process of Accepting Unwanted Change

Death of a loved one is certainly one of the most painful experiences a person can go through, and grief is a natural human reaction to loss. Before the mid 1900s, the way people coped with death was rarely studied, or even discussed, for that matter.

Until that time, death and dying were topics left for abstract philosophical discussions, and helping people to cope with these events was relegated to religion and religious leaders. The scientific community ignored any systematic investigation into how people coped with death. Traditional medicine also neglected the concepts of death, dying, and grief. Many doctors were uncomfortable with the subject because they felt a sense of failure when a patient died. This neglect was part of what has been called our "death denying society."

In 1969 a psychiatrist by the name of Elisabeth Kübler-Ross changed all of that with the publication of *On Death and Dying*. Dr. Kübler-Ross brought these subjects out into the open and presented details of the process of grief. According to Kübler-Ross, grief is not one emotional reaction but a complex progression of emotional and intellectual adjustments to being separated from a loved one. Until the publication of Kübler-Ross's book, most people thought of depression and grief as being the same state. According to Kübler-Ross, however, depression is one stage in the grieving process, and accepting unwanted changes involves other stages of adjustment. Denial, anger, bargaining, depression, and acceptance are the stages Kübler-Ross identified as comprising the complex process of accepting the death of a loved one or one's own death. Kübler-Ross was truly a pioneer in dealing with the subject of death, dying, and grief.

Kübler-Ross was not without her critics. Some psychologists resist looking at grief and the process of adjusting to unwanted change as "stages" people go through. They point out that many people do not necessarily go through all of the stages she proposed. They also note that many grieving people go back and forth between the stages. Other critics believe that deep, prolonged depression is more of a chemical imbalance than a response to loss. Actually, Kübler-Ross addressed most of these issues in her early writings, and her model of adjusting to unwanted change is as viable and meaningful today as it was when she first published her book. This model of accepting unwanted change is also pertinent to stroke survivors and their loved ones. As you will discover in the following discussion, the model can be applied to the three dimensions of loss discussed previously.

The Road to Acceptance

Before discussing the stages a stroke survivor goes through when attempting to adjust to permanent and irreversible losses, four important considerations need to be addressed. The "grief model" is not applicable to all patients, nor does it apply to all kinds of stroke-related losses. Special considerations must be made when applying this model to stroke survivors and their families.

First, to grieve over a loss a person must be aware of what has happened. This is a pertinent, if obvious, fact, especially concerning patients who are in a coma. A person in a coma is more than likely unaware of what has happened, so he or she is not going to grieve over loss of self, valued objects, or the psychological separation from loved ones. As discussed in Chapter 5, there are degrees of coma and awareness. A patient who has a partial awareness of what has happened may have only limited feelings of loss. The extent of the patient's awareness of what was lost dictates how deeply grief is felt.

Second, neurological factors can mask or eliminate the grieving process. For example, a stroke can cause euphoria, a heightened sense of well-being. Brain damage and/or a lack of oxygen can cause a person to feel unnaturally "high." When a patient is euphoric, he or she is unlikely to feel depressed or angry about what has happened, so the grieving response is either masked or eliminated in these people.

The third factor to be considered in the grief response is that the stroke survivor must have valued that which was lost. Some stroke survivors do not miss some or all of the things taken from them. For example, some people simply do not place a high value on communication. Talking and listening to others is seen by some as an intrusion into their privacy. Intimate discussions can make them feel uncomfortable. For some stroke survivors with one or more of the big three communication disorders, the stroke has given them an excuse for not having to engage in bothersome communication. Rather than grieving deeply over the loss of speech and language, these people welcome the change. Thus, they are unlikely to feel a sense of loss. Clinically, this reaction is called a *secondary gain*.

The fourth and final consideration in applying Kübler-Ross's stages of grief to survivors of stroke and the communication disorders that can result from them has to do with other ways people adjust to losses. There are other psychological ways to cope with major unwanted changes in life. The best example is religion. Some deeply religious people simply accept the changes as "God's will." The unwanted changes are regarded as a test or part of a plan. These people find acceptance and comfort in viewing life and adversity this way. Other psychological defense mechanisms besides the ones presented by Kübler-Ross can be employed to adjust to major unwanted changes. Some are more adaptable and successful than others.

Given the above qualifiers, most aware stroke survivors (and their loved ones) pass through most of the stages of grief proposed by Kübler-Ross. Not everyone passes through all of the stages, and sometimes stages are repeated. Sometimes the period of time spent in a particular stage is brief, and other times an individual gets stuck in a stage. The total time involved in the process of accepting unwanted change varies considerably. Most authorities on the subject of grief suggest that it takes between 6 and 12 months to adjust to a major loss, but it is perfectly normal for some people to take longer and for others to go through the process more rapidly.

As will be discussed in detail, when most stroke survivors are confronted with major losses in one or more of the dimensions, they pass through a period of denial.

The denial gives them time to mobilize less radical defenses. The stages of anger and bargaining happen because of the frustration associated with unwanted change. Depression occurs when the person becomes aware of the valued losses. More importantly, most patients and their families go on to accept what has happened and continue with their lives. One of the most valuable aspects of the grief model is that it shows the "light at the end of the tunnel." That light is the acceptance stage.

During the first three stages of Kübler-Ross's process of accepting unwanted change, the person is not completely aware of what has happened. This is especially true of the stage called *denial*.

"I Don't Boliovo It."
Denial is described as the "I don't believe it" stage of accepting unwanted change. Denial is a common psychological defense. When a person is confronted with something threatening, it is a natural human response to deny that it exists. To illustrate this point, "I don't believe it!" is one of the most common statements made by people when confronted with the news that a loved one has died. Blotting out reality is a psychological way of giving ourselves more time to begin to understand and accept what has happened. It is human nature's way of buffering the news until the person can mobilize other defenses.

Denial is a radical defense; it takes a lot of psychological time and energy to continue to blot out reality. Denial is also a perceptual defense. Even stroke survivors with major communication disorders can employ it because language is not essential to deny what is going on. Not only is denial a common defense; it is also the central factor of a lot of other defenses. For example, when people rationalize something, they must also deny some of their motives. The same is true for several other common defenses.

Three factors influence the rate and ease with which the stroke survivor passes through denial.

1. Knowledge of the situation. If the patient suspects the extent of his or her disabilities but is told very little, successful mobilization of other defenses to replace denial could be delayed.
2. Available time. If the patient has little time to adjust, as with the terminally ill, passage through this stage and the following ones is frequently more rapid than might otherwise be expected.
3. Personality and character before the stroke. Some people regularly use denial as their primary method of coping. This suggests a strong learned behavior. The past use of denial as a habitual coping style increases the likelihood that it will be used as the method of coping with the stroke.

Not only can the stroke survivor be expected to go through denial, but you and other family members may also experience this stage. Perhaps when you were first told of the stroke or saw what was happening, you denied it. You may still be engaging in denial, avoiding the reality that your loved one may never talk normally or walk again. This is not to say that hoping for the best or placing faith in God are the same as denial. Miracles do happen. But if doctors and other professionals agree that your loved one has obtained all of the recovery he or she is likely to achieve and you refuse to accept it, then you may be employing denial. The reality of the situation may be too great for you to handle, and denial may be employed to buffer the negativity.

In the short story, "Murphy's Inner World of Aphasia," at the beginning of this book, Murphy's wife, Beth, employed denial when he first had his stroke:

> *Beth saw the ambulance rush Murph off to the hospital. She was sure that this was just a minor and temporary problem. No way could this be happening to her. Murphy was too strong to fall victim to something like this. A feeling of calm surrounded her as she got into the car to drive to the hospital. There was relief in blotting from her mind the terrible things that were happening to her and Murphy.*

Murphy, too, fell in and out of denial during the first few hours in the hospital:

> *As Murph lay back, succumbing to the restraints, he felt calm; a sense of well-being surrounded him. As he stared at the hospital ceiling, he simply denied what had happened. He convinced himself that nothing bad was happening and if it was, it wasn't happening to him. He welcomed the break from reality, and he slipped into the sanctuary of sleep.*

"Why Me?"

Everyone becomes frustrated when they cannot avoid something negative. For the stroke survivor, there are many unalterable realities, and the anger and bargaining stages of accepting unwanted change are normal responses to them. The stroke survivor experiences constant frustration. The patient may be confined to a hospital when he or she would rather be at home or have to go to therapies when he or she would rather be with family members. Other frustrations include unwanted expenses, lack of privacy, painful treatments, separation from loved ones, loss of body functioning, and inability to communicate. Many patients feel a loss of control. Terminal patients would rather live than die. It is natural for people to become angry when these things happen.

Anger is the most common reaction to persistent frustration. Anger usually occurs when the person can no longer maintain denial. Sometimes the anger is so great that it becomes rage. However, even extreme anger or rage can be considered a step in the direction of acceptance because these emotions signal partial acceptance of what has happened or is going to happen. People deal with anger in a variety of ways. Some internalize it and others strike out verbally or even physically. Professionals, family members, and friends may become the brunt of the anger.

With patients who have a major communication disorder, accurate interpretation of their anger may be difficult. Because of the communication disorder(s), some patients may be unable to express the nature of their rage. Some patients in the anger stage may feign indifference or show resentment. More overt signs of anger may be seen in such things as throwing food, lack of cooperation, or bizarre behaviors. However, it is important to realize that many things can generate anger. You and others can do things that cause the anger. It is important to discover the cause of the anger and permit it to be expressed in acceptable ways.

Because of the stroke, you also may feel angry about the unwanted changes that have happened to you and your loved one. It goes without saying that the stroke can also have a frustrating negative impact on your life as well. Psychological separation, financial concerns, and major negative changes in your lifestyle may constitute some of the unwanted changes you must learn to accept. On that road to acceptance, it is natural to feel anger.

In the story "Murphy's Inner World of Aphasia," Beth also got angry when Murphy had his stroke. Anger set in when the realities of the situation became apparent.

> "Our first goal is to get him stabilized, and then we'll begin thinking about rehabilitation," Dr. Foster planned aloud. He wanted to go into more detail but felt the buzz of his cell phone. He checked the number and politely ended the conversation. As he walked off, Beth felt angry as the realities of the situation set in. She was angry with Dr. Foster for confirming the bad news and mad at herself for not doing something to prevent the stroke. She was also mad at Murphy for not taking better care of himself. All she could think was, "Why did this have to happen?" Beth was left alone in the crowded room, more alone than she had ever been.

Murphy's anger was directed at himself.

> The fall that Murph had taken into the family pictures a few days ago seemed like a distant nightmare. Murph's life had changed permanently. From Murph's perspective, all of the changes were unwanted. In an instant, he was transformed into a dependent, verbally impaired patient in a large, impersonal institution. Although he could see and touch Beth, his mate of 45 years, a wedge had been driven between them. He still felt the love, the fondness for her, but all

but the most basic expressions of his feelings were lost. Matt, Andrea, and the grandchildren visited him regularly, but there were painful silences and a lack of friendly chatter. He missed his old life sorely, and it angered him that so much had been taken from him. He certainly had not asked for the stroke, but he felt anger at himself for having it. He was angry at the whole situation. He was frustrated at being unable to change the situation, and that frustration also angered him.

Bargaining is also a response to frustration. It reduces frustration by allowing the patient to give the responsibility of the disorder to a higher authority, someone or something with superior power to deal with the evils of the stroke. Bargaining reduces the negative emotions associated with unwanted events that cannot be changed. Usually, the bargain involves giving up something of value for an exemption from the loss. By bargaining the individual attempts to delay or reduce the effects of the loss. The stroke survivor may bargain with God, physicians, nurses, and therapists. Many grieving patients bargain with themselves. Like people who respond with anger, the grieving person in the bargaining stage is partially aware of what has happened and is on the road to acceptance. It is a normal part of the grieving process.

Bargains struck with God include giving up something valued. The patient may bargain to never smoke cigarettes again, to stop drinking alcoholic beverages, or to go to church every Sunday if God will make the effects of the stroke go away. Bargaining with medical professionals involves searching for one "miracle" doctor or specialist who can use his or her skills to negate the stroke.

Bargaining also occurs with the speech-language pathologist. If the patient has a severe speech and/or language pathology, the bargain may be nonverbal. But higher functioning patients may verbally report the nature of the agreement to the therapist. It can be summarized as follows: "If I work hard and do everything required, then I will get all of my speech back (and all of the other aspects of being human implied by the capability to use speech)." Patients in this stage of psychological adjustment to the disorder may be highly motivated to engage in the therapies. They tend to work very hard to live up to their end of the bargain.

Bargaining permits the patient to focus his or her attention on complete recovery rather than to experience an appropriate awareness of limitations. It reduces frustration only because it lets the patient be unrealistic. Bargaining also involves denial. To bargain effectively, the patient must blot out the reality of the disorder and be unrealistic about the role God or others play in overcoming the disability. Patients who bargain with medical professionals are unrealistic about a specialist's abilities to negate the effects of a stroke. When patients bargain with themselves, they believe that the neurological damage can be reversed by willpower and determination alone.

You and other family members may find yourselves bargaining, too. Although finding the best rehabilitation center and the finest specialists to treat your loved one can certainly not be considered bargaining, being unrealistic about what they can do may be a sign of bargaining. The same is true of your expectations about therapies and treatments. Hoping for the best is not a sign of bargaining, but being unrealistic about your expectations can signal that you may still be struggling to overcome the inevitable.

Grieving Depression

When denial, anger, and bargaining have run their course and all attempts to overcome the losses have failed, grieving depression occurs. The patient feels a great sense of loss. Grieving depression occurs when patients become aware that they are permanently separated from a valued person, object, and/or function. In some patients, the depression lasts only a few days, but with others it may last for months. Some people do not pass successfully through this stage and become fixated in depression.

Grieving depression sets in when patients are aware of the losses and their defenses will not buffer or delay the reaction. Patients no longer deny what has happened and make no bargains. The anger felt previously subsides. The realities of what has been lost become apparent, and there is a deep sense of loss.

How long should grieving depression last? The answer to this question depends on many factors. The value of what was lost, the patient's awareness, his or her preexisting personality, and support from family and friends all determine the length of grieving depression. Even with the most significant of losses, the patient should have regular periods of normal emotions after three months or so. Brief episodes of depression can be triggered by pictures, thoughts, or sounds for years following the loss of a significant aspect of a person's life.

This type of depression is different from depression that results directly from brain injury or from a chemical imbalance (see Chapter 7). Grieving depression is a natural and expected occurrence in aware people who have lost something of value. Some authorities call the depression that results from brain injuries or chemical imbalances *psycho-organic* and grieving depression *reactive*. Of course, stroke survivors may have both types of depression, and they can create a vicious spiral of negativity, as Wendy noted about Murphy:

> *Wendy wanted Murph to be put on an antidepressant because he was too depressed, devastated by the recent events beyond a normal grief reaction. The injury to the cells of the brain and his inability to adjust to the unwanted events had combined to create a spiral of negativity. The poor guy just couldn't see the light at the end of the tunnel. Wendy would talk to Dr. Curzon about it.*

Depressed patients must always be monitored for signs of severe clinical depression, which requires medical intervention. In these situations, antidepressant medication can help break the negative spiral.

The transition from bargaining to depression often involves major changes in the stroke survivor's motivation. As was noted earlier, the patient in the bargaining stage may be highly motivated and enthusiastic about participation in therapies. While in grieving depression, however, the patient may not attend well to therapies. He or she may be lethargic and pessimistic, although some patients remain active while depressed. The patient appears preoccupied with the losses. For terminally ill patients, the depression is preparatory to separation from this world and all of the loved and valued aspects of it. In patients with severe speech and language disorders, the separation is also harsh.

Again, you and other family members and friends also may become depressed as the reality of the losses and unwanted changes becomes apparent. The effects of the stroke on your lives can also cause grieving depression. It is natural for you to feel depressed at the unwanted changes that have been caused by the stroke. The good news is that acceptance is around the corner.

Acceptance

If the normal and necessary grieving process runs its course, the patient enters the acceptance stage. Acceptance is the goal of grieving. Some people believe that being resigned to their fate is the same as accepting it, but resignation and acceptance are two different reactions, products of different psychological progressions. The person who is resigned to his or her fate may say: "I miss what I have lost, but there is nothing I can do about it so I'll just have to put up with it." Resignation is more of a result of suppression and repression than a product of the grief response. Accepting people accept their losses as neither good nor bad but just the way things are. They have placed the loss in a larger framework and are emotionally removed from it.

The accepting stage may be partial or complete. Partial acceptance occurs when the patient accepts only one or more dimensions of the loss. He or she may accept a paralyzed arm but remain unaccepting of aphasia. The terminally ill patient may accept death but remain plagued by negative thoughts about leaving dependent children. During early stages of acceptance, the patient may move back and forth between it and previous stages.

Just because a stroke survivor accepts his or her limitations does not mean that he or she will not continue to work in rehabilitation. The patient can accept the nature of the losses while remaining motivated to improve. The stroke survivor will continue to have the motivation to improve in those areas in which gains can still be expected. In fact, the accepting patient may be even more motivated and efficient at therapies than the patient who was bargaining, because the accepting patient can realistically assess the situation. He or she does not cling to unrealistic goals.

You and other family members and friends ultimately also can reach a stage of acceptance of your losses. You will learn to accept the permanent changes the stroke has wrought. The separation you feel from your loved one because of the communication disorder(s) will continue, but you will accept it. You will also accept the negative changes in lifestyle caused by your loved one's disabilities. By progressing through the stages of the grieving process, you can reach a state of acceptance of the unwanted changes you have experienced.

Helping the Grieving Process

Along the road to acceptance, things can be said and done either to help or interrupt the grieving process. No one likes to see their loved ones suffer, either physically or psychologically. Watching a stroke survivor try to overcome a permanent and irreversible loss is one of the most difficult things you can witness. It can be distressing to watch the patient engage in denial, anger, and bargaining over losses that are inevitable. Seeing your loved one in the grip of grieving depression can also cause you to want to do things to immediately ease the suffering. Although you can do nothing to change the reality of the losses your loved one has experienced, you can follow certain principles that will help the patient reach acceptance about what has happened. You can smooth the road to acceptance.

Allow Control

The psychological pain an individual experiences during the grieving process is partially due to his or her inability to alter the course of unwanted events. Frustration can be traced to the many unwanted alterations in the patient's life. But the feelings of helplessness that overwhelm the grieving patient can be reduced by allowing him or her to control certain aspects of his or her life. You and other family members and friends can easily find ways to allow the stroke survivor control, such as when and what to eat or when to go or not to go somewhere. Many decisions that are often made for the patient can be made by the patient instead, providing much needed control.

Provide Perspective

At times the stroke survivor may think there will be no end to the emotional pain he or she is feeling. The patient may feel caught up in a vicious cycle of loss and grief, especially during the awareness stage. Having a realistic perspective regarding the eventual acceptance of losses and the reduction of sorrow that will be found in the acceptance stage can be of immense help to the griever. Patients gain perspective when they discover more about the situation or events causing the suffering. Parents often provide perspective during adolescent crises by suggesting that "It is not the end of the world; you won't remember it in a month or so." You and other family members and friends should try to express to the patient that the grief and suffering *will* end. Explaining some of the psychological reactions described in this book will help the patient gain a larger, more constructive perspective.

Acknowledge the Losses

It is natural for people to avoid discussion of the losses with the griever. Although you may feel that you are helping the patient by not discussing or acknowledging the losses that have occurred, actually, this deprives the stroke survivor of the opportunity to express his or her grief. It is often helpful to the stroke survivor to have caring family members or friends serve as a sounding board. A stroke survivor, because of a communication disorder(s), will often have difficulty communicating his or her emotions, but this does not mean that he or she does not need to express them. You should encourage any type of constructive emotional expression by the grieving patient.

Do not feel rejected if the patient chooses not to discuss the losses and his or her feelings with you. Sometimes, because of emotional attachments and the roles played by family members, the individual may choose not to discuss or acknowledge the losses with close family members. He or she may feel more at ease displaying emotions with friends, acquaintances, or even strangers. Your loved one strives to maintain previously established roles with you and other family members and, of course, his or her decision should be honored.

Listen Quietly

When you are confronted with a grieving loved one's strong emotions, you may feel a need to explain, defend, or rationalize the losses. This is not necessarily disruptive to the grieving process. The stroke survivor may ask for suggestions and advice on how to deal with the situation. When the patient communicates his or her concerns and feelings about the losses, however, it is not always necessary to respond. Venting feelings and expressing thoughts are therapeutic in themselves, and just having someone listen is important. Remember, no one can remove the losses and the pain associated with them with a word or phrase. However well intentioned, these remarks may devalue the patient's thoughts and feelings.

Avoid Rewarding Denial

Rewarding denial can interrupt the course of grieving. Although denial is a natural defense, it should not be maintained for a long time. It is not to the patient's advantage for you to state or reinforce untruthful remarks. You should be open, honest, and tactful. Avoid both rewarding denial and brutally confronting the patient with the reality of the losses. When attempting to avoid rewarding denial, it is important not to overreact. Try to leave the patient with some degree of hope, which is an essential ingredient to recovery and maintenance of mental health.

Do Not Punish Anger

Anger is a natural and predictable consequence of loss. Expressions of anger by the patient should not be punished unless these expressions are destructive to the patient or to others. Anger that is nondestructive should be tolerated, understood, and, in some cases, encouraged. Rejection in the anger stage can result in chronic anger or in anger becoming directed inward. Stroke survivors with communication disorders are prone to inner direction of anger because the lack of speech and/or language may prevent socially acceptable ways of expressing it. Anger can be punished overtly or covertly. You can sometimes punish the patient's anger by avoiding him or her. Unintentional punishment may also occur when you require unrealistic tasks or express your disapproval with body or facial gestures.

Anger should be punished only if it becomes destructive. Try instead to redirect the anger. Provide the patient with objects that he or she can use to vent the anger harmlessly, or find another method by which the patient can express it. When anger is expressed inappropriately, it is important to let the patient know that although the anger itself is acceptable, the destructive expressions of it are not.

Avoid Bargaining

As already mentioned, providing hope is essential in helping patients reach acceptance. Stroke survivors must be able to perceive that progress is possible or they will lack the motivation to attempt recovery. However, providing false hope can result in a fixation in the bargaining stage of grief. Suggesting the possibility of total recovery when it is unrealistic is not recommended. Although bargaining can be temporarily advantageous to the patient, long-term bargaining will delay the patient's eventual acceptance and adjustment.

Do Not Provide Secondary Gains

The grieving stroke survivor may receive attention, sympathy, and frequent contact with others that he or she might not ordinarily obtain. This emotional support is important to progressing through the stages of grief and should not be discouraged. However, if the attention, sympathy, and frequent contact satisfy other psychological and emotional needs of the griever, they may interrupt the process of reaching acceptance. Satisfying these secondary needs can be seen as a form of dependence. For example, if a patient gets more attention from relatives because of a loss, and if this attention meets other psychological and emotional needs, he or she might resist moving through the stages of grief. The patient may have trouble giving up the role of griever because of the secondary gains.

Avoid Early Distractions

Distractions that occur early after the loss(es) may interrupt the grieving process. These early distractions allow the patient to avoid confronting the loss(es). Sometimes family and friends suggest that the patient become immersed in a hobby or work to "take his or her mind off the loss." During later stages of the grieving process, this may be helpful. However, overindulgence in such activities may be counterproductive to the eventual acceptance of the loss(es). The patient needs to take the time to become aware of them and of his or her reactions. The patient should be permitted the privacy necessary to adjust to the new facts and circumstances.

Provide Companionship During Depression

Depression is a natural reaction for the patient when he or she becomes aware of the loss(es). Many mental health experts believe that depression is a stage the patient must experience to gain ultimate acceptance of what has happened. This may be the first time during the grieving process that the patient is totally aware of his or her situation. Although it is natural for you to want to cheer up the patient, avoid superficial statements or acts that the patient might consider a devaluation of the pain he or she is experiencing. Just sitting silently with the patient can help reduce the patient's depression and feelings of loneliness by showing your concern for him or her.

The question may arise whether you should ask the patient's doctor for a prescription for an antidepressant medication to help combat the grieving depression. Antidepressants can help patients deal with the pain of the loss(es). The use of antidepressants to combat depression is a controversial subject, with good arguments on both sides. On the one hand, these medications are effective and have few side effects. Especially for patients with severe strokes and major communication disorders who are confined to nursing homes, it seems humane to provide them with medications to improve their emotional state. On the other hand, patients can only move naturally through the stages of grief if they are aware of what has happened and feel the sense of loss. Some medications may only postpone the process; they do not eliminate the grief. There are no easy answers to this dilemma. The patient's doctor is the first person you should contact about grieving depression. He or she will consider the patient's level and duration of depression and whether the antidepressant is necessary and medically advisable. You should also discuss the issue with the patient if his or her communication abilities allow it.

Loss is a natural and predictable consequence of living and so is the grief response. For the stroke survivor, these losses can include separation from loved ones, loss of self, and an inability to use and enjoy valued objects. Aware patients who do not have medical conditions that mask the response can be expected to pass through the stages of grief to ultimately reach acceptance. Along the road to acceptance, there are several things you and other family members can do to help your loved ones through the process. You, too, can expect gradually to learn to accept the changes that have taken place in your life, and this process may require you to experience the various stages of grief as well.

CHAPTER 11

Speech and Language Rehabilitation

When one is helping another, both are strong.—GERMAN PROVERB

Re-ha-bil-i-ta-tion (*re'ha-bil-i-ta-shun*): The Therapeutic Restoration of Abilities to Optimal Levels Following an Injury

It is natural to feel shocked and overwhelmed at first when a loved one has a stroke. Doctors, hospitals, X-rays, magnetic resonance imaging (MRIs), computed tomography (CT) scans, therapists, nurses, billing offices, waiting rooms, consent forms, and hundreds of other new experiences bombard your life. At times it feels as though everything is happening so fast that you have little time to think. After a while, as things settle down, you may start to wonder about the details of how rehabilitation works. It is natural to have questions about the who, what, why, how, and when of rehabilitation.

One of the first questions many family members and friends have about rehabilitation has to do with the very nature of brain damage: "If destroyed brain cells can never be returned to life, how is it that my loved one can be expected to recover some or all of the things taken by the stroke?" True, with our current medical knowledge, once a part of the brain has died, it can never be brought back to life. When one brain cell or millions of them have been deprived of oxygen for a sufficient time because of a stroke, they die and their death is permanent. Nothing known to medicine can bring dead brain cells back to life. But this does not necessarily mean that a body function, such as the ability to communicate, cannot be improved or even completely restored. Recovery of function happens all of the time, and this capability is the basis of speech and language rehabilitation. Although the death of brain cells is irreversible, partial or complete return of function is possible.

Self-Healing

If your loved one just had a stroke and is in the early stages of the rehabilitation program, you will be happy to know that his or her communication abilities are likely to improve on their own. Each day after the stroke has stopped evolving, your loved one is likely to get better. Some of the return of the patient's speech and language has nothing to do with the drills, exercises, teaching, behavior modification, and counseling provided by a speech-language pathologist. This unprompted improvement is called *spontaneous recovery,* which means that some recovery of a patient's communication occurs automatically rather than as a result of any medical intervention. Spontaneous recovery occurs in most stroke survivors, and that is why many patients automatically and without the benefit of therapy make some improvement in their speech and language.

Spontaneous recovery occurs for several reasons. Sometimes when a stroke occurs, there is a buildup of pressure in the brain. This pressure reduces the efficiency with which some parts of the brain do their jobs. Over time, the pressure subsides and those parts of the brain begin to function again automatically. Another reason for some automatic return of speech and language is that some brain cells are not destroyed; they are just "stunned." Eventually, the stunned brain cells return to normal functioning, as does some of the ability to communicate. Return of blood flow to the areas deprived of blood because of the stroke also can occur, and this, too, results in spontaneous recovery of speech and language. There are other reasons why spontaneous recovery occurs, but the fact remains that the brain, like other parts of the body, tends to heal itself. In the process of self-healing, many stroke survivors experience a return of some speech and language abilities. It is important to remember that spontaneous recovery does not necessarily mean the complete return of speech and language abilities. Although some communication abilities may return on their own, usually there is not a total spontaneous recovery of the ability to communicate.

Although spontaneous recovery is a blessing for stroke survivors and their loved ones, it is a curse for scientists because it makes research into which therapies can help patients much more difficult. It complicates efforts to determine scientifically which speech and language therapies are valuable because researchers can't be sure whether improvement seen in a group of patients is only the result of spontaneous recovery or due to therapy. Certainly, the blessing is much greater than the curse, but the problem of knowing which therapies are most helpful to a group of patients is a complicated matter. In fact, in the past some authorities believed that all recovery seen in stroke-related communication disorders was only the result of spontaneous recovery and not a direct result of therapy. The clear-cut value of therapy will be discussed later.

Competent Clinicians

The professionals who provide speech and language therapy to stroke survivors must meet rigorous standards established by the American Speech-Language-Hearing Association (ASHA). ASHA is a nonprofit organization that was founded in 1925. It has approximately 100,000 members and certificate holders. One of the main purposes of ASHA is to encourage the scientific study of the process of human communication. The organization also advocates for the rights and interests of persons with communication disorders.

ASHA sponsors national conferences, institutes, and workshops each year as part of its continuing professional education program. One of its main functions is to conduct an annual convention at which scientific reports, exhibits, short courses, and other educational and professional programs are offered. This convention is well attended by members of the profession. ASHA also publishes scientific journals to advance theories and research and to help members remain current in their diagnostic and therapeutic skills.

Certificates of Clinical Competence

ASHA provides practitioners with two certificates of clinical competence. A person can become certified in speech-language pathology and/or audiology. Although these two specialties are separate entities, they overlap. Because of the close relationship between speech and hearing, training in speech-language pathology also involves learning about audiology, and vice versa.

Currently, the highest level of education necessary to practice speech-language pathology is the master's degree, and applicants for either certificate must hold at least that level of education. ASHA also regulates the extent and nature of the training provided at institutions of higher education. All candidates must take a predetermined number and type of courses. Students take specific courses that address the different types of disorders they will treat and also general ones in psychology, education, health sciences, or related areas. In addition, the candidate must complete a minimum number of supervised clinical observations and practicum experiences. Practicum hours are obtained in specific areas and with different types of patients, all under the careful supervision of certified speech-language pathologists.

After completion of academic training and supervised practicum, the candidate for certification in either speech-language pathology or audiology must complete a clinical fellowship. This involves gainful employment, but with supervision provided by an already certified individual during the first 9–12 months of clinical practice. This activity is also regulated by ASHA. Before the certificate of clinical competence is granted, the candidate must also pass a nationally administered comprehensive examination. Beyond these extensive ASHA requirements, states also have licensing requirements for speech-language pathologists and audiologists.

All certified ASHA members must abide by an extensive code of ethics that details what is considered appropriate behavior by practicing clinicians and what is considered unethical. Its goal is to ensure that all speech and hearing disabled persons are treated competently, that every resource is used to help them, and that no one is subject to discrimination. The code of ethics specifically says that ASHA members must not provide services when reasonable gains cannot be expected to result from them. This specifically means that therapy cannot be provided to a patient when it is evident that it will not help. Although a reasonable prognosis can be given, speech-language pathologists cannot guarantee the results of their services.

The Value of Therapy

The value of speech and language therapy for patients with aphasia, apraxia of speech, and the dysarthrias has been studied for decades. This research has been in three general areas and has attempted to answer three research questions scientifically. First, does speech and language therapy cause more improvement in communication abilities than what can be expected due to spontaneous recovery alone? Second, do all patients benefit equally, or are there groups of patients with particular categories of disorders that improve more than others or do not improve at all because of treatment? Third, are specific types of therapies more beneficial than others in improving communication?

The first question, Does speech and language therapy cause more improvement in communication abilities than what can be expected due to spontaneous recovery alone? has been extensively researched. To answer this question, large groups of subjects have been tested, and information has also been obtained from patients and their families. The results are clear—these therapies do indeed help the majority of patients. In several large studies, researchers measured the gains in communication abilities within groups of patients who received speech and language therapy against the results attained by those in groups who did not receive therapy. The majority of these studies clearly support the value of therapy. They show that patients who receive therapy gain more and recover in broader dimensions than those who do not receive therapy. As a rule, the earlier therapy begins and the more frequently it is provided, the greater the gains.

Although self-reports from stroke survivors are subjective, they also indicate that therapy is beneficial. Most patients who have undergone therapy, and who have the communication abilities to answer questions about it, have said it helped them. These patients report that they benefited most in the psychological and emotional areas. Therapy helped their morale and general attitude about the disability. Surveys of stroke survivors' family members also support the value of speech and language therapy and indicate they believe the therapy helped their loved ones.

Researchers have also answered the second question, Do all patients benefit equally, or are there groups of patients with particular categories of disorders that improve more than others or do not improve at all because of treatment? Research conducted to date has found that severely involved patients, sometimes called *global aphasics,* are not as likely, *as a group,* to benefit from therapy. It is important to remember, however, that individuals within that group may still benefit from assistance and deserve the opportunity for a trial therapy. A patient should be considered severely involved or globally aphasic only after a relatively long time has passed since the onset of the stroke. Only patients who are neurologically stable should be put into the "severely involved" or "global" categories.

The third question, Are specific types of therapies more beneficial than others in improving communication? is an ongoing research question because new therapies and new variations of old ones are constantly being created and investigated. This ongoing research has also produced clear results. Certain types of therapies are helpful for specific types of disorders. For example, using a mirror for feedback purposes may help patients with dysarthria, while the use of a mirror does not necessarily help people with apraxia of speech. Studies have shown that swallowing therapy greatly decreases the risks of aspiration pneumonia and also is cost-effective. It costs less to give swallowing therapy and is better patient care for individuals who need it than to wait until they get aspiration pneumonia to treat them. In the category of aphasia, some patients benefit from being extensively stimulated. The more they are encouraged to communicate, the better they will do in therapy.

In summary, the value of speech and language therapy for stroke survivors has been studied extensively. The research is conclusive that specific types of speech and language therapy help most stroke patients improve their communication abilities, and the gains are greater than those due to spontaneous recovery alone. Stroke survivors make more improvement and improve in broader dimensions when they receive speech and language therapy. Another benefit of therapy is the emotional support it provides stroke survivors; therapy helps them approach the communication disorders in a positive and constructive manner and helps them with the adjustments they must make to the disability. The only exception is the category of global or severe aphasia. These patients, as a group, do not seem to benefit from therapy, although some individuals within this group have been known to make gains. There are exceptions to every rule.

Evaluating Communication Disorders in the Stroke Patient

When a person has a stroke and is taken to a hospital, several brain scans may be given. Some of them are done routinely and others are given only in special circumstances. The purpose of these tests is to help identify the type of stroke, where it is located within the brain, and the extent of the injury.

The ability to use machines to look inside the skull and examine the brain has advanced by leaps and bounds. A few decades ago, the only way to see what damage a stroke had caused was to use X-ray machines similar to the ones used to get a picture of a broken bone. Because these types of X-rays are not very precise, a neurologist—a physician specializing in the diagnosis and treatment of nervous system disorders—was often relied on to find out the specifics about the stroke. Nowadays, there are two machines that help neurologists and other physicians do their jobs with more precision and accuracy: CT and MRI scans.

One way to view the brain is by a CT scan. Another way of evaluating the nature and extent of a stroke is through MRI. There are also other ways to see inside a person's brain without surgery, but CT and MRI scans are the most commonly used. They are conducted by a physician called a radiologist, who specializes in the use of X-rays and other ways of scanning and getting an image of the inside of the body.

Another medical specialist who conducts extensive tests on a stroke patient is a physiatrist. This person is a specialist in physical medicine and rehabilitation and is often called on to determine, among other things, the stroke survivor's rehabilitation potential. A physiatrist is trained to make a judgment about how well the stroke survivor will do in a rehabilitation program and what therapies are warranted.

The primary or attending physician is the person who is formally and legally responsible for the patient's care throughout the stay in a medical care facility. This individual is often the stroke survivor's family physician and the doctor with whom you usually will have the most contact. He or she often orders tests and other procedures as part of the stroke patient's medical management, as well as makes referrals to other health care professionals.

As family members or friends of the stroke survivor, you need to understand the process of evaluating stroke-related communication disorders. Understanding is important if only for one reason—so that you will be able to ask the "right" questions about your loved one's speech and language abilities. Knowing the patient's communication strengths and weakness and acting appropriately around him or her require that you understand as much as possible about the evaluation process. In general, there are three reasons for testing and evaluating a stroke survivor's communication abilities.

1. Not all strokes cause communication disorders, so it is necessary to find out whether the patient's communication abilities have been compromised. Simply reading the results of the CT or MRI scan can give a good indication of whether a communication disorder will be present, although sometimes it takes time for the true extent of a stroke to show up. Occasionally, the patient's family and friends will believe that no communication disorder exists, when in reality the patient has one or more of the big three disorders. This is especially true of aphasia. Some stroke-related communication disorders, such as receptive or understanding deficits, surface only when the patient is pushed to answer complicated or detailed questions. For example, some people might assume that a patient understood what was said because he or she nodded correctly or remained silent when a statement was made. An aphasic patient can appear to understand what was spoken when, in fact, the information was not completely understood. With some stroke survivors, only through detailed testing can a communication disorder be discovered or ruled out.

2. Evaluation allows health care providers to profile gains made in the stroke survivor's communication abilities by comparing the initial evaluation, which is sometimes called the *basal*, with subsequent ones. Periodic evaluation of the patient's progress provides valuable information about which therapies are helping the recovery process and which ones should be stopped. Only through reevaluation can the clinician detect when the patient has made maximum gains and when to end therapy. As discussed later, these reevaluations need not be as formal or detailed as the initial one.

3. Evaluation provides valuable therapeutic information by categorizing the types of disorders so that they can be treated appropriately. After testing the patient's communication abilities, the clinician can use the information gained to design a program that will maximize the stroke survivor's strengths and minimize his or her weaknesses. One of the main principles of therapy is to use the stroke survivor's communication strengths to help improve his or her weakness. Only through periodic testing can these strengths and weaknesses be identified.

Recent studies on the communication disorders seen in stroke patients have shown that they change in nature and severity over time. This is particularly true of aphasia. It is not uncommon for a stroke patient's abilities to communicate to change dramatically. This change can occur not only in how well he or she speaks, writes, reads, and understands the speech of others but also in the very type of disorder. Over time, a patient may change from one diagnosis to another. This is partially caused by spontaneous recovery but also because of the therapy being provided. Because of the changing nature of communication disorders, it is necessary to discuss diagnostic categories and labels.

Categories and Labels

Health care professionals use medical terminology to facilitate communication between themselves and because the words usually have clear and precise meanings to medical professionals. These medical words are often Latin or Greek in origin or are based on the names of researchers, and they are not always easily understandable to people outside the health care professions. Sometimes, professionals forget that not everyone is familiar with medical terminology. They may say to family members and friends that a stroke survivor has "transcortical motor aphasia," "ataxic dysarthria," or "dyslexia with dysgraphia." The stroke patient's family and friends are often intimidated and confused when these words are used and not defined, and it is certainly true that meaningful communication does not take place. When you do not understand the technical and medical words being used, ask the health care professional to define them or, better yet, to describe your loved one's strengths and weaknesses. Communicating clearly is a simple courtesy on the part of the professional, and it is not unreasonable for you to request it.

Health care professionals should avoid labels when describing your loved one's communication disorders because they tend to pigeonhole patients unnecessarily. Because of the wide variety of stroke-related communication disorders and the vast number of symptoms, labels are often not an accurate description of a particular patient's abilities. Telling you what a patient can or cannot do, and describing rather than labeling these disorders, may take a little longer, but it provides you with a better understanding of what is happening. Compare the quality of information provided in the following two examples.

Example 1

The patient is a male who suffered a hemorrhagic stroke. The results of the speech and language evaluation indicate mild spastic dysarthria, moderately severe Broca's aphasia with agraphia, dyslexia, and homonymous hemianopsia.

Example 1 gives health care professionals valuable information about the patient and may be appropriate for a medical report because physicians and other professionals know what the words mean. However, even for specialists, labels tend to be too general and do not provide details about a specific patient. In the above example, the labels could have referred to many patients with a wide variety of communication strengths and weaknesses.

Example 2 refers to the same patient. His communication abilities are operationally defined and described in this example. Although some labeling is always necessary when discussing a patient, it can be reduced.

Example 2

The patient is a male who suffered a rupture of one of the main arteries leading to the speech and language centers of the brain. He slurs some pressure consonants, especially p and b, and has difficulty moving his tongue fast enough to produce speech normally. The area that controls planning and sequencing speech was damaged, and, as a result, the patient has difficulty getting his tongue to do what he wants except for some automatic utterances. He also has problems remembering words when trying to express himself. For example, when asked to describe a picture, he expressed himself in only 2-word utterances. The patient's writing is also impaired. Although he can copy letters and write his name, he could write only 2 of 10 words correctly when they were dictated to him. Primarily because he has vision deficits in the right sides of both eyes, he cannot read a paragraph and answer questions about it. However, he can read the names of 10 of 12 nouns in large print when he turns his head to the side to adjust for the vision problems.

Although it certainly takes more time and words to describe in lay terms what a patient can and cannot do, this practice ultimately provides more information and improves communication between specialists and the stroke survivor's family members and friends. The important thing for you to remember is to not settle for medico-jargon when health care professionals discuss your loved one's communication abilities with you. Simply ask them to define the terms or describe what your loved one can and cannot do rather than to give labels. It is never inappropriate to ask for clarification when you do not understand the specialist's words. You always have the right to ask for explanations in terms you can understand.

Formal Speech and Language Testing

There are many tests available to assess a stroke survivor's communication ability. Some tests are more comprehensive than others and many are geared to specific types of disorders. A speech and language clinician may choose to give one test or to use sections from several tests to get a profile of the patient's communication abilities. Some clinicians do not use formal tests because they prefer to assess a patient's communication abilities using their own battery of questions and exercises. What follows is a review of the kinds of information that may be obtained for each of the big three stroke-related communication disorders.

Testing for Dysarthria

When testing for dysarthria, the clinician is assessing the effects of muscle paralysis or weakness on the patient's ability to speak. The goal is to decide how much the muscle paralysis or weakness has affected the patient's physical ability to make sounds, syllables, words, and phrases. The results of the test provide specific information about how well the patient's speech can be understood and give detailed information about which part of the speech production mechanism is impaired. Generally, these tests evaluate the following parts of the speech production mechanism.

1. **Breathing for Speech Purposes.** Because people talk on compressed air coming from the lungs, the patient's breathing strength and coordination are evaluated. It is also important to decide whether the stroke has impaired the ability to let the air out of the lungs gradually and smoothly during speech.
2. **Voice.** If the stroke affected the patient's voice box, the dysarthria evaluation discovers whether the vocal cords can vibrate. If vibration is present, an assessment of the patient's voice quality is made. Does the patient now talk with a harsh, hoarse, or breathy voice quality? Is speech produced loudly enough? Has the stroke affected the patient's pitch range?
3. **Articulation.** This aspect of the evaluation looks at how well the tongue and lips are able to move and shape the air coming from the lungs. Some of the questions that testing will answer include: "Does the tongue go to one side of the mouth when it is protruding?" "Can the tongue, and particularly its tip, move to the top of the mouth during speech?" and "How fast can the tongue move during speech?" The clinician also assesses the specific sounds produced in error and the types of mistakes that are made. (This is discussed in more detail later.)
4. **Nasality.** Sometimes a stroke can affect the soft palate's ability to close off the nasal chambers during speech. When patients have problems moving the soft palate, they may sound too nasal. During this aspect of the evaluation, the clinician looks to see if the soft palate lifts or elevates when the patient says, "Ah." Occasionally, the soft palate lifts when the "ah" is said, but it moves slowly or sluggishly during speech.
5. **Rate and Rhythm of Speech.** Because of paralysis or weakness of the speech mechanism, some patients talk too slowly. Some types of dysarthria also cause speech to be too fast or cause bursts of rapid speech. Besides assessing the patient's rate of speech, the dysarthria evaluation also looks at the stroke survivor's use of emphasis, pauses, and inflections.

At the conclusion of the dysarthria evaluation, the speech-language pathologist knows the extent of the effects of muscle paralysis or weakness on the patient's physical ability to produce sounds, syllables, words, and phrases. Beyond knowing what aspects of the speech production mechanism are impaired, such as breathing, voice, and articulation, the clinician will have a list of sounds produced in error and be able to determine how well the patient can be understood.

Testing for Apraxia of Speech

Apraxia of speech impairs the stroke survivor's ability to perform complex or skilled speech acts. The problem is not that the muscles used for speech or the nerves attached to them are weak or paralyzed. Apraxia of speech is a programming deficit in which patients have problems getting their mouths to do what they want during speech. In some mild cases of apraxia of speech, the disorder goes away spontaneously a few days after the stroke.

When testing for apraxia of speech, the speech-language pathologist's objectives are to find out whether the disorder exists and if so, to what extent, and to gather information on how to provide therapy to combat it. There are several formal tests for apraxia of speech, most of which look at how well a patient can repeat what has been spoken or read progressively longer words. Although there are other aspects to the evaluation of apraxia of speech, having the patient repeat sounds, syllables, words, and phrases is useful.

Many clinicians also distinguish between oral apraxia and apraxia of speech during this evaluation. Like apraxia of speech, oral apraxia involves purposeful and voluntary actions of the muscles of speech, but only during nonspeech activities. During the evaluation for oral apraxia, the clinician looks at how well the patient can move his or her speech structures during activities such as licking the lips, puckering, protruding the tongue, and so on.

At the conclusion of testing for apraxia of speech, the speech-language pathologist will know whether and how severely the stroke has impaired the patient's ability to purposefully program and sequence speech movements. The clinician also has information about the patient's programming and sequencing abilities for nonspeech acts. As you will learn in the therapy section, the patient's ability to program nonspeech movements can sometimes be used to help stroke survivors relearn how to program speech acts.

Testing for Aphasia

Of the big three communication disorders, aphasia is the most complicated and time consuming to evaluate because it can disrupt all avenues of communication: reading, writing, speaking, gesturing, and understanding the speech of others. Each avenue of communication must be evaluated separately and placed in a framework that reflects the totality of the individual's language disorder. When testing for aphasia, both the way the information is presented to the patient (spoken or written) and the patient's output (gesture, writing, or speech) are considered in the scoring. Some tests simply record the patient's performance as correct or incorrect, while others have more complicated scoring systems.

The test or tests chosen by the clinician also reflect his or her philosophy of treatment. As with the tests for dysarthria and apraxia of speech, some clinicians administer only one test of aphasia, while others use their own battery of questions, exercises, and subtests. The aphasia evaluation is usually divided into receptive and expressive subtests. Receptive evaluations address reading and understanding the speech of others, while tests of expressive language are concerned with writing and speaking. The use and understanding of gestures are also assessed. Although aphasia tests vary considerably, most of them assess the following avenues of communication.

1. **Reading.** The reading subtests of the aphasia evaluation assess how well the patient can read both silently and aloud. Some patients have problems understanding single letters and words. Finding out how well a patient can match written words to pictures or objects is an important part of this subtest. Reading evaluation also may involve the patient's comprehension of sentences, paragraphs, and pages of information.

2. **Understanding the Speech of Others.** Questions answered in this section of the evaluation include, "How well does the stroke survivor understand spoken words?" "Does the patient follow short, simple verbal requests?" "How well does the stroke survivor understand complex questions and statements?" The tests for finding out the nature and severity of understanding problems involve asking questions that range from the simple and noncomplex to the complex and detailed. During spontaneous recovery, some patients who have problems understanding the speech of others improve rapidly. This is especially true of patients who have only mild difficulty understanding the speech of others.

3. **Writing.** The subtests that look at writing problems consider a wide range of deficits. Some aphasic persons with writing problems cannot copy geometric forms such as squares, triangles, and circles. Other patients have problems spelling and writing words and short sentences. Higher level types of writing problems usually are apparent when the patient cannot write when the examiner dictates the words. It is important to remember that these types of writing problems are not the result of hand or finger weakness or the awkwardness of using the nondominant hand. They are problems with expressing thoughts through written language and with recognizing and reproducing symbols.

4. Speaking. The subtests that evaluate a patient's speaking problems look at how well he or she can say progressively longer utterances, repeat what has been spoken, define words, and describe pictures. Determinations are made about how fluent the speech of the patient is and how aware he or she is of errors. Types of naming errors are evaluated, such as using words with associated meanings, using words that rhyme with correct words, and making random mistakes. The grammatical correctness of the expressions is also evaluated. One of the main questions asked during this aspect of the evaluation is, "Does the patient talk in 'telegraphic speech?'"

Many clinicians also look at how well the patient functions in real-life situations. Either by observing the patient or giving a questionnaire, a determination is made about the person's actual use of language in day-to-day situations. Role playing can also be used to assess a patient's communicative abilities in typical daily living activities.

Testing for Swallowing Problems

Some patients with one or more of the big three communication disorders also have problems chewing and/or swallowing their food. Many of the speech muscles are also the ones used for eating, although it is possible for a patient with a chewing and/or swallowing problem not to have speech difficulty.

Swallowing problems are usually checked out in a "bedside" evaluation and also by a special kind of X-ray. The bedside evaluation looks at several types of problems that are usually indicative of a swallowing disorder, such as the presence of dysarthria, lack of a gag reflex, difficulty moving the tongue, or vocal cord paralysis or weakness. The X-ray is called a video swallowing study, sometimes called a *modified barium swallow*, and it presents a moving picture of the patient's chewing and swallowing. The speech-language pathologist is usually present during this X-ray to observe where the problem occurs, for example, in the mouth, back of the throat, or at the level of the voice box, to decide which therapies are helpful.

Additional Evaluation Information

No speech and language evaluation would be complete without noting the patient's pertinent medical status and getting information about medications he or she is taking. It is important to get as much information about the patient's personality characteristics, medical history, and social situation as possible. One of the most crucial determinations to make is whether the patient is depressed, anxious, or has other psychological problems due to the stroke. The presence of any of the complications discussed in Chapter 4 should also be noted. Of particular significance is the presence of exaggerated emotions, panic attacks, difficulty shifting thoughts, and perceptual problems. For the patient who speaks more than one language, it is necessary to know the first language, which language is spoken in the home, and the language preferred by the stroke survivor.

Although a formal speech and language evaluation is usually conducted before therapy is provided, remember that the evaluation process is ongoing. The health care team must regularly evaluate the patient's abilities and deficits so that adjustments can be made in therapy. Most stroke survivors improve and change during the recovery process, making periodic reevaluations necessary to monitor these changes. These reevaluations need not always be as formal or detailed as the initial one, but ongoing assessment of the patient's communication strengths and weaknesses is important. The team must also note other changes that may occur during therapy, such as changes in medications and alterations in psychological, medical, social, and family situations. Reevaluations are necessary to decide when therapy is no longer warranted because the patient has achieved his or her potential.

Philosophy of Treatment

The primary goal of speech and language rehabilitation is to help the stroke survivor regain as much of the ability to communicate as possible. Always remember that research conclusions about the factors affecting recovery often apply to large groups of patients, but there will always be individual exceptions. In addition, some factors are supported by a large body of research, while others have been identified only through clinical observations or studies conducted with a small number of subjects. Although the factors contributing to a stroke survivor's maximum recovery are probably variables that apply to most patients, they are not absolute rules. When reading about these variables, you should remember that they relate only to patients when all other things are equal. When one or more of these variables (and many others not listed here) are combined, the recovery equation changes. Following is a list of the many factors affecting recovery that have been reported in books, journals, or scientific conventions.

1. **Extent of Brain Injury.** In general, patients with larger areas of brain injury are less likely to make good gains than those with small amounts of brain damage.
2. **Location of the Brain Injury.** Patients who have damage to specific areas in the speech and language centers (and the tracts leading to and from them) tend to have more difficulty than those whose stroke affected adjacent areas.
3. **Type of Stroke.** Patients who have a ruptured blood vessel generally recover less than those who have the plug type of stroke.

4. Age of the Patient. Patients who are extremely advanced in age are less likely to do well in rehabilitation than younger stroke survivors.

5. Complication. Certain complications such as extremely high levels of anxiety, difficulty shifting thoughts, panic attacks, perceptual disorders, and so forth interfere with speech and language rehabilitation potential.

6. Sick and Feeble. Patients who have many medical problems generally do not do as well as healthier patients.

Each patient's unique combination of level of motivation, family support, and learning style also must be considered in a treatment program. When it comes to any therapy, the patient's motivation to recover is a vital ingredient, and this is particularly true of speech and language therapy. After all, a therapist can only help patients to help themselves. A patient with a strong desire to overcome the disability works hard at therapy and will do better than one who is unmotivated.

Family members often ask, "Can motivation be created or increased in patients who have low levels of it?" This critical question has many implications for the patient, family members and friends, and for the entire rehabilitation process. Unfortunately, there is no clear answer. For some patients, rewards, encouragement, and support can be used to increase and encourage their desire to work hard at rehabilitation. For other patients, it seems nothing can be said or done that will increase their motivation. Some of the many reasons for this variability in motivation include the effects of the brain injury, medications, and the patient's personality type.

When attempting to improve patients' motivation, there are four important considerations. First, for motivation to increase, patients must believe that progress is likely. They must be aware that the work, energy, and time commitment will pay off. Second, patients must believe that their efforts in rehabilitation will result in meaningful and important gains. Third, patients must be provided with measurements of progress so that they can see the results of their labor. Finally, patients must have the encouragement and support of everyone close to them. Although it is unlikely that these considerations will cause a completely unmotivated patient to change into one who is highly motivated, they are necessary to maintain and strengthen a patient's willingness to participate in the rigors of rehabilitation.

The power of support from family and friends cannot be overstated. Support plays a direct and significant role in the patient's recovery of speech and language abilities. When the patient has regular contact with loved ones and communicates with them, therapy occurs. When the communication is appropriate, positive, and rewarding, the interaction with family members and friends provides the patient with valuable learning experiences. Regular contact with loved ones can also ward off or reduce depression, anxiety, and other psychological factors that hinder therapy.

Different learning styles should be considered in therapy. Not everyone is good at "book learning" and some intelligent and successful people have "street smarts" as opposed to "school smarts." Some people learn well on a one-to-one basis, while others learn better in groups. Some individuals respond better to teachers who are direct and matter-of-fact in the way they present information, and others learn best by an unstructured trial, error, and experimentation approach. Even the time of day set aside for therapy should be considered whenever possible. Some people do better and think more clearly in the mornings, while others are night owls. One stroke survivor may make more gains in long therapy sessions, while another may do better in short ones.

One final aspect in the philosophy of treatment must be discussed. It is perhaps the most important consideration—the patient's psychological frame of reference. Philosophers, psychologists, and educators recognize two frames of reference in people. The first is an *external frame of reference*. People who have a predominantly external frame of reference believe that much of the good and bad that happens in life is the result of external factors. They look to people and things outside themselves for the causes and effects of life events and experiences. They believe that mystical or spiritual forces, or that society, cause the events and experiences in their lives. These people tend to feel awash in events they cannot control. In contrast, a person with an *internal frame of reference* believes that, although external events influence life, much of what happens is self-directed. A person with an internal frame of reference chooses to accept responsibility for many life events and especially for how he or she reacts to them. Although most people have different frames of reference about different aspects of their lives and at different times in their lives, most people also fall into one group or the other. The stroke survivor's frame of reference should be considered, or at least acknowledged, and adjustments made when possible and necessary to facilitate recovery.

The Role of the Speech-Language Clinician

The speech-language pathologist provides several important services to help the stroke survivor make the maximum recovery gains possible. The type of communication disorder a particular patient has is important in determining the clinician's role. Some disorders require a lot of drills with individual one-to-one contact, while other speech and language pathologies require that the patient attend group therapy sessions and/or do daily homework assignments. The speech-language pathologist will provide the following services to most stroke survivors at some point in their rehabilitation programs.

   1. **Structured Program of Therapy.** The clinician provides a structured program of therapy that addresses the patient's specific speech and language

pathology. Based on the results of the initial speech and language evaluation, the patient's communication weaknesses are targeted for remediation, which is updated periodically by reevaluations. A gradual progression, a step-by-step sequence of drills, exercises, and learning objectives, is designed to move the patient from deficient performance to normal or near-normal abilities. The clinician makes judgments along the way to decide whether the patient has succeeded in achieving the goals set and if it is time to move on to the next level. The progression allows the patient to first achieve objectives that are prerequisites for later stages of therapy.

2. **Feedback about Progress.** The speech-language pathologist must quantify the patient's communication progress. For the stroke survivor to make maximum gains, he or she must know which activities are helpful and the extent of the communication improvement that is being made. This feedback is needed on a daily, weekly, and monthly basis. When the clinician provides objective measurements of the patient's gains in ability to communicate, the patient is given valuable reinforcement. Combined with the rewards that go along with the ability to communicate more effectively, this feedback provides needed encouragement for the patient to continue with the therapy activities. To maintain high levels of motivation to continue with therapy, stroke survivors need to know that they are improving and reaping the benefits of their efforts.

3. **Support, Rewards, and Encouragement.** Particularly for patients with severe communication disorders, the speech-language pathologist provides crucial encouragement and emotional support. Sometimes a patient may feel overwhelmed by all of the negative changes that have occurred. It is comforting to have regular contact with a person who sees other patients with similar disorders. When the clinician focuses on things that can be done to overcome or reduce the communication disorder(s), the stroke survivor feels that there is hope and a direction to recovery. This gives the stroke survivor a feeling of empowerment over the stroke and the disabilities caused by it.

4. **Family Counseling.** Communication disorders resulting from strokes affect not only the stroke survivor, but they also have a dramatic impact on family members and friends. Because family members and friends have frequent contact with the patient, they can also be important variables in the treatment program. Knowledgeable, caring, and proactive family members and friends can supplement and enhance speech and language therapies by providing stimulation, rewards, encouragement, and a positive and constructive approach to the disorder(s). Conversely, when family members do not understand the communication disorder(s) faced by a loved one, they can do and say things that are counterproductive to the goals of

therapy. Family counseling by the speech-language pathologist can help to ensure that family and friends are positive factors in the patient's recovery.

5. **Advocacy Services.** If the stroke only resulted in a mild communication disorder, most patients are able to advocate for themselves to see to it that their needs are met and that they are treated well by others. Unfortunately, because of severe communication disorders some patients cannot use the power of speech to advocate for themselves. This inability to communicate can result in fewer and less effective services and treatments than those that more able patients receive. This is particularly true of patients confined to nursing homes or other extended care facilities. Because the speech-language pathologist understands the nature of the patient's communication disorder(s), he or she can serve as an advocate for the stroke survivor, making sure that the patient is treated well and competently by the people caring for him or her.

6. **Referral.** The speech-language pathologist is responsible for ensuring that all of the services the patient needs are available. If the stroke survivor has medical, psychological, or social needs that are not being met, it is the clinician's responsibility to make appropriate referrals. These referrals can be made directly to the professionals or agencies involved, or they can be brought to the attention of the stroke survivor's physician and/or family.

In summary, as part of the health care team, the speech-language pathologist provides the stroke survivor with a structured program of therapy that specifically addresses the type and severity of the communication disorder. Feedback about the patient's progress combined with support and encouragement help keep the patient motivated and progressing. Family counseling helps to ensure that family members and friends are positive influences on the patient. In addition, the clinician may advocate for the patient when necessary to make certain that he or she is treated well and fairly. Appropriate referrals are also made when the stroke survivor needs the assistance of additional professionals or social agencies.

Therapy for the Dysarthrias

Because there is more than one type of dysarthria, there is more than one type of therapy. As a rule, there are specific treatments for flaccid or spastic speech muscles and therapies that can help muscles that move too fast or too slow or that are ill-coordinated. The speech clinician looks at the impaired area of the speech production system and provides appropriate therapies. One patient may need to work only on tongue movements, while another may need to work on breathing muscles and the voice box. Some patients may have to do drills to strengthen and improve the range of motion or to gain more coordination over the whole speech production system: breathing muscles, voice box, tongue and lips, and the soft palate. Some stroke survivors have two or more different types of dysarthria simultaneously that affect different aspects of the speech production system. Some types of dysarthria change over time, too. Therefore, different types of therapies must be provided, sometimes simultaneously, for different parts of the speech production system.

Because stroke survivors with dysarthria often make specific types of sound production errors, it is helpful to consider the way speech-language pathologists look at articulation disorders. Articulation errors are separated into the following types: distortions, omissions, and substitutions. A distortion is the substitution of a nonstandard sound for a standard one. The best example of a distortion is the presence of too much nasality. For example, the *p* sound typically is not produced with the nasal resonance created by the soft palate in a lowered position. And when an individual produces the *p* sound with the nasal feature present, he or she is said to produce it with distortion-nasal. When the patient produces a sound that the clinician cannot identify, the sound is considered a distortion. Sounds may be distorted in the initial, medial, or final positions of words.

Omission occurs when an individual does not produce a sound. For example, when *abbit* is uttered for the word *rabbit,* the individual has omitted the *r* sound in the initial position. Omissions also occur in the medial and final positions of words.

When some other recognizable sound is produced instead of the appropriate one, a substitution occurs. For example, an individual may substitute the *w* for the *r* in the initial position and create the word *wabbit* for *rabbit.* A *w* for an *r* in the medial position would result in the articulation of the word *cawot* for *carrot.* A substituted sound is not the same as a sound that is added to a word. An added sound is one articulated in a word in addition to all of the correctly produced sounds; it is neither a substitution nor a distortion. These added sounds often occur in apraxia of speech.

Although therapies must be adapted to specific patients, certain activities are useful in improving the speech of many stroke survivors with dysarthria. The following drills, exercises, and changes in the way a patient speaks often help dysarthric patients compensate for the specific type of weak, paralyzed, or ill-coordinated speech muscles they have.

1. **Slowing the Rate of Speech.** In most activities, the faster a person does something the less precise he or she is at doing it; hence the old adage, "Haste makes waste." The faster you try to wash dishes, mow the lawn, or paint a house, the less care and precision go into it. The same principle holds true for speaking. The faster a person talks, the less precisely each individual sound is made. When speaking becomes faster than about 600

words a minute, most people become unintelligible. For many stroke survivors, reducing the rate of speech helps them adjust for muscle weakness or paralysis of the speech system. Slowing the rate of speech helps the stroke survivor relearn how to produce each individual sound clearly and precisely. As the patient progresses in the rehabilitation program, he or she can begin to talk progressively faster once again.

2. **Exaggerating Individual Sounds.** Speech can often be improved significantly by exaggerating each individual sound. Although the patient may find it difficult to get into the habit of exaggerating each sound while talking, after a while it becomes second nature, and the more the patient exaggerates the sounds, the better speech becomes.

3. **Clearly Producing the Final Sounds of Words.** In normal speech, there is a tendency to produce the first sound of a word more clearly than the sounds that occur in the middle or at the end. When the stroke survivor with dysarthria is encouraged to produce the final sounds of a word as clearly as he or she does the other ones, speech improves, sometimes dramatically.

4. **Opening the Mouth More Widely.** A singer opens his or her mouth more widely to allow the voice to radiate more effectively. For a stroke survivor with dysarthria, it is also sometimes helpful to learn to open the mouth wider when speaking. This allows the patient to produce sounds more clearly and reduces the tendency to muffle speech. Opening the mouth more widely also helps the patient to remember to slow his or her speech and to exaggerate each sound.

5. **Speaking Louder.** Speech has to be of sufficient loudness to be understood. No matter how clearly or precisely the sounds are made, speech will fall on "deaf ears" if it is not loud enough. Sometimes just having the stroke survivor sit or stand with an erect posture helps increase loudness.

6. **Working on Specific Sounds.** For many dysarthric patients, the sounds made when the tongue reaches the top of the mouth are the most difficult to make. Particularly troublesome are those sounds produced at the top and front of the mouth, such as *t, th,* and *d.* As a result, the speech-language clinician may want the patient to do specific exercises to strengthen and improve the movement of the tongue. Most of the time, these exercises are speech drills, but sometimes nonspeech activities are used, such as trying to touch the nose with the tongue or sticking the tongue out as far as possible. However, it is usually best to give the patient speech exercises rather than nonspeech ones because speech exercises transfer more naturally to speaking situations.

7. **Setting Standards.** Sometimes just having the patient try harder to produce speech clearly will result in significant improvement. One way of do-

ing this is to set up a number system that reflects the patient's increased efforts. A scale of 1 to 10 works best. On this 1 to 10 continuum, the number 5 represents the normal, easy, effortless way people usually make their sounds. The number 1 is speech that cannot be understood and that is produced in a slurred, distorted manner. The number 10 represents per . . . fect . . . ly . . . ar . . . tic . . . u . . . la . . . ted . . . sp . . . ee . . . ch in which every sound is made with the absolute amount of precision that is humanly possible. Setting the goal of an 8 or 9 standard, and praising the stroke survivor for trying to reach it, results in higher levels of speech precision, as well as providing a way of measuring and rewarding improvement.

8. **Other Therapies.** The dysarthric patient's voice, respiratory support, nasalization, and rhythm of speech are other areas that may need improvement. The speech-language pathologist may have the stroke patient work on getting the voice box to produce voice or to improve the quality of the sound coming from it. Dysarthric patients may need to learn how to reduce the amount of nasal resonance and/or to improve the rhythm of speech. Some dysarthric patients may benefit from *augmentative communication devices* such as computers to improve communication. Several therapies can help patients to achieve these goals.

The goal of the speech and language rehabilitation program is to help the stroke survivor learn to produce speech as clearly as possible. During this time, the patient may make the maximum amount of effort and attend intently to the therapies. Sometimes when the patient ends therapy, however, he or she will not continue to put the same amount of energy, attention, and effort into speaking clearly. It is natural for performance levels to drop off when therapy ends. This is sometimes called *regression to the mean.* One of the principles of dysarthria therapy is that if the patient achieves a high level of success in direct therapy, he or she will not drop back too far when the therapy ends. Therefore, dysarthria therapy should produce the very best speech possible during the course of therapy so that when the patient's performance naturally drops off after therapy concludes, he or she will still be left with improved speech.

Dysarthria therapy is a lot like physical therapy. The speech-language pathologist does many of the same things a physical therapist does to strengthen muscles, improve range of motion, and improve general functioning. The main difference between physical and speech therapy has to do with access to the muscles. Whereas it is relatively easy for a physical therapist to grasp and help move a patient's arm or leg, it is another thing to work with a weak or paralyzed tongue, soft palate, or vocal cord. Because of the accessibility problems, speech-language pathologists must be creative and resourceful when dealing with speech muscles and in choosing therapies.

Therapy for Apraxia of Speech

Stroke survivors with severe apraxia of speech often have problems programming the movements of the breathing muscles, voice box, mouth, and tongue. In severe cases of apraxia of speech, many patients cannot coordinate them to get any speech to come out voluntarily and purposefully. Some patients may have a few automatic utterances such as a sound, word, or short phrase, but in severe cases of apraxia of speech, there is often no ability to speak.

Therapy for patients with severe apraxia of speech often begins with the basics. The first thing the patient must be taught is to purposefully direct the airstream from the lungs to the speech mechanism. One way clinicians teach this skill is by having the patient blow into a tissue or handkerchief. Getting the air to flow through the mouth for speech purposes is the first step. The next step, getting the patient to produce sounds with the voice box, is done using feedback. One way is to place the patient's hand on the clinician's voice box when voiced sounds are made, then place the hand on the patient's throat. Sometimes, the vibration feedback is enough to get the patient to produce voice. Some clinicians use a stethoscope for feedback. By placing the stethoscope so that the patient can hear both his or her own vocal cord vibrations and those of the clinician, the patient can sometimes learn more control over voicing. Building from these basic steps, the speech clinician then gradually and systematically helps the patient relearn voluntary control of speech production.

Therapy for mild and moderate cases of apraxia of speech also involves helping the patient relearn voluntary control of the speech production mechanism, but the focus of the therapy is usually on the tongue. If the patient can read, control of the articulators can be taught using letters and words as cues. If a patient is aware of errors and is self-corrective, that is, if he or she knows when a mistake has been made and can correct it, then reading aloud is good therapy and can be done independently. Patients who do not know when a mistake has been made or cannot correct on their own need a therapist to help them learn purposeful speech.

One of the determinations made during the evaluation of apraxia was whether the patient has oral apraxia. Recall that oral apraxia is like apraxia of speech except that it occurs for nonspeech oral movements. The patient without oral apraxia can lick the lips, protrude and elevate the tongue, and make other nonspeech movements voluntarily. This ability is important because when a patient can purposefully move his or her articulators, these movements can be used to learn speech placement. For example, if a patient can voluntarily bite the lower lip, he or she can then be taught to do this to help make the f and v sounds. Many patients with apraxia of speech who have little or no oral apraxia can benefit from this approach. Using hand gestures can also help patients learn to start purposeful utterances. For example, the patient might learn to say "I" or "I want" while touching his or her chest and then bring the hand into a fist. These hand gestures can be used to prompt a purposeful utterance.

Automatic utterances can be used to help with purposeful speech. Sometimes stroke survivors can be taught to produce automatic utterances purposefully and to expand them. For example, if a patient says "Darn it" automatically, he or she can be taught to say "Darn it, Mary" or "Darn it, I want water." Also, by using distractions and relaxation, many patients learn to be less purposeful in their speech and consequently gain more automatic utterances. For example, if the patient is taught to think about how the voice box feels when it vibrates or how the tongue feels when it moves from one position to another, the patient learns feedback and may also gain more automatic speech.

Some patients with apraxia of speech can sing common songs. In many ways, they resemble people who stutter when they talk but do not do so when they sing. Often, by using common, simple songs such as "Row Your Boat," "Happy Birthday," or "America the Beautiful," the patient with apraxia of speech can sing the words in the song and then be taught to say them without the melody. Common statements and requests can also be prompted by having the patient learn them to a melody.

The primary objective for apraxia of speech therapy is to help the patient regain control over voluntary and purposeful speech acts. Simply put, a patient is taught to gain control over his or her speech mechanism. Of course, when these patients have aphasia as well as apraxia of speech, as often happens, the job becomes much more complicated.

Therapy for Aphasia

Therapies provided for aphasia patients are usually intensive and prolonged. Sessions are generally conducted for one or two hours a day. Less frequent therapy is provided to patients confined to a nursing home or extended care facility or when they are seen as outpatients.

Frequently, because of muscle weakness or paralysis, the aphasia patient is required to change from writing right-handed to using the left hand. Some clinicians also encourage left-handed writing because it is believed that writing left-handed causes the patient to use more of the right side of the brain that has unimpaired brain cells. Naturally, this therapy would depend on the location of the brain damage.

When a stroke survivor has aphasia, the therapy provided depends on which avenues of communication are most impaired, the severity of the disorder, the presence or absence of motor speech deficits, and the presence of other complications. Added to the variability of the disorder is the fact that each individual with aphasia has unique levels of motivation, family support, learning abilities, and psychological makeup. This requires the speech-language pathologist to design a highly individualized program of aphasia therapy for each stroke survivor. A variety of workbooks, tapes, computer programs, flash cards, and books are available to the speech clinician to treat these patients. Many materials focus on a particular type of deficit.

Recall that aphasia rarely impairs only one avenue of communication, although some forms of expression and understanding may be more severely impaired than others. The goal of aphasia therapy is to use the avenues of communication that have remained most intact to help improve the more impaired ones. For example, if a patient has minimal problems with reading abilities, then the clinician may use reading aloud to help improve the patient's ability to remember words for expression. By reading aloud, the patient can relearn expressive vocabulary.

As mentioned previously, patients with global or severe aphasia may not be able to benefit from treatment, whereas some stroke survivors with mild word-finding problems can be expected to recover normal communication. Patients with severe receptive problems, for instance, the inability to understand anything written or said, are difficult to treat because of the communication barriers between the clinician and the patient. Such a patient-clinician communication barrier makes it difficult to design and conduct a therapy program.

Often, patients with aphasia also can have one or more of the motor speech disorders discussed in Chapter 3. Apraxia of speech and/or one or more of the dysarthrias often occur simultaneously with aphasia. When this happens, the speech-language pathologist must design a treatment program that addresses all of the communication deficits and makes allowances for specific problems created by the motor speech disorders. For example, because patients with apraxia of speech and aphasia may not be able to repeat what is spoken to them, using repetition as a form of therapy must be avoided. The clinician will not be able to use repeating what is spoken to help the patient relearn language until later in the program, if at all. Sometimes patients with severe dysarthria cannot be understood, not because of a language problem but because of muscle weakness or paralysis. This makes it difficult for the clinician to monitor the patient's word-finding accuracy.

The presence of complications (see Chapter 4) also requires an individualized approach to aphasia therapy. Reading aloud, working on monetary values, and working on writing exercises must be avoided or adjustments made if the patient has difficulty shifting thoughts. If a patient tends to get stuck on one idea or mental set, then this complication must be dealt with first and adjustments made in other therapy activities. Aphasia therapy must also be individualized for patients who have panic attacks, exaggerated emotions, and so forth.

For patients with aphasia, there are virtually hundreds of objectives and thousands of ways of achieving them. Aphasia therapy involves a variety of teaching, counseling, and behavior modification approaches, and the goals of sessions are individually designed, because some patients are likely to go into nursing homes, others will return home, and yet others will be able to resume jobs. An infinite number of subtle variations can be made to individualize each session to a particular patient's learning style. To give you a basic understanding of the goals of aphasia therapy, the general goals and objectives in each avenue of communication are listed below.

1. **Reading Problems.** When working on reading problems, the patient tries to attach meaning to letters, short words, longer words, two words together, and short, simple written sentences. More complex reading objectives include having the patient read short, simple paragraphs and answer questions about them. Higher level reading objectives are designed to help the patient read and understand short stories.

2. **Writing Problems.** Patients with severe writing problems are taught to grasp and control a pencil; copy large geometric forms such as triangles, circles, and squares; and to make individual letters. Other objectives include having the patient learn to write his or her name and the names of family and friends. Higher level activities involve writing words, sentences, and short paragraphs. Writing when the clinician dictates something is one of the highest goals.

3. **Math Problems.** The goals are to get the patient to do simple arithmetic problems and to understand monetary values. First, the patient must relearn the meanings of numbers, coins, and paper money. Then the stroke survivor relearns how to do simple, elementary school types of problems and to make simple change. Higher level activities include doing more complex math problems and making change for higher denominations of money.

4. **Problems Understanding the Speech of Others.** Patients with severe problems understanding the speech of others sometimes must begin at the one-word level. Pictures or objects are placed on the therapy table and the clinician tells the patient to point to or grasp the appropriate picture or object when its name is said. Sometimes the clinician must physically place the patient's hand on the picture or object and say the word several times. As the patient improves, more pictures and objects are used. Later, the clinician uses longer utterances and commands for the patient to follow. Role playing, games, and drills are used to get patients to understand dialogue.

5. **Expressive Language Problems.** For patients who use telegraphic speech, sentence expansion activities can be helpful. For example, when the patient responds to a question such as "How are you?" with a simple, short response of "Fine," the clinician can give a cue or prompt to expand it. The patient is cued to say "I am fine" or "I am doing fine, thank you." Sentence completion exercises, in which the patient fills in the left out word in statements such as "Red, white, and _____," "The United States of _____," and "Knife, fork, and _____" can help the patient be more expressive. Pictures and written flashcards can be used to help the patient retrieve words and phrases.

For some patients who speak jargon, special consideration must be given to denial. Some jargon aphasia patients will not acknowledge that they have a communication disorder. When the clinician brings it to their attention, they completely or partially deny that it exists. Obviously, a person must recognize that he or she has a problem before it can successfully be dealt with. When working with these stroke survivors, it is necessary to bring the presence of the disorder to their attention. This must be done gradually and gently and be accompanied by praise and rewards for confronting the disability. Every time the patient is confronted with his or her disability, ego strengthening statements should be provided. Brutal confrontation about the disability should be avoided.

Aphasia is a language disorder and as such all aspects of language must be addressed. The rules by which sounds are made into words and words are strung into sentences are important aspects of language therapy. These must be considered on both the expressive and understanding levels. However, much of what is done in aphasia therapy has to do with the semantic aspect of language: words and their meanings. Most aphasia therapy is vocabulary work. During expressive communication, the stroke survivor must either relearn the meanings of words or learn how to recall words easily and fluently.

There is one overriding rule in vocabulary work: The words chosen for expression should be relevant and important to the particular stroke survivor; the words targeted for therapy should be individualized to a patient's life. Words such as *level, square, joist,* and *plumb-bob* are important for an individual who has an interest in carpentry, whereas *calls, puts, options,* and *price-to-earning ratios* are words that would be important to a stockbroker or a person with interest in the stock market. Words that are spoken infrequently and that are unimportant to day-to-day activities should be given a lower priority in therapy. As a rule, vocabulary development should begin egocentrically and work outward. This means that patients should first learn words that are close to them, such as body parts, clothing, family names, food items, and room objects, and gradually work outward into the environment.

Therapy for Swallowing Problems

The patient's physician, a registered dietitian, and the speech-language pathologist work together to develop swallowing objectives. In addition, an occupational therapist may be involved in helping the stroke survivor relearn how to hold eating utensils, move, and lift food to the mouth. Nurses and nursing aides become involved in the swallowing therapy when the patient starts to meet nutrition needs orally rather than through tubes or an IV. Swallowing therapy usually consists of three parts.

First, the speech-language pathologist may want to adjust the texture of foods and the thickness of liquids. Some patients can tolerate only naturally thick or artificially thickened liquids. Naturally thick liquids include some soups, sauces, and gravies. Thin liquids can be thickened by adding the artificial thickener that has no taste and can be added to coffee, tea, water, soup, and other inherently thin liquids. The amount of thickness is controlled by the amount of it added. Food textures are usually adjusted by the kitchen staff under the direction of a registered dietitian. Many stroke survivors with a swallowing problem will start with pureed food, which has been put in a blender and made into a near-liquid form. Higher on the ladder of texture are chopped and soft diets. The temperature of foods and liquids is controlled, too, because either hot or cold foods and liquids can be tracked more easily in the mouth and throat than tepid ones. This helps the patient monitor the swallow.

The second element of a program of swallowing therapy involves positioning of the patient. Some stroke survivors with swallowing problems have fewer problems eating if they are sitting up, while others do better when leaning a little forward or backward. The goal is to let gravity help with the swallow. Sometimes, having a patient swallow while his or her head is turned can help protect the airway.

Carefully timing the swallow and "clearing" activities are the third part of most swallowing therapies. When learning to swallow normally, the patient is taught to chew and contain food and then to move it carefully to the back of the throat for swallowing. Many patients are instructed to take a breath before the swallow and not to let it out until after the swallow is over. This allows time for the food or liquid to get past the voice box and into the stomach, thereby reducing the risk of breathing it into the lungs. Some patients also benefit from clearing activities such as pushing the air out of the lungs with a voiced sound, such as "ah," at the end of the swallow, which further prevents seepage of liquids and food particles into the lungs. Many patients find it helpful to produce one or more dry swallows after the one that carried the food or liquid. This further helps to direct the liquid or food through the appropriate tube and clears the passages to the lungs.

Most stroke survivors with swallowing problems regain some or all of the ability to swallow. Unfortunately, a small percentage of patients must get a permanent tube placed in their stomachs. This tube, sometimes called a *peg tube,* allows nutrients to be placed directly into the patient's stomach.

Speech and language therapy is often hard work. It is not "work" in the sense that it is physically demanding. After all, it does not take much physical energy to talk; a person could talk continuously all day and not generate enough energy to boil a cup of water. Instead, therapy is hard work because it requires careful attention to detail, concentration, and patience. It often involves drills, drills, and more drills. When it comes to speech and language, "practice makes perfect." Perhaps a better way of saying this is that "Speech and language practice makes for the best recovery possible given the extent of the brain injury caused by the stroke."

One of the most important ingredients in any speech and language rehabilitation program is the relationship between the clinician and the stroke survivor. The patient and the clinician work closely together during speech and language therapy. The often close physical contact and the activities of correcting and improving someone's speech and language are very personal and make speech and language therapy rewarding for both the clinician and the patient. It is satisfying for a clinician to help another person regain the ability to communicate. It is rewarding for the patient to improve and to reap the benefits of this marvelous human ability— the ability to communicate. In any close working relationship, both parties must respect the rights of the other. The following "Aphasic Patient's Bill of Rights" was designed to state clearly the patient's rights going into a therapeutic relationship. It was first presented at a convention of ASHA in 1986.*

---

*D. Tanner, "The Aphasic Patient's Bill of Rights," paper presented at the Annual Convention of the American Speech-Language-Hearing Association (Detroit).

The Aphasic Patient's Bill of Rights*

Preamble

I am an individual with a speech and language disorder. The disorder may be mild and only cosmetically affect my ability to communicate or it may be severe and completely eliminate my ability to represent my thoughts and feelings with speech and language. My disorder can be complicated by sensory, perceptual, cognitive, and psychiatric disturbances. I may be mobile, homebound, or confined to a nursing home, medical care facility, hospital, or rehabilitation center. Regardless of my deficits, I am entitled to the human dignity afforded to noncommunicatively disabled individuals. Although my fundamental human rights are protected by the Constitution of the United States of America and other rights are extended to me by the policies and procedures of facilities and organizations, because of my communicative deficits, I require the following:

Our Relationship

Upon your acceptance of me as a patient, you assume three responsibilities. First, you are to provide the best clinical services of which you are capable. You are to use all of the knowledge, skills, and resources available to help me minimize this disability. Second, by accepting me as your patient you agree to serve as my advocate in situations in which I, my family, or my court-appointed guardian cannot represent my wishes. In those situations, you will use your powers of speech and language to defend and protect me from attempts to deprive me of human dignity. Third, you have an obligation to provide significant people who come into contact with me your appraisal of my specific impairments and strengths. You will provide me with the benefit of the doubt regarding the status of those abilities that you are not absolutely certain have been impaired. Although I value and respect your professional position, you are employed by me. As such, my wishes will prevail regarding the course of therapy and all other considerations affecting me. If I am considered legally incompetent, my guardian will serve as my advocate, but this Bill of Rights will stand as a guiding principle for your interaction with me.

Unconditional Positive Regard

You have the responsibility to treat me with unconditional positive regard. You may not like or approve of the things I say or do, but you have the responsibility to value me as a human being. You will project unconditional positive regard to me verbally, nonverbally, and in all aspects of our relationship. In addition, because I may not be able to protest

*Dedicated to the memory of Mr. "Chuck" Huston.

forced interaction with people who do not maintain positive regard for me, you will serve as my advocate in those situations. You will ensure that I am protected and insulated from individuals who do not extend to me this basic human consideration.

Common Courtesy

I have the right to all of the common courtesies extended to the verbal population. I have the right to be addressed formally as Mr., Mrs., Ms., or Miss. I expect to be greeted in a pleasant and respectful manner. You shall engage in the social graces with me. I may not comprehend the words you speak, but I can appreciate the extension of common courtesy.

Grooming

I have the right to proper grooming. I shall be given adequate time to prepare myself for public interaction. If I am incapable of grooming myself due to paralysis or other impairments, I shall be assisted in becoming presentable. You have the responsibility not to transport me out of my room or home without addressing my right to proper appearance. Additionally, you will serve as my advocate to ensure that I will be presentable at all times.

Privacy

I have the right to privacy. I am entitled to periods alone or with relatives and friends. I have the right to have these times uninterrupted. I also have the right to refuse visitors. You have the responsibility to attend to my wishes regarding these matters and to protect my privacy.

Mobility

Although I may be confined to a wheelchair, I have the right to determine my movement. I have the right to be asked or encouraged to participate in decisions regarding mobility. You will not allow me to be shuffled from place to place without first informing me of the destination and, in some manner, obtaining my approval.

Emotions

I have the right to genuine, albeit in some cases exaggerated, emotions regarding my predicament without having them ignored or intellectualized as inappropriate. My emotions about this disability are appropriate to me, and others should appreciate and respond appropriately to them. You have the responsibility to accept my emotions as genuine and to respond to them in an understanding and compassionate manner.

Personality

I have the right to my unique personality. As long as my behaviors are not destructive, I have the right to tolerance, understanding, and appreciation of my unique personality characteristics. You have the responsibility to ensure that I am provided the same degree of personality tolerance extended to members of the verbal population.

Therapy

I have the right to be treated as an adult. Therapy materials designed for children are demeaning to me. You have the responsibility to ensure that therapy materials are appropriate for my age, sex, interests, and disabilities.

I have the right to be informed of the prognosis for my recovery as a result of the therapy you provide to me. If I am incapable of understanding these reports, you have the responsibility to share the prognosis with my physician, family, and/or court-appointed guardian.

I have the right to refuse therapy. A verbal person's wishes regarding therapy would be honored and I have the same rights.

I have the right to be made aware of the purposes of therapy techniques in those conditions in which I am capable of comprehending all or part of them. We are partners in my treatment, and you should attempt to communicate to me the objectives of a particular therapy. If behavior modification is used, I shall be made aware of the nature and purpose of the system. Foods, institutional privileges, and other reinforcements may be used only with my (or my family's or guardian's) prior consent.

Quality Institutional Services

I have the right to prompt and considerate institutional services. Because "The squeaky wheel gets the grease," I may be denied the quality services provided to individuals with intact powers of speech and language. You will serve as my advocate to ensure that I am treated fairly and provided quality services while I am disabled.

CHAPTER 12

Questions and Answers

All of us, at certain moments of our lives, need to take advice and receive help from other people—ALEXIS CARREL

No matter how comprehensive a book is, there are always certain topics not covered that may be of interest to family members. Many of these issues are specific to a particular patient. Some questions might arise about unusual or rare aspects of communication disorders resulting from stroke. Your doctor or other health care professional is the best resource for these concerns. However, following are examples of questions that have been asked by family members and friends of communication disabled stroke patients. These questions, and their answers, are provided in an attempt to cover issues and concerns not directly dealt with in previous chapters.

Q: *A friend of mine suffered a serious stroke and is completely unable to communicate. He is in a nursing home. My friend was a high school teacher for 20 years. Before the stroke, he always insisted that his students and casual acquaintances address him as "Mr. Erickson." Now that he is in the nursing home, everyone calls him "Bob." I know that before the stroke, he wanted only close friends and family members to be on a first name basis. I believe this bothers him. What do you suggest?*

A: Mr. Erickson has the right to all of the common courtesies extended to the verbal population. He might not be able to understand the specific words, but he certainly can appreciate the intent. You should talk to the nursing staff, physicians, and therapists and explain the situation. Ask them if they could extend this courtesy to your friend, and thank them in advance for their cooperation. When you are visiting him and observe someone being too familiar, correct them by referring to "Mr. Erickson." Do this in a pleasant and friendly manner. You might also put a note up in his room that tells people of his preference.

Q: *My husband was recently transferred to a rehabilitation center. He had a stroke about two weeks ago and is now ready to undergo intensive therapies. Before the stroke, he always took pride in his appearance. He would never leave the house without carefully selecting and matching his clothes and he was careful about grooming. His friends nicknamed him "Dapper Dan." Since being admitted to the rehabilitation center, he has an intensive schedule of physical, occupational, and speech therapies. The problem is that when the nurses, aides, and therapists transport him to different sections of the rehabilitation center, they often do it when he is sloppily dressed, his hair is unkempt, or he is unshaven. This problem might seem insignificant to many people, but I know it bothers Dan. Is this a common and necessary practice with stroke patients?*

A: No, this is not a common problem nor is it necessary. Unfortunately, it does occur, especially in busy rehabilitation centers and nursing homes. Sometimes there is neither the staff nor the time to attend carefully to these things. It is probably unavoidable some of the time, but it should never be standard practice. Before a patient is transferred to a different part of the facility, he or she should be appropriately dressed and groomed. Verbal patients can insist on this, but patients with stroke-related communication disorders may not be able to express their concerns. Therefore, I suggest you talk to the director of nursing about this. It may require that Dan be awakened earlier in the morning to provide time for these matters. You should also mention this to the occupational therapist. Dressing and grooming could become goals of his occupational therapy. Occupational therapists call this an "activity of daily living" (ADL). Soon, Dapper Dan may learn how to do some of these activities for himself.

Q: *My wife suffered a stroke a few months ago and is unable to talk normally, although she is improving. She lives at home with me and has learned to communicate with hand gestures and limited speech. We get along fine at home, but when we go to town she gets embarrassed, especially when she is unable to express her thoughts verbally. Yesterday, at a restaurant my wife appeared to be embarrassed when she ordered lunch. How should I deal with this kind of situation?*

A: I'm sure the server felt awkward as well. Most of us feel awkward when communication breaks down. One way of preventing embarrassment is for you to order for your wife. Although this is not the best way to increase her independence, it may be the only solution given her communication problems. This is the best option if the embarrassment felt by your wife makes her less likely to get out of the house and to do pleasant things. Another way of dealing with the situation is to explain to the server that your wife suffered a stroke and has trouble talking, and that she might need more time to complete her order. Whatever the solution you choose, it is important to discuss this issue with your wife. Let her know that communication disorders are a part of life and that strokes have happened to many people. Though her feelings are natural, having a communication disorder is not something to be embarrassed about.

Q: *My father lives in a sheltered living center. Most of the patients come and go as they want. The problem is that Dad will not go to a nearby store without me although he wants to go there often. I think it is because of his communication disorder. I'd like to visit him every day and walk with him to the store, but I'm too busy with my work and family. Do you have any suggestions?*

A: Sheltered living centers, day programs, and supervisory nursing facilities all provide excellent services to patients with minor disabilities. Your father's requests for you to go with him to the nearby store might be a roundabout way of asking you to visit him more often. It may also be a reflection of his fear of being in a situation in which people might not be able to understand him and perhaps take advantage of him financially. I suggest you go to the store and meet with the manager. Explain the situation and ask if he or she can help. The manager can inform the clerks of your father's communication problem and give them your telephone number in case he has problems while at the store. You should also suggest to your father that he take with him only the amount of money necessary to buy what he needs.

Q: *Something my mother does is driving me crazy. She had a stroke a few weeks ago and since then she gets extremely upset. During the past week, she has been trying to tell me something important. For the life of me, I cannot understand the question. She starts off saying, "You must, now, must be done, . . ." and then trails off into words and phrases that don't make sense at all while she is gesturing wildly. The more I try to guess what she is talking about, the more upset she becomes. What should I do?*

A: This awkward game of "charades" is a common problem. Many stroke survivors with communication disorders attempt to express complex thoughts and find they are unable to complete them. Sometimes, it seems the harder they try, the worse their speech becomes. Family members, friends, nurses, doctors, and other people often find these failed attempts to communicate extremely frustrating. Unfortunately, there is no easy solution to this problem. One method that has proven helpful is to strive to keep the patient relaxed and calm. Studies have shown that patients who are relaxed are able to talk more easily. If it looks as though your mother will continue to be unable to express this important question or idea, you should try to diffuse the situation. In a kind but firm voice, inform your mother that it is futile to continue speaking, but that you will come back to the idea later. Hopefully, by then she will be able to be more functional in her communication.

Q: *My son suffered a stroke at a young age. He was left with very little speech and has been receiving speech and language therapy. At first during therapy, he liked the speech-language pathologist, and together they made improvements in his ability to speak. They seemed to get along well until recently. Now my son often refuses to go to outpatient therapy and when he does go, he won't work hard. He seems to have lost confidence in the clinician. I feel that he can make more gains in his ability to talk, but I don't know what to do. What do you do when the patient-therapist relationship is strained?*

A: Express your concerns to the speech-language pathologist. The clinician may not know that there is a problem. Sometimes, a clinician can simply run out of ideas to keep the therapy activities interesting and relevant. At larger medical facilities, there is often more than one speech-language pathologist available to do outpatient therapy. You, your son, and the clinician should discuss the problem and, if necessary, reschedule outpatient therapy with another clinician. Don't worry about hurting anyone's feelings. This problem is more common than you think. Speech-language pathologists are professionals and will place the patient's needs first and foremost.

Q: *I am unable to visit my mother in the nursing home because I can't drive. She will be 90 years old this month and is unable to talk because of global aphasia. I worry that because she can't communicate, she is being neglected by the staff. I fear that doctors, nurses, and therapists won't take the time to anticipate her needs. Unfortunately, there are no other family members in the vicinity to visit her regularly. How can I be certain that she is being treated as well as the other patients?*

A: Your mother's global aphasia has severely damaged her ability to communicate. She does not have the ability to read, write, speak, or understand the speech of others. If she is truly globally aphasic, neither can she use hand gestures well enough to express thoughts and feelings. It is natural to be concerned about her welfare because patients who can ask for help are more likely to get it. However, you can take comfort that most nursing homes meet or exceed stringent rules about patient care. If you become concerned that the quality of care for your mother is less than it should be, notify your mother's attending physician. If your mother is receiving speech-language services at the nursing facility, the speech clinician can also serve as advocate to see that her needs and wants are met. Use the telephone to talk regularly with the director of nursing or the social worker about any concerns you may have. Also, share important information with the shift nurse. Even little things, such as the kinds of television shows your mother prefers to watch, food likes and dislikes, and sleeping habits, should be shared with the nursing staff.

Q: *I am a partially retired business executive and still consult part time with my previous employer. A few months ago, I had a minor stroke that has resulted in slurred speech. Therapy helped me overcome the speech defect, and I can consult at the office and even give speeches without slurring my sounds very badly. My face and tongue are still weak, and I also lack sensation on the left side of my face. My biggest problem is that I drool and it is extremely embarrassing. Any suggestions?*

A: Drooling is a common component to strokes that impair the tongue, face, and lips. Some patients describe the lack of sensation as similar to what happens when a dentist deadens a tooth. Drooling can also result from inattentiveness (sleep drooling) and swallowing problems. One method of eliminating this source of embarrassment is to ask your wife, a friend, or a colleague to cue you every time you need to wipe your mouth. The cue can be a subtle hand gesture such as pointing to the side of the mouth. It can also be an audible signal such as clearing the throat. When you get the cue, you can wipe your mouth or swallow and avoid the embarrassment of drooling.

Q: *I am very angry. My wife had a serious stroke about five weeks ago and is completely unable to talk, read, or write. However, she understands everything I say to her. Yesterday, the speech-language pathologist asked that I be present when he did a test. Time after time, the therapist asked my wife to point to a square, circle, or triangle or to lick her lips. When my wife was not able to do these things, the therapist would ask her to do other things that were equally hard. This made me extremely angry. What can I do to stop this?*

A: For many reasons, anger is one of the more common emotions experienced by family members of the stroke survivor, and sometimes the anger stems from all of the unwanted changes that have happened to a loved one. People are frustrated at the situation, and anger is a natural reaction. Unfortunately, sometimes this anger is directed toward health care professionals. Of course, professionals can do things that can cause justifiable anger, but this does not sound like such a situation. Sometimes, a speech-language pathologist will ask a family member to observe the testing of a patient. In part, they do it to show the family member that he or she may have unrealistic ideas about what the stroke patient can do. Although it is possible that your wife does understand everything that it is spoken to her, it is also very likely that this is not the case. Ask for a meeting with the speech-language pathologist and discuss your concerns with him openly. Meanwhile, give some thought to the possibility that you are angry because the test showed that your wife does not really understand much of what is said to her.

Q: *My sister's stroke left her with Broca's aphasia. When she tries to talk, she has trouble remembering what words to use. Sometimes, when she can remember the word she wants to say, she stutters it. Often, I know the word she wants to say. Should I supply the word for her or let her continue to stutter on it?*

A: The speech of a Broca's aphasia patient sometimes sounds like stuttering, but they are two different types of communication disorders. There is no clear-cut answer to whether you should supply the word for your sister. The main thing you should do is ask her if she wants your help in these situations. If you don't get a clear answer from her, follow these guidelines. First, give her plenty of time to find the correct way to say the word. Do not hurry her. Make certain that she knows you will take the necessary time to listen to her, and be relaxed and calm. Second, if you are certain you know the word she wants to say, give her a few hints, such as the first sounds of the word. If this doesn't help her, then supply it and watch her reaction. Note whether she appears relieved or disappointed by your help.

Another guideline for dealing with these issues comes from communicating with people who actually do stutter. Compare the difficulty of saying a word with carrying an object. If someone is carrying a light object with little effort, help with it would not be welcomed. It might even be resented. However, if the object is big and cumbersome, he or she may appreciate the help. Look at the degree of difficulty your sister is having. If it is a minor problem, a word that will eventually be spoken clearly with little trouble, she probably will not appreciate the help. However, if her attempts to say a word are far from the way it is correctly spoken and she is clearly struggling, your help may be appreciated.

Q: *I understand that when patients have receptive aphasia, they have problems understanding speech and possibly also problems with reading. These problems exist because of the areas of the brain that have been damaged. I know all of that. My question is, "Why do some of these people talk in nonsense?"*

A: This is a very good question and one asked by many family members. It is true that in most cases of receptive aphasia, the expressive parts of the brain are not damaged by the stroke. There is no general agreement about why some of these patients talk in jargon or nonsense. Some authorities believe that the brain operates as a whole and that one part is dependent on the others. Thus, damage in one area indirectly affects other areas. Other authorities believe that jargon speech comes from the patient not being able to monitor carefully his or her speech output. Receptive aphasia patients may not understand their speech output any better than they understand the speech of others. Because of the language problem, patients express nonsense words because they can't monitor and correct. Another reason given for jargon aphasia has to do with a disrupted vocabulary. Because of the stroke, patients' words and their meanings have been disrupted and patients may simply be expressing these mixed-up ideas. The final reason is psychological. After a while, you would expect patients to realize that they aren't making sense and to stop talking altogether. This would be a reasonable thing to do when no one understands what they are trying to say. Some authorities believe that this persistent nonsense is psychological, a result of denial. Patients refuse to accept the fact that they are not making sense. Most likely, the jargon speech in some aphasia patients is the result of some or all of the preceding reasons.

Q: *A friend of mine has aphasia. Before the stroke, he was fluent in three languages: English, Spanish, and French. I am also fluent in Spanish and English. Which language should I use when talking to him?*

A: In a few cases, strokes and other types of brain injuries render one language lost while another is left relatively intact. Although this preservation of one language over another is rare, it does occur. The language you probably should use when talking with your friend is the one typically used by both of you before the stroke. Hopefully, if your friend is getting speech and language therapy, it is in the language most used and practiced. If this is not so, contact the speech clinician and discuss the situation with him or her.

Q: *Why do some patients with aphasia confuse "Yes" and "No" when you ask them a simple question?*

A: Some aphasic patients are disoriented because of a stroke, and thus they are confused when they answer a simple question. Other patients may not understand your question. In many cases of aphasia, the patient incorrectly says "Yes" for "No" and vice versa because these words are similar. Both are one-word responses to closed-end questions. Confusing "Yes" and "No" is similar to the mistake a patient makes when he or she says "Car" for "Truck," "Pencil" for "Pen," or "Up" for "Down." They often say "Yes" or "No" while nodding the opposite answer. If you have to choose between the verbal response and the head nod, go with the head nod. It is more likely to reflect the individual's true wishes.

Q: *My mother has verbal apraxia. Sometimes she does a good job of getting her words out. Other times, she is unsuccessful. We encourage her to try harder, and we cheer her on as she tries and tries to say the words correctly. Are there any other things we can do to help her say the words?*

A: Verbal apraxia is also known as apraxia of speech. It is a speech programming problem for purposeful and voluntary types of utterances. The area of the brain responsible for getting the muscles of speech to work correctly has been damaged. As a result, your mother knows what she wants to say but cannot say it. Part of apraxia of speech is the fact that automatic speech is sometimes said easily and clearly. This is because automatic speech is said with little forethought; it is less purposeful. Because automatic, non-purposeful speech is easier to say than purposeful and thoughtful utterances, telling your mother to "try harder" is probably not a good thing to do. It may cause her to be more conscious of speech, thus making it more purposeful and difficult. The best thing to do is to encourage her to use the trial and error approach. She should not force speech but keep trying different articulation placements until she gets it right.

Q: *Since my stroke, I have noticed that I now have a hoarse voice. It is also deeper in pitch. Can laryngitis be caused by a stroke?*

A: Laryngitis is the swelling or inflammation of the mucous membranes of the larynx. The word means "swelling of the larynx." One of the main symptoms of laryngitis is a hoarse voice quality. Many conditions can cause hoarseness, including smoking, overuse of the vocal cords, infections, and tumors. Hoarse voice quality can also be caused by a stroke that results in spastic muscles. Because of the rigid, tense muscles, the vocal cords cannot vibrate easily. Sometimes, a tube placed in a patient's throat to keep the airway open results in hoarseness because of the irritation it caused to the throat. I suggest you discuss this concern with your physician. He or she can find out the cause of the hoarseness and recommend the correct treatment.

Q: *Every time I enter my mother's nursing home room, she cries and cries. It takes a long time for her to stop sobbing. When I mention my children, she starts crying all over again. The crying is very upsetting to me. The nurses say she is "emotionally labile" and that the crying will eventually go away. What should I do until then?*

A: First, you should understand that your mother probably feels strong emotions when you come into the room and the crying is a response to that. The crying may also be an emotional response to the mention of her grandchildren. Emotional lability is not inappropriate crying; it is exaggerated.

Your mother has lost some control over her crying; she cries too much and too easily. However, you should recognize that her feelings and emotions are appropriate given her circumstances and perspectives. The nurses are correct; in time your mother is likely to gain more control over crying. Meanwhile, when she cries, try to distract her into thinking and talking about more uplifting and happy topics. You should also discuss this problem with her physician. Her doctor may want to prescribe medication that will help her to gain more control over the crying.

Q: *I believe my father is getting Alzheimer's disease. He had a stroke a few months ago and has been living with us at home. Yesterday, when the telephone rang he started to go to the door to open it. A few weeks ago, the opposite happened; he answered the telephone when someone knocked at the door. Is this one of the signs that he is losing his mind?*

A: Actually, the behavior your father displayed was an indication of a disorder known as auditory agnosia, which is a perceptual deficit in which the patient forgets the meaning and significance of sounds. It is relatively rare, but it can happen because of a stroke and other types of brain damage. Common sounds that we are accustomed to hearing every day such as horns honking, birds singing, children playing, and telephones ringing are confusing to the person with auditory agnosia. There is usually nothing wrong with the patient's hearing; it is perception that is impaired. Your father hears these sounds, but he has forgotten what they mean or confuses their meanings. Although these types of things can also occur due to Alzheimer's disease and other disorders, when they are the only symptoms, they are more likely a perceptual disorder and not an indication that he has dementia.

Q: *I think the hospital staff has misdiagnosed my mother. They think she has problems swallowing and I know she doesn't. They said something about her having an "NPO." I brought her in a vanilla milkshake yesterday and she loved it. She didn't have any choking or coughing. Who should I tell about this?*

A: You should bring this situation to the attention of the shift nurse as soon as possible. While it is possible that the hospital staff has misdiagnosed the swallowing problem, it is more likely that she does indeed have this problem. The designation of NPO means that she shouldn't take anything orally, and this includes milkshakes. The absence of choking and coughing does not necessarily mean that she has a good swallow. Coughing is nature's way of protecting the airway from foreign substances. Some stroke patients have silent aspiration. This means that they appear to have a normal swallow because they do not cough or choke. In reality, because of numbness, weakness, or paralysis of the swallowing mechanism, they don't have the protective reflex of coughing. Part of the vanilla milkshake could have gone into her lungs, which can lead to pneumonia. The hospital staff should be told of the situation immediately.

Q: *My wife had a stroke about three weeks ago. Since then she has been in a coma. I have tried and tried to wake her up, but nothing seems to work. I read in the newspaper about a man who was in a coma for years and then woke up. How long do you think it will be until she wakes up?*

A: Over the years, there have been several articles in newspapers about patients who have awakened from long-lasting comas. Scholarly research has also shown that this sometimes occurs. However, the comparison of waking up from sleep and awakening from a coma is not a good one because being in a coma is different from being in a deep sleep. There are many psychological and physical differences. There are also different types and levels of coma. Without knowing the specifics about your wife's condition, it is impossible to speculate accurately about when, or if, she will come out of the coma. You should discuss this concern with her physician.

Q: *My brother is in the intensive care unit and has aphasia. I have noticed that the television is left on most of the day and night. Is this to stimulate him?*

A: Having the television on in the patient's room to provide stimulation might be the idea behind this common practice. However, I don't believe it is a good one, especially for patients with communication disorders. The sounds coming from a television are artificial. Often, they consist of canned laugh tracks, superficial dialogue, and loud commercials. I believe this can confuse more than stimulate many patients, especially those with understanding deficits. Some patients can even become desensitized to real speech. I also think it interferes with rest and sleep. I suggest that the television be turned on only when the patient wants to watch a program and should be turned off at other times. Of course, if your brother is capable of indicating his wishes, they should be respected.

Q: *The rehabilitation team is working on improving my father's memory. Dad is having a hard time remembering little things like the days of the week or the time and date. They have given him a memory notebook and sometimes he uses it. Other times he forgets to bring it along. Do you have any suggestions?*

A: Memory notebooks are very helpful for some patients with memory problems as long as they remember to take it with them. It may be helpful to attach the notebook to your dad's watch, wallet, or belt with string or tape. This will help him remember to bring it along and use it. There are also electronic devices available to assist with memory.

Q: *My father had a stroke a few months ago. Since then I have been with him at every meal to help him eat. I know he has aphasia and that all avenues of communication have been impaired. But why does he occasionally put the knife in the coffee and try to use it like a straw? Sometimes he also tries to cut his food with the spoon. Is this part of aphasia?*

A: No, it is not part of aphasia. You don't need language to be able to know how to use eating utensils. This problem may be related to a vision deficit. If this is the case, make sure that he is wearing his glasses when he eats. It also might be that the stroke affected his vision and a new eye examination is required. Sometimes, patients who confuse eating utensils and other objects have visual perceptual disorders or thinking problems that require special therapies.

Q: *Should every patient who has a stroke be given antidepressants?*

A: Current antidepressant medications have few side effects and can do a remarkable job in elevating the spirits of depressed stroke patients. This has led some authorities to suggest that they should be prescribed for anyone who has depression. However, I don't believe this is a good idea for everyone who experiences a bout of depression. Many cases of depression lift on their own. Additionally, depression can arise from loss, and depression is a natural and necessary stage of the grieving process. I certainly agree that patients who have serious or prolonged depression should be provided with counseling and/or antidepressants. I disagree that medication should always be given as the quickest and easiest solution to a psychological problem. It is important to discuss this with the physician and that a health care professional assess the nature and extent of the stroke patient's depression and prescribe appropriate treatment.

Q: *My mother is in a nursing home because of a severe stroke. She cannot talk very well and spends most of the time in bed. Her diet consists of puree foods and liquids. She has both upper and lower dentures that she has used for many years. Although she does not need to chew, do you think she should wear her dentures anyway?*

A: Yes. Unless there are medical reasons for her not using dentures such as sores, choking, or breathing problems, she should wear them just as she did before she had the stroke. There are three reasons for this. First, if she stops using her dentures for a long period, the fit between them and her gums can change. This will make them feel uncomfortable and foreign when she does wear them. Second, wearing her dentures will help her appearance and make her feel more comfortable with the way she looks. Third, if she has problems speaking and getting her needs and wants met, dentures are important. Many sounds require the tongue to contact the teeth or to push air between the teeth. For the best speech possible, she should wear the dentures. However, it goes without saying that if she prefers not to wear them, her wishes should be honored.

Q: *A friend of mine had a stroke a few months ago. Since then he has been talking to an animal that does not exist. He says there is a dog in his room, and I find him talking to it all of the time. When I tell him that there is really no dog in his room, he gets upset and argues with me. Should I try to talk him out of these delusions?*

A: First, it is necessary to distinguish between delusions and hallucinations. A delusion is a thought disturbance, a belief that is untrue but rigidly held by the person. A common delusion is one of grandeur, in which a person may believe he or she is a superior human or a supernatural savior of the world. When a person erroneously believes that he or she is in extreme danger or at the mercy of powerful forces, he or she has a delusion of persecution. A person who hallucinates, on the other hand, perceives things that do not exist. He or she sees objects that are not there, hears sounds and smells odors where none exist. Some people feel sensations that do not occur, such as bugs crawling on them. Delusions and hallucinations often occur together. As you can see, your friend appears to be hallucinating that there is a dog in his room.

    I suggest you discuss the situation with your friend's doctor. He or she can prescribe medication that can reduce or eliminate these disturbances. The doctor may also want to refer your friend to a psychiatrist or a psychologist, too. Meanwhile, I recommend that when your friend talks about his hallucination you do not debate or argue with him about it. Hallucinations can be powerful forces in a person's life. You usually cannot talk a person out of them and should not attempt to do so.

Q: *What can be done for a stroke survivor who always has a dry mouth and is not supposed to have food or liquid?*

A: First, discuss this with his or her physician. Some medications can cause a dry mouth and the doctor may have an alternative to the one causing it. Second, discuss the situation with the patient's nurse or speech-language pathologist. Flavored wet swabs can be used to moisten a patient's mouth, or he or she may be able to tolerate a small amount of ice chips despite the NPO label. Be certain to get permission from the doctor, nurse, or speech-language pathologist before giving the patient anything orally.

Q: *My wife is legally blind and used the Braille method to read. Since she had her stroke, she cannot read by Braille anymore. That is her only problem with communication, She talks, writes, and understands the speech of others as well as she did before the stroke. Why can she no longer read like she did before?*

A: There could be several reasons for her inability to read using the Braille method. Given that she has no other problems with communication, it is likely that she either has numbness in her fingertips or a perceptual disorder known as tactile agnosia. Because of the numbness in her fingertips, she cannot feel the raised letters and thus cannot read. Tactile agnosia is a perceptual deficit in which, although she can feel the raised letters, she has lost the ability to perceive them correctly. A woman with tactile agnosia would not be able to distinguish car keys from money when she places her hand in her purse. The same would hold true for a man's ability to know the difference between a comb and a pocketknife when he puts his hand in his pants pocket.

Q: *My mother recently had a stroke and now has a trach. She understands what I say and writes me notes when she wants something. Are there other ways she can communicate with me?*

A: A "trach" is a "tracheotomy," an operation to open an airway into the windpipe through the neck. It is usually temporary, but during this time it may be difficult or impossible for the patient to communicate because the air coming from the lungs does not go through the patient's mouth. There are different types of trach tubes, and some allow the ability to communicate. I suggest you discuss this situation with your mother's doctor to see what can be done with the existing trach to permit speech or whether substituting a different type is advisable.

Q: *My friend has aphasia. Before the stroke, he was hard of hearing and wore two hearing aids. Now, when I visit him in the nursing home, I frequently find that his hearing aids do not work because the batteries are run down or that the aids have been left in his dresser. Because he has aphasia, are the hearing aids unnecessary?*

A: Your friend's hearing aids are as important now as they were before the stroke. Even if your friend has global aphasia and all avenues of communication are severely impaired, his ability to hear environmental sounds such as the radio, television, music, birds chirping, or the sound of thunder are still important if only for psychological reasons. If the batteries are dead, you can purchase new ones at most drugstores or the nursing home can supply them. Sometimes, because of a stroke a patient may need another hearing aid evaluation. Discuss the situation with the director of nursing or the social worker.

Q: *My wife had a stroke five years ago. At the time, we lived in a rural community in which there was no speech and language rehabilitation available. Recently, we moved to a large city, and I wonder if she could now benefit from therapy? Can a person who had a stroke a long time ago still benefit from therapy?*

A: Yes, it is possible that your wife could still benefit from a formal program of speech and language rehabilitation. The best bet is for you to discuss this with your doctor or to call a rehabilitation hospital and ask for an evaluation for rehabilitation potential. The medical evaluation will be conducted by a physiatrist, who is a specialist in physical medicine and rehabilitation. Also, a speech-language pathologist will probably conduct a complete speech and language evaluation. The results will indicate whether your wife would benefit from therapy.

Q: *My husband was a concert pianist before his stroke. His only problem is that he has aphasia. He will be going home soon. Will the aphasia affect his ability to play the piano?*

A: There have been several studies on aphasia and its effects on artistic skills. What does the loss of language do to the ability to play a musical instrument, paint, or sculpt? Unfortunately, there is no clear answer to this question. It depends on the severity of the aphasia, the type of artistry, and how accomplished the artist was. Some aphasia patients retain most of their artistic abilities, while others lose all but the most basic skills. Some studies have shown that the more accomplished the musician, the more a language disorder impairs his or her abilities. This has led some authorities to speculate that language is important, if not essential, to high-level musical abilities.

CHAPTER 13
Profiles in Recovery

A strong positive mental attitude will create more miracles than any wonder drug.—Actress and stroke survivor PATRICIA NEAL

The stroke patient and his or her family can learn a lot from others who have overcome or successfully adjusted to stroke-related communication disorders. While no two strokes or the communication disorders caused by them are identical, there are common trials and tribulations experienced by many stroke survivors and their families. What is most important, there are often uplifting success stories showing the courage, determination, and resourcefulness of stroke survivors and their families in meeting the challenges of this major life-altering event. Some of these success stories involve only one aspect of the stroke-related communication disorder while others concern an all-encompassing spiritual, religious, and psychological adjustment philosophy. What follows are six case studies about stroke-related communication disorders and how patients and their families coped with them. While these profiles are based on real persons and actual events, I have taken the liberty of changing names, places, and some factual aspects of them to preserve the privacy of these remarkable people. Literary license has also been taken for readability and descriptive purposes, and some profiles are composites for illustrative purposes. However, these profiles can give you valuable information about how others have met the challenges of strokes and the communication disorders caused by them.

Stroke Survivor "Christine," Husband "Darrel," and Son "Alan"

Emotional Lability

Read pages 57–60 about emotional lability and the "triggers" that can set off bouts of crying.

Like many stroke survivors, Christine could not remember the moments immediately before the stroke nor collapsing at the dining room table. Neither could Christine remember being lifted onto the stretcher or the ride to the hospital with the ambulance siren screaming for cars to get out of the way. Although Christine was conscious, she did not register the panicked look on her husband's face as she was poked, prodded, and punctured by emergency room personnel. Only vague recollections remained of being slid into the narrow metal tube while powerful magnets helped technicians visualize her healthy and damaged brain cells. Finally, when the diagnostic ordeal was completed, Christine was pronounced "stable" and moved to the intensive care unit for monitoring. She lay on her back, intermittently escaping into sleep, while high-tech instruments connected to her nose, arm, finger, and chest beeped, hummed, and buzzed. After what seemed an eternity for Darrel, the doctor came into the waiting room and reported that Christine had suffered a stroke. Although it was too soon to pinpoint the exact part of Christine's brain damage, he said it likely involved the left hemisphere and the areas associated with movement of her right hand, leg, and side of her face. The doctor also matter-of-factly said Christine could have problems with her speech.

The doctor was right; Christine's stroke affected her ability to walk, use her right hand and arm, and to speak. Eventually, she was transferred to the rehabilitation wing of the hospital and spent several months learning to walk with a quad-cane. The physical therapists helped her learn to stand with minimal assistance and to use the four-legged cane as a source of balance. Wobbly though she was, Christine achieved semi-independence and could get from one place to another. Her right hand was weak and for a while, she wore a plastic splint to keep it from pulling into a tight contracture. With the help of occupational therapists, and despite spastic hand and arm muscles constantly pulling against themselves, she gradually relearned the ability to eat and to dress herself.

"Spastic dysarthria" was the medical term given by the speech-language pathologists for Christine's difficulty speaking. Fortunately, her ability to use and understand language was unimpaired by the stroke, but unfortunately, spastic speech muscles initially made many of her utterances unintelligible. Her voice was raspy and speech sounds were slurred and indistinct. The speech-language pathologist was as resourceful as the other therapists, and by the end of her stint in rehabilitation, Christine's speech was understandable. If Christine remembered to speak slowly, exaggerate speech muscle movements, open her mouth widely when talking, and enunciate very clearly, she could be understood by most people who took the time to listen carefully to her labored speech. Oh, there were problem speech sounds such as the "t" "d," and "th," but with practice, practice, and more practice, she conquered the tongue elevations necessary to produce them clearly. By the time Christine was discharged from the rehabilitation unit, she felt prepared to walk, eat, dress, and speak with relative independence. What Christine was not prepared for were the bouts of crying, the downright sobbing episodes that were set off so easily. Of all the challenges she faced by virtue of the stroke, dealing with emotional lability was the biggest one of all.

Initially, Darrel and Alan thought that Christine's frequent crying was simply a normal and appropriate reaction to the unwanted events associated with the stroke. Difficulties walking, dressing, eating, and talking would make anyone feel like crying. Being confined to a rehabilitation unit for weeks and being away from home and loved ones would sadden anyone. The frustration, fear, and anxiety that are understandably a part of a dreadful stroke would depress even the most upbeat and light-hearted people. Nevertheless, it was her first "day pass" from the rehabilitation unit, and the visit to Alan's home, that showed Christine's crying went far beyond what was normal. The sight of Alan's young twins running to greet their grandmother set off a bout of crying for Christine that she was unable to stop. The crying lasted nearly 30 minutes and stopped only when the twins left the room. When they returned, Christine again began to sob uncontrollably. Darrel and Alan thought something was clearly awry, and when they returned to the rehabilitation unit, they asked the speech-language pathologist about it.

According to the speech-language pathologist, emotional lability is the exaggerated emotionality that occurs in many patients who suffer brain damage to the part of the brain known as the motor strip. Lability, not to be confused with "liability," literally means "unstable" and "prone to a breakdown." According to the speech-language pathologist, emotional lability is a result of brain damage and the emotions associated with the stroke. In the past, some specialists considered emotional lability to be an "inappropriate" response to a patient's predicament. However, most authorities now recognize that the emotions are appropriate, but exaggerated. Some stroke patients also laugh too easily, but because there is more to be sad about, crying is far more common.

The speech-language pathologist agreed that Christine had severe emotional lability. By the time Christine was discharged from the rehabilitation unit, she would have several bouts of extreme crying per hour. The emotional lability was so severe that it interfered with her speech intelligibility, caused hoarseness, and gave the impression to strangers that she was suffering from dementia. Being out-of-control emotionally was distressing to Christine, but Darrel and Alan found it particularly anxiety provoking to see their wife and mother cry incessantly. Something needed to be done about this severe case of emotional lability.

Christine was scheduled for outpatient speech therapy three times per week. Although the goals of therapy included improved speech production, the primary goal was to find a way to deal with the emotional lability. During a conference, Christine, Darrel, Alan, and the speech-language pathologist decided to first address the crying through therapy and then through medications if necessary. The speech-language pathologist suggested using the "Three P" therapy as a guide for minimizing or eliminating the emotional lability. The crying would be dealt with by addressing "predisposing" factors, "precipitants" that set off the crying, and those things that "perpetuated" the behavior.

The first "P" in treating Christine's emotional lability addressed those factors that predisposed her to bouts of crying. What in Christine's life made her susceptible to the negative mood swings and emotional lability? The speech-language pathologist concluded that the primary predisposing factor was Christine's brain damage, which they could do nothing to change. The good news about the predisposing factor was spontaneous recovery. Most patients naturally recover abilities and functions lost or impaired by the stroke. According to the speech-language pathologist, Christine would likely become less predisposed to crying episodes as time passed. However, other general factors may predispose her to crying such as not sleeping well, stress, lack of exercise, and poor diet. Although these general factors were hard to control, Darrel, Alan, and the speech-language pathologist agreed that Christine needed plenty of sleep, reduced stress, more exercise, and a healthy diet. They would do what they could to effect these positive changes in Christine's life.

The second "P" in the treatment equation concerned the precipitants of emotional lability. What environmental or thought "triggers" set off the bouts of crying? In Christine's case, certain words and images were the primary precipitants of crying. Emotional images, such as the sight of her twin grandchildren, would trigger the crying behavior. Additionally, certain words when spoken by others or by Christine herself would cause the crying. Words such as "stroke," "nursing home," "paralysis," and "grandchildren" would spark the bouts of crying. While Darrel, Alan, and the speech-language pathologist agreed that completely avoiding these emotional sights and words was impractical, they would be sensitive to these emotional triggers and gradually expose Christine to them.

The third "P" addressed in the treatment of Christine's emotional lability was the perpetuating factors. What caused the crying jags to continue for so long and what could be done to reduce the severity and duration of the episodes? Christine gave important information about reducing the length and severity of the emotional lability. She noted that, while she was crying, if she directed her attention to a positive or neutral image, the crying subsided. Consequently, during some of her crying spells, Darrel, Alan, and the speech-language pathologist encouraged her to look out of a window, stare at a painting or picture, or to shift her attention to a pet or another neutral or positive image. Through trial and error, it was found that shifting attention in such a manner reduced not only the severity of the crying, but also how long it lasted.

Addressing the predisposing, precipitating, and perpetuating factors of emotional lability ultimately was successful in treating Christine's bouts of crying. By minimizing the predisposing factors, doing away with as many precipitants as possible, and reducing the perpetuating components associated with Christine's emotional lability, she ultimately could control and manage her crying spells, and without medication. Certainly, spontaneous recovery was involved in her improved emotional responses, but the "Three P" therapy also played an important part.

Stroke Survivor "Allison" and Husband "Stephen"

Homonymous Hemianopsia and Visual Neglect

Read pages 67–68 for a discussion of visual field deficits.

Allison has always been a beautiful woman, and according to her husband Stephen, far too young to have suffered a stroke. Her face, with its high cheekbones, perfect nose, and full lips, is adorned by flowing, jet-black hair. Allison's remarkably large eyes, topped by perfectly sculpted eyebrows, contrast beautifully with her alabaster skin. It was not unusual for men to stare at this vision of loveliness, but seeing how she had applied makeup only to the left side of her face brought a startled look from Stephen and others in the occupational therapy room. According to her neurologist, Allison's stroke affected the vision centers of her brain, and resulted in visual field deficits, a type of cortical blindness. The medical label for the blindness in the right sides of both eyes is "right homonymous hemianopsia" and the failure to attend to that part of her visual field is "right visual neglect."

That same day, Stephen was twice more made painfully aware of her visual field deficit and neglect. Most patients eat in the large rehabilitation dining room with the help of their family members and friends. Rehabilitation patients are encouraged to eat in the dining room to enjoy the socialization, rather than having solitary meals in their rooms. Stephen sat to Allison's left side as food service aides distributed the meals. Although hospital food has a poor reputation, at this rehabilitation facility, the meals are really quite tasty. A plate with mashed potatoes, peas, and meat loaf thoroughly drenched in gravy was placed in front of Allison. Coffee, water, napkins, and utensils were also placed in their proper places. Allison began eating with gusto, and when she was done with the meal, it was as if there were an imaginary line drawn from the top to the bottom of the plate. Only the potatoes, peas, and meat loaf on the left side of the plate had been consumed. In addition, Allison did not touch the coffee because it was on the right side of the table. Allison showed no concern for the unusual behavior and appeared oblivious that only half of the meal had been eaten.

After dinner, Stephen wheeled Allison back to her hospital room and helped her into bed. As she lay on her back, Stephen began talking to her. He stood on the left side of the room and spoke of their son's new job. Allison listened intently to Stephen. Then, Stephen casually walked to the right side of the room to arrange flowers on the bed stand, and Allison followed him with her large eyes. As Stephen crossed the middle of the room and entered Allison's right visual field, she stopped visually tracking him. Her eyes would not move past the midline of her body to the right side of the room. She did not turn her head to compensate for the blindness and seemed to disengage from the conversation. When Stephen entered her right visual field, it was as if he no longer existed. For Stephen, the strange events of the day, the makeup, meal, and now Allison's inability to attend to him when he was on the right side of her visual field was just too much. He went to the nursing station and asked the speech-language pathologist who was writing notes in a chart if she had a few moments. Stephen needed to know more about Allison's strange behavior and whether she would return to normal. Most important, Stephen wanted to know what could be done to improve Allison's visual acuity and awareness.

The speech-language pathologist told Stephen that she was already working on the visual field deficits. Allison's vision problems were also affecting her abilities to read and write. When a written page was placed in front of her, and she was asked to read it, Allison would read only one-half of the words. Like the imaginary line drawn from the top to the bottom of the plate during mealtime, a border separated the right and left sides of the page. Allison was oblivious to the words on the right side of the page. When writing, Allison also did not violate the imaginary line; she would write only to the middle of the page. The speech-language pathologist told Stephen that she was encouraging Allison to "cross midline" during reading and writing exercises. Stephen asked the speech-language pathologist why Allison refused to acknowledge the right side of her world.

According to the speech-language pathologist, a partial psychological explanation for Allison's avoidance of her right visual world involves the coping mechanism of avoidance. Allison avoided looking to the right affected side of her visual field because that is where negative and threatening things have happened to her. The right side of Allison's body was paralyzed, and by avoiding looking in that direction, she maintained psychological wholeness and integrity. Although her blindness was completely the result of the brain damage, Allison's neglect was, at least partially, psychological.

The next morning, Allison, Stephen, and the speech-language pathologist began an intensive program for the homonymous hemianopsia and visual neglect. After Allison was placed in her wheelchair by the nursing aides, the therapist and Stephen began transporting her to the therapy suite. Actually, therapy began with transportation as they took their time and slowly moved through the long hospital corridors. Stephen walked in front of Allison and to her right. He would capture her attention and then point to an object or structure in her right field of vision. The speech-language pathologist would gradually turn the wheelchair to the right until Allison would attend to the object or structure. When she made eye contact with it, both the therapist and Stephen praised her for visually crossing midline. Variations of this activity were the primary therapies for Allison's homonymous hemianopsia and visual neglect. Psychologically, the most important ingredient to the therapy was for Allison to feel comfortable and secure when prompted to cross midline and that praise and support be given for her confronting the visual field deficit.

Over the next few weeks, Allison learned to cross visual midline and to attend to people and things in the right side of her world. Through gradual steps during eating, applying makeup, reading, writing, and during transport, Allison eventually learned to confront her fears. Her compensating for the blindness by crossing visual midline was done, in no small measure, because of the support and encouragement of Stephen and the speech-language pathologist.

Grandfather "Earnest" and his Extended Family*

Religious Healing Ceremony

Read Chapter 7 for a discussion of stroke and depression.

There is no shortage of missionaries on the Navajo Indian Reservation, and they can be very persuasive. Many of Earnest's clan converted to Christian religions of various denominations, and it seemed fewer and fewer of his people were members of the Native American Church. For Earnest, it was sad that so few people spoke Navajo, lived in hogans, and had a connection to the roots of the noble Diné people with such a remarkable history. He had spent his life on this huge reservation, tending to his herd of sheep, growing maize, and rasing a large family. Even after the death of his wife, Earnest refused to move from his beloved hogan to one of the government tract housing units in Kayenta, Arizona. His traditional hogan, with the door facing magnificent sunrises, sits atop a plateau with a panoramic view of Monument Valley and the commanding red rock formations. Earnest was a traditional Navajo and proud of it. At 77 years of age, Earnest prided himself on being a hard worker and a fine carpenter. One day while helping a relative shingle a tool shed, Earnest suffered a stroke. He was rushed to Farmington, New Mexico, where doctors stopped the bleeding inside his brain and saved his life. The stroke caused aphasia and weakness on the right side of his body. After three weeks in the rehabilitation unit, Earnest's family arranged a healing ceremony and obtained a weekend pass from the hospital. The miracle of modern medicine would be supplemented by the Peyote Way.

It was challenging for the English-speaking examiner to evaluate Earnest's aphasia. There are very few Navajo speech-language pathologists, and even fewer who are bilingual, so the evaluation session required an interpreter. During the evaluation, Earnest was cooperative, polite, and in true traditional Diné way, soft-spoken, lacking of eye contact, and several times, he would gesture by using his lips and chin to show the general location of an object. His youngest daughter, a student at Diné College, was fluent in Navajo and English. However, during the evaluation, it was necessary to adjust the assessment protocol to adapt to the unique

---

*(What is reported here does not divulge sacred rites of the Native American Church. Permissions were obtained for a nonmember observer, and there was a representative from tribal government present to ensure appropriate witnessing of the ceremony.)

nature of the Navajo language. For example, when testing for wordfinding problems, the examiner would ask Earnest to look at several photographs and provide the names of relatives, expecting the interpreter to say, "He said that was "Robert" or "Lucy" or "Ruby." However, the interpreter explained that Earnest would say their relationship in the family or clan, rather than their names, a common way for traditional Navajos to refer to relatives. Another adjustment had to be made for the tonal nature of Navajo because it appeared that Earnest was stuck saying a grandchild's name. When shown a picture of one grandchild, he appeared to be repeating the same name immediately after being shown a picture of another child. The interpreter noted that their names were very similar, and it was primarily the pitch rise and fall on the final vowels of their names that signaled different children. Earnest appeared to benefit from therapies, but there was heavy reliance on the interpreter who attended each session. There were inherent difficulties in quantifying gains and structuring treatment because of the language issues. For Earnest, one of the worst aspects of the stroke was depression; he was clearly clinically depressed.

The Navajo Indian Reservation extends into Arizona, New Mexico, and Utah, and the Peyote Healing Ceremony was held in a remote region of its eastern border. It is called the "checkerboard area" because private and reservation lands appear checked on a map. The large eight-sided wood hogan with its door facing the east easily accommodated the churchgoers and the all-night ceremony. Earnest eagerly anticipated the religious service, and when the time came, he sat at a place of honor in front of the congregation.

When the church members entered the hogan, they walked around the interior in a clockwise manner, symbolizing a person's travel from birth to death. They greeted Earnest and sat cross-legged in a circle on blankets or sheepskins. The "healing way" ceremony lasted for nearly 14 hours with a wood stove providing heat for the 24 churchgoers. Coals were taken from the wood stove and placed on the ground, and throughout the ceremony, cedar chips were placed on them to produce the sweet-smelling smoke that served as a purifying agent. The services were conducted in Navajo by a special medicine man, a "Roadman," holding high esteem in the community. At the beginning of the ceremony the Roadman explained the purpose of the ceremony. He said that Earnest's communication disorder was caused by him falling out of harmony with nature.

On the floor of the hogan, a mound of dirt was formed into a quarter-circle, representing Earnest's life travel and called a "moon circle." A peyote cactus button was placed on the moon circle and represented his place on the road of life. The peyote used by the participants in the ceremony was provided as a powder and placed in a tea. The container of peyote tea was placed next to the moon circle and was taken by the church members four or five times during the ceremony. The use of the peyote cactus among some Navajo Indians is an important element to their religious and healing beliefs. The drug mescaline, a stimulant and hallucinogenic, is derived from peyote, and is associated with taking God into the body. To believers, peyote helps transform them into a state of physical, mental, and spiritual well-being and helps make the Great Spirit and other supernatural forces more apparent.

During the service, prayers sung in Navajo were offered by members of the Church and directed at the Great Spirit and lesser Gods for the benefit of the patient. The idea was to coax them into helping Earnest again become one with nature and to cure his illness. Hand-rolled tobacco-mix cigarettes were used as a medium in which the words were conveyed by the smoke to the Great Spirit. A flute was used to signal to the Gods that prayers were forthcoming, and there was singing of traditional Native American songs accompanied by the rhythmic beat of several drums and rattles. Church members sang in perfect harmony. The prayers were sincere efforts by Earnest's friends and family to persuade the Great Spirit to help him. That cold winter night in a remote region of the Navajo Indian Reservation, the ancient songs, rattles and flutes, drum beats, and prayers resonated throughout the enchanting high desert plateau, and Earnest basked in the traditional Navajo way. The ceremony ended at sunrise with the congregation singing the beautiful "Morning Song." For breakfast, several large bowls of traditional Navajo food were served communal style to the members. As the faithful left for their homes, Earnest and his family thanked them for their attendance and bid them farewell.

As with all religious customs and rituals, it was difficult objectively to assess the result of the Peyote Healing Ceremony on the patient's speech and language abilities. At the conclusion of the ceremony, there was no demonstrable improvement in his communication abilities. However, there was a dramatic change in Earnest's adjustment to the aphasia. He was much more positive about his illness, and the depression he was experiencing appeared to lift. Monday, Earnest returned to the rehabilitation unit and continued the therapies.

Multiple Stroke Survivor "Verne" and Wife "Nancy"

Memory Problems and Higher Level Mental Processing Deficits

Read pages 77–84 for a discussion of memory loss and problems learning new information.
Verne and Nancy married late in life. Verne was 84 when his wife of 64 years died an awful death from Alzheimer's disease. Nancy, three years younger than Verne, lost her longtime husband to a heart attack 10 years earlier. Six weeks after the death of Verne's wife, they were married in a small ceremony. At the wedding, Nancy confided to her sons and daughter that since the death of their father, her life

was empty and she looked forward to sharing the twilight years with Verne. Besides, she said, "I need someone to care for." After a brief honeymoon, Verne and Nancy began life anew.

Both Verne and Nancy were born on farms and spent their lives tending to cattle, horses, and sheep, and working the good earth. Perhaps, it was the hard outdoor work, healthy farm living habits, or just the luck of the draw, but Verne and Nancy began their life together in good physical and mental health. Both strong-willed and fiercely independent, the not-so-young newlyweds divided their time between their Idaho farm homes in the summer and an Arizona vacation home in the winter. Together, they had four years of wedded bliss, and then several strokes challenged their independence and self-reliance.

The drive from summer Idaho to winter Arizona is about 700 miles, and during the first four years, Verne and Nancy gladly drove the distance. Despite the pleading of their children not to set off by themselves, offers to drive them, and comments that they would enjoy the commercial airline flight much more, the two octogenarians insisted on doing the driving themselves. Their children were understandably concerned about their safety and the safety of others on the road. Nevertheless, for Verne and Nancy, the Idaho-Arizona road trip was symbolic; it represented their independence and life together. No amount of coaxing, cajoling, and concern would change their minds.

One day while they were in Arizona, Verne fell in the shower. All was normal for Nancy that Sunday morning until she noticed that Verne's shower was taking too long. She went to the bathroom and saw him lying on the floor. With some help from Nancy, he could get up, dress, and go to the dining room for breakfast. At the table, Nancy began to suspect that Verne's fall was caused by more than slippery soap. The right side of Verne's face sagged, and he had difficulty lifting his right hand. When he spoke, his speech was slurred. When Nancy could understand his speech sounds, the words were inappropriate. For example, when he wanted the sugar passed to him, he ask: "Fast pepper." After breakfast, Nancy had to help him to his favorite chair and noticed that he had "wet himself." It was then that Nancy called 9-1-1. Verne had always hated hospitals, and at first, refused to get into the ambulance. However, with pleading from Nancy, he finally consented. That evening, Verne returned home with the diagnosis that he had suffered two strokes in the past, and that day, he had likely experienced a ministroke. Although the doctors at the hospital wanted to keep him there for further study, he insisted on returning home: "I do not want to die in a hospital." Over the next few weeks, Verne improved but remained frail and needed assistance walking. Nevertheless, Nancy feared it was Verne's deteriorating memory and mental abilities that were likely going to end their life together.

Recently, Verne's significant hearing loss had gotten worse. Years of tractor-work on the farm had taken a toll on his hearing. The likely cause of the hearing loss was the haybaler. Perhaps the most noisy contraption on the farm, this machine lifts rows of alfalfa into chomping and compressing jaws, ties knots of thick twine around the bales, and spits them out in neat rows. When baling hay, the noise can be deafening. Since the ministroke, Verne had refused to wear his hearing aids. Apparently, either the way they felt in Verne's ears or the way they amplified room noise was irritating. Also, since the ministroke, Verne had lost some of his recent memories, although distant past recollections remained intact. He also had difficulty following instructions. Of course, it was difficult to tell whether his problems following simple instructions were a result of the hearing loss or the ministroke. What was most distressing for Nancy and Verne's family was his confusion. Verne would get lost easily, sometimes in very familiar places. As summer approached with the scheduled return to Idaho, Verne and Nancy's family discussed the options. They reached an agreement that it would be best for all if Verne were placed in a nursing home. With Nancy's deteriorating health, nursing home placement seemed like a logical thing to do. When Nancy was told of the decision, she stated with firm resolve: "He is not going to a home while I am still alive."

People do not realize how difficult it is for children of elderly parents to properly care for them. A lifetime of respecting and obeying parents makes defying their wishes a very difficult proposition. Clearly, given Verne and Nancy's ages, and the obstacles they faced, a nursing home would give Verne the best care. And continuing the Arizona-Idaho car trips was out of the question. But what to do? Nancy was adamant that Verne was not to go to a nursing home and that she would care for him.

"Where there is a will there is a way" and after weeks of telephone conferences, meetings, and e-mails, Verne and Nancy's sons and daughters agreed to respect their parents' wishes. It was unanimously agreed that continued driving was dangerous, so their cars were disabled. This was met with anger and disapproval from both Verne and Nancy, but their safety, and the safety of others, was nonnegotiable. Family members would drive them to and from their Idaho and Arizona homes. A visiting nurse was hired to daily help them with cooking, dressing, and other daily living activities. Family members and neighbors arranged schedules where they would check on them regularly.

When dealing with these types of issues, often there is not a clear-cut decision that would be best for all concerned. Verne and Nancy's family decided to respect their parents' wishes. Much like Verne and Nancy had been with their children decades ago, their sons and daughters placed love and family highest on their list of life's priorities. Certainly, all involved faced a future of hard realities, but they would meet them with courage and determination.

Stroke Survivor "Joan" and Husband "Carl"

Post-Stroke Clinical Depression-Anxiety Disorder

Read Chapters 7 and 8 for a discussion of stroke-related depression and anxiety disorders.

Joan's reason for pursuing a psychology degree and becoming a clinical psychologist was partially to understand her own bouts of depression. They started in her teenage years and, as she learned in graduate school, are more common in women than men. She also learned that depression and anxiety go hand-in-hand in many persons. During Joan's career, she helped hundreds of patients navigate through their depression. She was a good clinical psychologist, a great listener, and it was sadly ironic that after she suffered her stroke, she fell into a deep state of depression and anxiety. Even worse, the stroke took her ability to express herself; she could tell no one about the dark cavern of despair into which she had fallen. Joan cried easily, was listless, lethargic, and sometimes agitated. Her face showed the depth of the psychological pain. Fortunately her husband, Carl, saw the nonverbal signs and symptoms of the affective disorder and became proactive in dealing with it. Two weeks after the stroke, he requested a psychiatric consultation. After the psychiatric examination was complete, the doctor sat down with Carl and discussed the results and recommendations.

According to the psychiatrist, diagnosing depression-anxiety in patients with severe aphasia is difficult and far from an exact determination. Their communication disorders interfere with, or in Joan's case, completely eliminate the ability to report thoughts and feelings. Consequently, mental health professionals heavily rely on friends and families for insights into what the patient is likely experiencing emotionally. Carl was surprised to learn that depression is the "common cold" of mental illness; about 10 percent of the population get clinically depressed every year. The doctor gave Carl a quick rundown on what is known about stroke-related depression-anxiety.

According to the psychiatrist, the depression-anxiety in most stroke survivors is not appreciably different from the types of mental health problems seen in persons without brain damage. Studies have shown that depression and anxiety in stroke survivors are similar to the psychiatric disorders seen in persons who do not have brain damage. However, it has been found that patients with larger areas of brain damage do not suffer from depression and anxiety as much as those with less brain damage. Additionally, 50% of all stroke survivors will have depression-anxiety that is long lasting. Joan's stroke caused brain damage that is relatively small but in an important area for expressive communication purposes.

The psychiatrist explained that the site of the brain damage plays a role in whether a patient will have depression-anxiety and how severe it will be. If the stroke occurs in the right hemisphere of the brain, patients are more likely to have the opposite of depression-anxiety, for example, apathy, cheerfulness, or even euphoria. Joan's stroke was on the left side of her brain, and in the frontal lobe, giving depression-anxiety a 70 percent probability of occurring. For reasons the doctor could not explain, many more women than men suffer these types of strokes.

Given what was known about Joan's stroke, the psychiatrist said that a firm diagnosis could not be given that she was clinically depressed and anxious. However, in these types of cases, it is better to assume the patient is suffering from depression-anxiety than to believe otherwise. With the current knowledge about depression and anxiety disorders, unnecessary suffering can be prevented for many stroke survivors. With that said, the doctor outlined a course of treatment for Joan's depression-anxiety.

The doctor immediately placed Joan on an antidepressant. There are several types of antidepressants used to readjust the brain's chemistry. The type of antidepressant prescribed to Joan caused an increase in a particular chemical in the brain by slowing its natural elimination. This medication would also help with Joan's anxiety. While all drugs have side effects, the new generations of antidepressants have very few of them. However, Joan would be watched carefully for signs that she was reacting negatively to the drug therapy. Unfortunately, it would take several days and possibly weeks for her to feel the full effects of the medication. The doctor told Carl that while antidepressants are modern miracle drugs, they are not a quick fix for Joan's depression-anxiety. Joan's stress levels also needed to be addressed.

The role excessive and prolonged stress plays in depression-anxiety has long been known. People who experience high levels of stress for long periods are vulnerable to depression-anxiety. Even positive stress like marriage, moving to a new city, or a job promotion can cause depression. Negative stress such as the loss of a job, death in the family, and illness are linked to depression. According to the doctor, Joan's stroke, hospitalization, and her physical problems are all major stressors. One of Joan's biggest stressors is the frustrating type of communication disorder she suffered. Joan has a "nonfluent" type of aphasia, meaning it is frustrating. Frustration leads to anger, and anger that is inner directed can, over time, cause depression. In Joan's case, the frustration and anger are likely turned inward because she cannot express her thoughts and feelings.

In nonfluent aphasia, the patient has trouble remembering names for expression. A frustrating aspect of nonfluent aphasia is the "tip-of-the-tongue phenomenon." As the label suggests, it is having trouble remembering the name of something or someone; there is a "sense of knowing" but the word still cannot be recalled. Another frustrating aspect of nonfluent aphasia is "apraxia of speech." In apraxia of speech, the patient has trouble getting her tongue, lips, and other speech structures to say the word. In her mind, Joan knows the word she wants to say but cannot say it or mispronounces it. Because the stroke did not damage her understanding centers, Joan knows when she makes a mistake and she struggles to correct it. Unfortunately, with apraxia of speech, the harder she tries to correct the mistake, the more difficult it is to speak. Having problems remembering and pronouncing words are major sources of stress for the stroke survivor.

Being out of control is also stressful. A stroke survivor with nonfluent aphasia has verbal impotence. Two types of verbal impotence occur in expressive aphasia. First, not being able to move speech muscles voluntarily is a form of verbal impotence. Many times, when Joan tries to create a speech sound or to utter a word, her speech muscles will not move properly or at all. Second, being unable to stop a muscle from moving is a type of verbal impotence. Often when Joan would attempt to speak, her speech muscles would go to the wrong position, and she would be unable to stop the movement. An even more disturbing aspect of verbal impotence is "automatic speech," which often occurs in expressive aphasia. When Joan voluntarily and purposefully tries to say something, she often cannot speak. However, when no forethought is given to what she wants to say, she sometimes can automatically say certain words and even phrases. This vast difference in speech production abilities can be puzzling and distressing for aphasic patients. And of course, because swear words are often said automatically, they spring from Joan's mouth easily. According to Carl, the automatic cursing is especially distressing for Joan because she was never a vulgar or crude person. Not being able to perform a body function that in the past was done easily and automatically is threatening to a person's sense of self and wholeness. Verbal impotence is stressful, interferes with a sense of well-being, and casts a depressive cloud over normal living.

One way of reducing the speech-related stress for Joan, and to help combat her depression-anxiety, was to create an environment where perfect or normal speech is not expected. Joan, always a hard worker and someone who confronted her problems head-on, spent much of her time struggling to remember names and to get her speech mechanism to work properly. She constantly had words "on the tip of her tongue," and when she could recall them, fought to say them. Not only was expressive aphasia stressful for Joan; it was also distressful for listeners. There was always tension in the room. Conversations with Joan frequently became awkward games of charades.

To reduce the constant speaker stress, all listeners communicated to Joan both verbally and nonverbally that they did not expect perfect and normal speech. Joan's visitors created a relaxed, comfortable environment where simply being with her and sharing time together was most important. When Joan obviously wanted to say something important, and was unable to do so, listeners communicated that they would come back to it later; it was not a big deal that she could not talk now. The speech-language pathologists also created a nondemanding type of speaking environment and taught Joan how to relax. Interestingly, reducing Joan's speaking anxiety had a positive effect on her ability to speak. Because speech was less purposeful and voluntary, and Joan was relaxed, she recalled words more easily and was more successful when trying to say them.

Three weeks after the psychiatric consultation, Joan was well on the long road to recovery. Eventually, she could have basic communication with loved ones and bask in the nonverbal companionship. What was most important, Joan's depression lifted. She had a positive attitude about rehabilitation and what the future had to offer. Although Joan did not make a complete recovery from the stroke, over time, she learned to live with the speech and physical limitations it caused without clinical depression-anxiety.

Stroke Victor "LeRoy"

Acceptance

Read Chapter 10 for a discussion of loss, grief, and accepting unwanted change.

For LeRoy, the *Serenity Prayer* said it all: "God grant us the serenity to accept the things we cannot change, courage to change the things we can, and wisdom to know the difference." Never one to sidestep a challenge, LeRoy confronted his massive stroke straight on. His courage, determination, and hard work following the stroke were an inspiration to all. LeRoy's life as a minister and his faith in God had prepared him for life's challenges, and this medical setback was to be no exception. The congregation of the small church expected nothing less of him. LeRoy would be victorious over this stroke.

"Global Aphasia" was listed on LeRoy's chart and defined him for all who read it. Other labels for his stroke-related communication disorder include "Irreversible Aphasia" and "Severe Expressive-Receptive Aphasia." The massive stroke had caused severe damage to the major speech and language centers of the left hemisphere of his brain. LeRoy's communication disorder cut across the board. Other than occasionally being able to say "Uh" and "Kayla," he could neither speak, read, write, nor understand the words spoken by others. Although LeRoy could use and understand simple gestures, elaborate use of them for communication was beyond his capabilities. For a minister whose life revolved around the spoken and written word, aphasia had landed a devastating blow. The stroke had ravaged LeRoy's commanding power of language and isolated this kind, caring preacher man from his loving congregation.

At first, LeRoy denied all that had happened to him. Although the denial was not complete or present all of the time, this psychological defense was God's way of easing the shock of it all. In denial, there were minutes where LeRoy was oblivious to what the stroke had taken from him. Denial buffeted the pain of separation caused by the communication disorder. Denial made LeRoy believe the medical problem was minor and temporary. Denial was like a protective door allowing the reality of the massive stroke to enter his mind when the time was right. Thank God for denial.

As time passed, denial gradually dissolved and anger reared its ugly head. LeRoy, who was a kind person by nature, found himself angry with the whole situation. He was angry that he could no longer talk, walk, or dress himself. It angered him that his life had changed so dramatically, and without time to prepare. What was most disturbing to LeRoy was that he found himself angry with God for letting the stroke happen in the first place.

The frustration that led to his anger also caused LeRoy to bargain. Though he could not put his thoughts into words, at some level, LeRoy bargained with himself, the rehabilitation staff, and God. If he mustered his strength and determination, he bargained, he could prevail over the stroke. If he worked hard in the therapies, he would be fully rehabilitated. If LeRoy recovered, he promised, he would be a better servant to God.

For LeRoy, the denial, anger, and bargaining were attempts to overcome the losses caused by the stroke. His mind was still working out the reality of the situation; he was trying to decide if the losses were real and permanent. What is most important, LeRoy was trying to overcome the stroke and the disabilities it caused. Denial, anger, and bargaining were all natural psychological reactions most people have to these types of things. As long as they were appropriate in degree and duration, these psychological defenses were positive coping mechanisms used by people to adjust to unwanted change. During these attempts to overcome his losses, LeRoy, like most stroke survivors, did not slide smoothly through the steps to acceptance. Sometimes he was angry or bargaining, and other times he returned to denial. LeRoy occasionally backslid psychologically.

When denial had run its course, the anger had subsided, and there were no more bargains to be struck, LeRoy slipped into a deep grieving depression. The grieving depression was not the result of LeRoy's brain chemistry gone awry. It was knowing that he was permanently separated from people, abilities, and things that he had loved so dearly. Sadly, it was during grieving depression that LeRoy felt the full value of that which the stroke had taken. He felt depressed at the loss of his physical abilities, many of which he had taken for granted. Simple physical acts of getting out of bed and walking were now beyond his reach. Symbolically, this once-independent man of God could not even stand on his own two feet.

Also gone was LeRoy's calling in life. The stroke had taken his God-given ability to communicate with his parishioners. When his parishioners would visit, the previously rich verbal exchange was now relegated to nonverbal awkwardness. Gone were the compassionate discussions about right and wrong, love and hate, good and bad, saints and sinners, and the meaning of it all. Gone was the spiritual rush of turning faith into action. Gone was the comfort of words that calmed the restless soul and elevated the spirit. LeRoy also desperately missed the trappings of his religion. The church, altar, sacrament, sights, smells, and sounds of his religion were now only memories of a better past. But by far, the most grievous loss LeRoy suffered was the inability to pray. The devil stroke had taken the intimate words shared by this man and his God. As LeRoy lay on his back staring at the cold, sterile ceiling of his nursing home room, he sank into the depth of despair. Hopelessness and helplessness saturated his heart and soul. He could find no consolation in knowing that humans are no strangers to grief; loss of all the worldly treasures has been around since Adam and Eve. It is a cross for all to bear.

As time passed, the grieving depression gradually subsided. At first, hours would pass without the deep sense of loss, and later, days and weeks of glorious acceptance came into LeRoy's life. It was not than LeRoy was resigned to his fate for resignation is nothing more than tolerance of adversity. In acceptance, LeRoy realized that his losses were a part of God's grand plan. Several months after his stroke, LeRoy finally realized that God had not forsaken him. In acceptance, LeRoy basked in the pleasure of knowing that he once was the recipient of God's wonderful gifts, rather than being depressed by the loss of them.

To some, the stroke LeRoy suffered and the losses it caused were the devil's work: vicious, brutal, and so unfair. This servant of God had spent his life doing good, and with one fell swoop, the stroke had taken away all that was important to him. Some may say that LeRoy was a stroke "victim" and that evil had prevailed. Some people may believe that stroke and communication disorders are punishment for past sins. Some people are shortsighted about these things. But, LeRoy's life was the totality of his experiences. The bond between him and his maker was far too strong to be destroyed by mere brain damage. LeRoy's acceptance of the unacceptable has truly made him a stroke "victor."

The Silent Tongue (aphasia)

by
Kathleen Gerety, R.N.

The words you do not hear the tears you cannot see
Are hidden within my nucleus, this is my new identity
I am alike dry earth, shriveled and worn
With no nurturing to the soul
And I am quite helpless, in my world no longer whole.

So bear with me and try to creep inside this silent tent
My ills have bereaved my spirit
My soul is discontent.

Please do not look at me . . . as if I am not here
Please do not speak to me . . . as if I cannot hear
Although I can't express myself with this muted speech of mine
My needs are very important it's difficult to define.
Please be polite and patient . . . maintain my dignity
My mind is tired and weary with this disability
I sit in silence in my room I cannot say "Good Morning Sun"
The words are tangled in my mind
Like twisted branches on a vine.

Those who speak in silence have a fervor
We . . . Who talk so freely don't understand or know
Take a walk into a garden, see the flowers row on row
Their colors are bright, their life is sweet
And we hear words of passion in the *silent way* they speak.

Murphy's Inner World of Aphasia: "Beth's Story"

On this dark interstate highway, losing yourself in thoughts of roads not taken is so easy. The ever-present engine purr, whine of steel-belted tires meeting pavement, and the monotony of roadside reflectors sculpt thoughts of long-forgotten days of yore. As Beth drives the Bounder through the dark expanse of southern Arizona, she knows that decisions she made so many years ago mattered. With Murphy sound asleep in the back of the motor home, Beth recalls the lines of a Robert Frost poem she was forced to learn when she was a young school girl:

Two roads diverged in a yellow wood,
And sorry I could not travel both
And be one traveler, long I stood
And looked down one as far as I could
To where it bent in the undergrowth;

When Murph asked for her hand in marriage, he promised that life with him would never be boring, a vow that has turned out to be an understatement. Modestly, even to herself, Beth admits that there were more handsome, more sophisticated, more polished men vying for her hand, but Murph's cockiness and promise of a lifetime of excitement tipped the marriage equation in his favor. The stroke and aphasia he suffered so many months ago are proving to be the biggest challenge yet, and yes, life is far from boring.

As the motor home purrs through the empty night, Beth realizes that the guilt she felt about Murphy's stroke no longer tugs at her conscience. She finally knows, on that important emotional level, that she is not responsible for the plug of something or other that blocked the blood flow to his brain. Strokes happen, and as Dr. Foster said, perhaps nothing could have been done to prevent this life-changing event. Murphy suffered from high blood pressure for several years, but he was exercising, eating better, and religiously taking his medication. Besides, the stroke was not a burst blood vessel that high blood pressure often causes; it was an obstruction. Sadly for Beth, Murphy, the children and grandchildren, the plug was in the left side of his brain, and it deprived blood to the all-important speech and language centers. As so often happens with strokes affecting speech and language, Murph's right side is also weak; but with the assistance of a quad cane, he can slowly get around. A green freeway sign passing overhead shows that the next gas station is 50 miles yonder, and Beth checks the fuel gauge. Relieved that it shows more than half a tank of expensive gasoline remaining, her thoughts briefly return to that terrible morning when Murphy collapsed into the bedroom dresser, knocking the family pictures to the floor. Curiously, she recalls that her first concern was for the broken glass and the potential of cuts, as her mind tried to process the terrible event that was unfolding before her eyes.

As Beth continues down the road of remembrance, she thinks of her life with Murphy as divided by that disastrous night: before and after aphasia. Certainly, before aphasia, life with Murph was not a cakewalk, and neither was it always an uphill climb. Their early years were full of the stressors all young couples experience as roles, responsibilities, and routines are established. Back then, people married for life, and Beth and Murphy needed time to establish the rules of the lifelong partnership. Beth was thankful that Murphy was a communicator; he was never one to hide from her and life in a beer bottle or a televised baseball game. Murphy, at least before the stroke, was not a speechless spectator on life's journey. Although not always pleasant, their communication was open, fair, and giving, and what is most important, they both knew how to listen. The war separated them physically for a time, but they were never far removed from each other's thoughts. Beth never told Murph she kept every war letter in a secret cranny in the very bedroom dresser where the aphasia began. During the worst of times in their relationship, she would often read them, silently and alone in the sanctuary of their bedroom, as if those letters were an antidote to the poison threatening their marriage.

They say married couples argue about three things: children, money, and sex. The birth of their children, Matt and Michelle, brought more responsibilities and Murphy and Beth rallied to the occasions. Especially when the children were young, Murphy rarely questioned Beth's rearing habits. When he disagreed, he did so privately and discreetly. Beth feels blessed that both children were really no more trouble than most, and even during the trying teenage years, home life was usually tolerable. Looking back, she realizes just how rich their home was in communication. The bantering, arguing, laughing, crying, planning, and even the shouting embodied the energy of their family. And the "Love ya" farewells, so naturally uttered as children ran for the school bus, expressed the depth of it all. Communication with the children gradually matured as they grew into young adults. Beth and Murph's directing and protective assertions diminished as the children came of age, and they welcomed Matt and Michelle as adults in the relationship. Beth and Murphy's communication also evolved with fewer unnecessary words spoken, relying more on mental telepathy to anticipate everything from romance to the passing of a saltshaker. When brainstorming, they appreciated the importance of throughly considering an idea without prematurely dismissing it. "Let's run it up the flagpole and see if anyone salutes it" was a common cliché they used when exploring options. Aphasia has now reduced their rich communication to the basics, and it has been many months since Murph has been able to express himself about the important things in life. Beth fancies the harvest moon hanging from the rural Arizona sky and the scent of farmers' crops being readied for market. She pilots the huge recreational machine with confidence and skill while Murphy sleeps quietly, gently rocked by the continuous sway of their temporary home on wheels.

Beth wonders if any couple, other than the suffering super-rich with their silver spoons jammed in their mouths, ever have enough money. Beth knows that Murph always felt guilty for the constant lack of money they endured despite her frequent assurances that things were manageable financially. It made matters worse that one of her young suitors had since acquired vast wealth and publicity. Men of Murph's generation took bread-winning seriously, and it didn't matter to Murph's self-esteem that Beth's successful suitor was never a serious factor in the mating equation. The aphasia and the tremendous stroke-related out-of-pocket medical expenses no doubt contributed to Murph's severe clinical depression. Thanks to God, loving family support, therapies, and antidepressants, "happy pills" as the children call them, Murph's spirits have since lifted, at least somewhat. The antidepressants certainly have improved his take on life, but the reality of life after stroke still frequently rears its ugly head. Fortunately, Murph was always an optimist, and even in the depths of his melancholy, Beth could see flickers of his enduring spirit in that silent cavern of despair.

Since Murph's stroke, they have yet to reconnect intimately. They were never a couple to couple incessantly nor did they display public shows of affection, PSAs as their children characterized them, but they shared a closeness no one else needed to know. It was a physical bridge, but the words they whispered were as much of their love as anything physical. Unlike love in the classic movies of the 40s and 50s, seldom did fireworks light up the sky nor did symphonies crescendo to their union. Sadly, since the stroke, Murphy has turned away from Beth's soft caresses, apparently shamed by his stroke-ravaged body. And what truly saddens Beth to this collapse of the intimacy bridge is that, try as she may, she cannot make him understand that he does not repulse her. Beth also understands that on a deeper level, Murph is just not ready to resume that part of his life. Beth has always been patient about these things, and she will wait until the time is right. After all, when she had her disfiguring breast surgery, Murphy had been there until her self-concept and self-esteem could adapt to the loss. It would be wrong to say that ending their physical intimacy is no big deal, but an exaggeration to deem it an insurmountable obstacle. Beth checks the speedometer to be certain that the auto control is keeping the Bounder at the speed limit. For Beth, getting a speeding ticket at her age would be embarrassing and confirm the neighbors' suspicion that the motor home is too much for her to handle. "Nonsense" she retorted at the bon voyage party, "I have driven school buses with much more precious cargo and never dented a fender." Beth knows that she has never been one mindlessly to step to any drummer's beat as she recalls the second stanza of her favorite poem:

> Then took the other, as just as fair,
> And having perhaps the better claim,
> Because it was grassy and wanted wear;
> Though as for that the passing there
> Had worn them really about the same,

Murphy's stroke and aphasia have dramatically changed their marital roles, something Beth admits is not necessarily a bad thing. Before aphasia, Murph took care of negotiating mortgages, bargaining with car dealers, trying to get the best value from appliance salespeople, and obtaining credit cards with the lowest interest rates. Beth took care of the usual day-to-day purchases and gladly deferred to him on the other things, tasks she considered unpleasant. However, six months ago, Beth was thrown into the mix of disagreeable when their old pickup would not start. In the past, few things were more distressing for Beth than questioning a mechanic's claim that expensive car repairs were necessary. Before the aphasia, Murphy fluently spoke the language of grease monkeys and rarely was he gouged by them. At the auto repair shop, Beth was certain she would not fare well when the mechanic droned on and on about the need for wires, plugs, timing belts, regulators, something called an "alternator," and the thousand dollar price tag it all would cost. He was obviously proud of his special vocabulary, and she was told of the needed parts and labor in a manner typical of a physicist explaining nuclear fusion to a preschooler. Beth surmised what pre-aphasic Murphy would do, and she decided to question the need for each part. Soon it became apparent that a new battery would return the pickup to running status. The mechanic, obviously distressed that a woman would have the audacity to question his vast knowledge of things mechanical, cautioned her that it was just a matter of time until the other repairs would be necessary. He reminded her of the breadth and girth of his mechanical prowess. Beth recalls thinking to herself that everything is just a matter of time, and what matters is how people spend their time. She decided that if the pickup became undependable, she would trade it in on a newer one rather than to replace it part-by-expensive-part. The pickup has run just fine since the battery replacement, and Beth smiles when she thinks of driving it from the repair shop, and the mechanic's frown barely hidden beneath grease smudges.

Using a small lever on the armrest of the driver's seat, Beth adjusts the right rearview mirror and reflects that the worst of the aphasia-times happened immediately after Dr. Foster discharged Murph from the rehabilitation center. Murphy was clearly happy to be released from the confines of the cold impersonal institution, and to be embraced by the warm familiarity of his home of 40 years. After the welcome home party, and family and neighbors finally vacated the premises, Beth and Murph sat quietly in the living room. There was an awkwardness to the moment, much like strangers feel on an elevator while making small talk. Murph would occasionally give her that slanted smile she had grown accustomed to in the hospital, and several times he telegraphed shortened utterances Beth could not clearly decipher. He apparently wanted to express something very profound. They danced the dance of aphasia, and in the end, communication failed them. It was an extremely frustrating moment, and for the first time in their relationship, Beth was strangely uncomfortable around Murph. She was not uncomfortable with Murph per se; she was ill at ease with her thoughts about the future and dealing with his disabilities. She sensed that Murph was shamed by his childlike speech. She sensed he shuddered at the thought of another bout of incontinence and the necessity of adult diapers. She sensed that Murph felt diminished as a man and that he dreaded being a lifelong burden. She sensed that Murph feared for the future and would welcome an end to it all. And what disturbed Beth most about this awkwardness was that she sensed Murph might be right. Fortunately, Beth recalls as she passes a lumbering cross-country tractor-trailer truck with an insufficient hill-climbing engine, her appraisal of the situation was unduly pessimistic. She whispers the third stanza of Robert Frost's immortal refrain:

And both that morning equally lay
In leaves no step had trodden black.
Oh, I kept the first for another day!
Yet knowing how way leads on to way,
I doubted if I should ever come back.

The doctors call it spontaneous recovery, and it occurs in most stroke patients. It is the natural tendency of the body to heal itself, and when combined with therapies, many patients improve significantly in their physical and communication abilities. Fortunately, Murphy was one of the lucky ones, and his walking and talking improved over time. His expensive wheelchair is now parked in the guest bedroom, at least for now. Most helpful for Murphy, and millions like him, is the Americans with Disabilities Act. Nowadays, there are plenty of handicapped parking spaces, ramps, and specially constructed elevators and bathrooms. Thanks to that landmark legislation, disabled people are far less handicapped and can continue to participate fully in life despite their limitations. Beth and Murphy have been pleasantly surprised to find that other travelers, for the most part, are also kind and patient with the disabled. Food servers, ticket takers, ushers, and other service people also take the time and have the necessary patience when dealing with Murphy's new life-challenges.

Beth has been careful to walk that fine line between expecting too much and too little of her post-stroke husband. Expecting too much sows the seeds of frustration and failure, and what is even worse, ultimately, are blows to his frail self-esteem. Beth knows Murph is talking as well as he can and that hurrying him, or demanding communication perfection, disrupts the process even more. On the other hand, expecting too little of Murphy condemns him to a lifetime of victimization and promises unrealized. Each day, Beth walks that tenuous fine line.

As Beth returns the Bounder to the right lane, she ponders the decisions she and Murphy have made since aphasia entered their lives. They could have become victims to the stroke and aphasia, given up, and succumbed to the inevitable. Beth could have studied brochures of nursing homes and assisted living centers, and sought relief from her uncommunicative burden. For pessimists, that would certainly be the most sane course of action for a woman her age and her stroke-victim husband. Murph could have refused therapies and resigned himself to the multitude of losses the aphasia hath wrought. After all, everyone knows there comes a time to accept disabilities rather than mindlessly trying to overcome them. The children and grandchildren could have turned back from their aphasic patriarch, the flimsy bridge of communication connecting them, and bid their father and grandfather farewell. They could have heeded the advice of friends and family and gone through with the sale of the Bounder. This marvelous traveling machine could be in the hands of a different couple traveling life's roads. Perhaps, the philosophical mechanic was right; it really is just a matter of time, and the "sooner the better." Then, just perhaps, the mechanic was wrong on both counts.

Beth knows she and Murph were never easy victims; they have always confronted life's challenges with determination and persistence. Unlike so many hapless victims sharing their heartaches on daytime talk shows, proud of their failures and eager to share them with national audiences, Beth and Murph have always stood up to adversity. They never easily retreated when the going got tough. Beth knows that accepting the losses aphasia brought to their lives is different from being resigned to them. Stroke and aphasia are major life events, but at least for Beth and Murphy, they are not sufficient to detour them from enjoying the many roads yet to be traveled in the sunset of their lives. Beth again checks the fuel gauge and realizes that there still is plenty of gasoline to get them to parts unknown. The freeway sign shows a historical detour to a town called "Tombstone" and a daily re-enactment of a gunfight at an OK Corral. The signal light beeps, beeps, beeps as the Bounder exits the well-worn freeway and Beth recites aloud the final stanza of Robert Frost's famous ode to roads not taken:

> *I shall be telling this with a sigh*
> *Somewhere ages and ages hence:*
> *Two roads diverged in a wood, and I—*
> *I took the one less traveled by,*
> *And that has made all the difference.*

Resources

Aphasia Support Group Resources

National Aphasia Association support found at
http://www.aphasia.org/index.php

American/Canadian support group listings found at
http://www.aphasia.org/acg.php

Scotland/Ireland/London support group listings found at
http://www.bbc.co.uk/health/conditions/stroke/usefulcontacts_index.shtml

France, Italy, Australia support group listings found at
http://www.ydac.on.ca/R&p/RP0803_3.html

Aphasia Support Groups and Associations*

Alabama
Aphasia Support Group
Mercy Medical, 101 Villa Dr., Daphne, AL 36526

Arizona
Thunderbird Samaritan Stroke Support Group
Easter Seals Society, Thunderbird Samaritan Hospital, 5555 W. Thunderbird Rd.,
Room 1-B, Glendale, AZ 85306

Ahwatukee Foothills Stroke Support Group
Ahwatukee Foothills Samaritan Health Center, 4530 E. Ray Rd., Phoenix,
AZ 85044

John C. Lincoln Stroke Club
Cowden Center, 9202 N. 2nd St., Phoenix, AZ 85020

The Stroke/Aphasia Via Linda Group
Via Linda Senior Center, 10440 East Via Linda, Scottsdale, AZ 85258-1000

*(Source: National Aphasia Association and the Rehabilitation Institute of Chicago)

Aphasia Support Group
HealthSouth Scottsdale Rehabilitation Hospital, 9630 E. Shea Blvd., Scottsdale, AZ 85260

Stroke Support Group
HealthSouth Scottsdale Rehabilitation Hospital, 9630 E. Shea Blvd., Scottsdale, AZ 85260

Sun Cities Aphasia Group
Easter Seals Society, Sun Health Community Education Center, 13632 N. 99th Ave., Sun City, AZ 85351

Arizona State University Aphasia Groups
Dept. of Speech and Hearing Science, P.O. Box 870102, Arizona State University, Tempe, AZ 85257-0102

Carondelet St. Joseph's Communication Group
St. Joseph's Hospital, 350 N. Wilmot, 4th Floor Rehab Conference Room, Tucson, AZ 85711

University of Arizona Aphasia Groups, Aphasic Clinic, 1131 E. 2nd St., University of Arizona, Tucson, AZ 85721

Arkansas
Stroke Support Group of Northwest Arkansas
St. Mary's Hospital, Rogers, AR 72756

California
Aphasia Community Group
Cedars-Sinai Medical Center, 150 N. Robertson, Beverly Hills, CA 90211

Pat Martin Stroke Support Group of Contra Costa County
Mt. Diablo Medical Center, Concord, CA 94520, or John Muir Medical Center, 1601 Ygnacia Valley Rd., Walnut Creek, CA 94596

Stroke + Head Injury Support Group
Washington Hospital, Washington West, Anderson Auditorium C, 2000 Mowry Ave., Fremont, CA 94538

Communication Recovery Groups
St. Jude Medical Center, 101 E. Valencia Mesa Dr., Fullerton, CA 92835

CSU Hayward Aphasia Group
California University - Hayward, Speech, Language & Hearing Clinic, MB# 1097A, Communicative Sciences and Disorders, Hayward, CA 94542

Interpersonal Skills - Stroke Support Group
College of Marin, Disabled Student Services Program, 835 College Ave., Kentfield, CA 94904

Long Beach V.A. Stroke Group
Long Beach V.A. Medical Center, Speech Pathology (126), 5901 E. 7th St., Long Beach, CA 90822

Stroke/Aphasia Support Group
CA Heights United Methodist Church, 3759 Orange Ave., Long Beach, CA 90807

Aphasia Community Group
Cedars-Sinai Medical Center, South Tower, Rm. CCR A or B, 8700 Beverly Blvd., Los Angeles, CA 90048

Stroke/Aphasia Support Groups-Stroke Association of Southern California
2001 South Darrington Ave., Suite 308, Los Angeles, CA 90025

Veterans Stroke Support Group
VA Outpatient Clinic, Speech Pathology (126), 150 Muir Rd., Martinez, CA 94553

Aphasia/Stroke Support Groups
Newport Language, Speech & Audiology Center, Inc., 26137 La Paz Rd., Suite 104, Mission Viejo, CA 92691-5309

Aphasia Center of California
200 Grand Ave., Oakland, CA 94610
Website: www.aphasiacenter.org

Caregivers Stroke Support Group for Women
Stroke Recovery Center, 2800 E. Alejo Rd., Palm Springs, CA 92262-6253

Sharing & Caring Support Group
Stroke Recovery Center, 2800 E. Alejo Rd., Palm Springs, CA 92262-6253

Peninsula Stroke Association Support Group Network
Peninsula Stroke Association, 3801 Miranda Ave., VAPAHCS, Bldg. 6, Rm. A-162, Palo Alto, CA 94304

YESS (Young Enthusiastic Stroke Survivors)
Sharp Rehab Center, 2999 Health Center Dr., San Diego, CA 92123

Stroke Club, Stonestown Family YMCA
Senior Annex, 3150 20th Ave., San Francisco, CA 94132

Stroke/Communication Group
City College of San Francisco, John Adams Campus, DSPS Dept., 1860 Hayes St., San Francisco, CA 94117. *Note: Must call to register; this is a Group Speech Therapy Course.*

Stroke Support Group
Meets 3rd Friday of month
73 Broad St., San Luis Obispo, CA 93401

Express Yourself
Aphasia Group of Santa Barbara, Santa Barbara Cottage Hospital, Burtness Auditorium, 320 W. Pueblo St., Santa Barbara, CA 93101

The Pathfinders Communication Skills Group
Center for Students with Disabilities, Santa Monica College, 1900 Pico Blvd., Santa Monica, CA 90405

West Contra Costa County Stroke and Aphasia Support Group
Doctors Medical Center, 2000 Vale Rd., San Pablo, CA 94805

Stroke Support Group
HealthSouth Tustin Rehabilitation Hospital, 14851 Yorba St., Tustin, CA 92780

Conejo Valley Stroke Support Group
Los Robles Hospital Outpatient Center, 4415 S. Lakeview Canyon, Westlake Village, CA 91361

Sacramento Valley Peer Counseling, 1013 2nd St., Woodlawn, CA 95695

Colorado
Conversation Groups
Speech Language Hearing Sciences, University of Colorado-Boulder, Campus Box 409, Boulder, CO 80309

Broomfield Stroke Support Group
Broomfield Senior Center
280 Lamar St., Broomfield, CO 80038

Stroke Survivors Support Group of Fremont County
Pueblo Bank & Trust, Canon City, CO 81212

Sky Cliff Center-Stroke Support Group, First United Methodist Church, 4600 Hwy. 86, Castle Rock, CO 80104

Washington Park Aphasia Group, Washington Park Community Center, 809 S. Washington St., Denver, CO 80209

CNI Support Group
Colorado Neurological Institute, 501 E. Hampden Ave., Aspen Room, Englewood, CO 80110

Young Stroke Survivors Group, N. Colorado Therapy Center, 2780 28th Ave., Greeley, CO 80631
(People of all ages are welcome.)

Eagle County Stroke Club
P.O. Box 152, Gypsum, CO 81637

Young Stroke Survivors
Easter Seals Bldg., 5755 West Alameda Ave., Lakewood, CO 80226

Rocky Mountain Stroke Association
5666 S. Bannock St., Littleton, CO 80120

Montrose Memorial Stroke Support Group
Montrose Memorial Hospital Rehab. Center, 800 S. Fourth St., Montrose, CO 81401

Stroke Survivors Support Groups of Pueblo
710 1/2 E. Mesa Ave., Pueblo, CO 81006-1023

Spanish Peaks Stroke Support Group
Trinidad State Nursing Home, Chapel, 409 Benedicta Ave., Trinidad, CO 81082

Courageous Communicators
Lutheran Medical Center, PM&R Dept. (2nd floor), 8300 W. 38th St., Wheat Ridge, CO 80033

Connecticut

Lawrence & Memorial Hospital Aphasia Support Group
Pequot Health Center/Rehabiliation Department, 52 Hazelnut Hill Rd., Groton, CT 06340

Stroke Support Group
Ahlbins Centers for Rehabilitation Medicine, 226 Mill Hill Ave., Bridgeport, CT 06610

Aphasia/Stroke Support Group
Spector Rehab. Assoc., P.O. Box 107, Colebrook, CT 06021

Greenwich Hospital Aphasia Support Group
Greenwich Hospital, 5 Perryridge Rd., Greenwich, CT 06830

The Aphasia Club
Hartford Hospital, 80 Seymour St., Hartford, CT 06106

Communication Enrichment
Hospital for Special Care, 2150 Corbin Ave., New Britain, CT 06053

Stroke Support Group
Hospital for Special Care, 2150 Corbin Ave., New Britain, CT 06053

Aphasia Group
Southern Connecticut State University, Center for Communication Disorders, Davis Hall, 501 Crescent St., New Haven, CT 06515

Stroke Support Group
Stamford Rehab Hospital, Shelburne Rd. at W. Broad St., Stamford, CT 06904

UCONN Aphasia Groups
UCONN Speech and Hearing Clinic, Storrs, CT 06268

Delaware
Beebe Medical Center Stroke Support Group
Lewes Senior Center, 310 Nassau Park Rd., Lewes, DE 19958

New Castle County Stroke Club
Easter Seals, The Jewish Community Center, Garden of Eden Rd., Wilmington, DE 19803

District of Columbia
Howard University Stroke Group
Howard University - Speech & Hearing Clinic, C.B. Powell Building, 525 Bryant St., NW, Washington, DC 20059

Providence Hospital Stroke Support Group
Providence Hospital, Wellness Institute, 1150 Varnum St., NE, Washington, DC 20017

Stroke Survivors Support Group
Iona Senior Services, 4125 Albermarle St., NW, Washington, DC 20016

Florida
Morton Plant Rehabilitation Stroke Support Group
Morton Plant Rehab Center, 400 Corbett St., Belleair, FL 33756

Stroke Support Group
Florida Atlantic University, Communication Disorders Clinic, 777 Glades Rd., Boca Raton, FL 33431-0991

Young Stroke Survivors Group
Heartlands of Boca Raton, 7225 Boca Del Mar Dr., Boca Raton, FL 33433

The Bethesda Memorial Hospital Stroke Support Group
Clayton Conference Center, 2815 S. Seacrest Blvd., Boynton Beach, FL 33435

Stroke Support Group
Blake Medical Center, Dolphin Room, 2020 59th St. West, Bradenton, FL 34209

Communication Club
Stroke Services/Rehab, Morton Plant Mease HealthCare, 430 Morton Plant Way, Suite 101, Clearwater, FL 33756

SCAMP (Stroke Club at Morton Plant)
St. Myrtle Ave., Clearwater, FL 33756

The Aphasia Interactive Support Group
Florida Hospital - Deland, 701 W. Plymouth Ave., Deland, FL 32720

Young Peoples Stroke Club
HealthSouth Sunrise Rehab Hospital, Outpatient Rehab Center & The Bridge, 1007 W. Commercial Blvd., Ft. Lauderdale, FL 33309

Aphasia Therapy & Groups: Mark J. Witkind & Associates Speech & Hearing Services Consultation Care Center
Mailing Address: 425 Hardee Road, Miami, FL 33146-3510

North Collier Aphasia Support Group
North Collier Outpatient Rehab Center, 11181 Health Park Blvd., Suite 106, Naples, FL 34110

North Bay Rehabilitation Support Group
Morton Plant North Bay Hospital, 6600 Madison St., New Port Richey, FL 34652

Stroke of Hope Club, Inc., Aphasia Groups
860 U.S. #1, Suite 106, North Palm Beach, FL 33408

Stroke Club of Marion County
Marion County Extension Agricultural Center Auditorium, 2232 N.E. Jacksonville Rd., Ocala, FL 34470

The Aphasic Support Group
Memorial Rehabilitation Center - Peninsula, 264 S. Atlantic Ave., Ormond Beach, FL 32176

Aphasia Community Support Group of Sarasota
Outpatient Neuro Center - Sarasota Memorial Hospital, 4th Floor, Room 4A, 1700 S. Tamiami Trail, Sarasota, FL 34239

The Stroke of Hope Club, Inc. & Aphasia Group
Indian River County Affiliate, Sebastian United Methodist Church, 1029 Main St., Sebastian, FL 32958

Sun City Center Stroke Group
Kings Point Club House in Kings Point, Sun City Center, FL 33573

Aphasia Communication Group
Florida State University, Dept. of Communication Disorders, LL Schendel Speech & Hearing Clinic, 131 Regional Rehabilitation Center, Tallahassee, FL 32306-1200

Stroke Support Group
The Neuro Rehab Outpatient Facility, 1305 E. 6th Ave., Tallahassee, FL 32308

University Hospital Stroke Club
Conference Room, 7200 University Dr., Tamarac, FL 33321

Aphasia Group at University of South Florida
Communication Disorders Center, PCD 2036, 4202 E. Fowler Ave., Tampa, FL 33620

Tampa Aphasia Support Group
2906 W. Price Ave., Tampa, FL 33611

Road Ahead Stroke Support Group
Florida Hospital Waterman, 1000 Waterman Way, Tavares, FL 32778

The Stroke of Hope Club, Inc.
Indian River County Aphasia Group
Community Room, Indian River Mall, 6200 20th St., Vero Beach, FL 32966

The Aphasia Group Section of Golden Rule Stroke Club
Sun Bridge Health Center, 6414 13th Rd. S, West Palm Beach, FL 33415

Winter Haven Hospital Aphasia Support Group
Winter Haven Hospital, 200 Avenue F NE, Winter Haven, FL 33881

Georgia
Aphasia Conversation Group at G.S.U.
Georgia State University Speech, Language and Hearing Clinic, 30 Pryor St.,
8th Floor, Atlanta, GA 30303

Atlanta Aphasia Association, Inc.
Emory University, Emory Center for Rehabilitation Medicine, Rm. 101, 1441
Clifton Rd., Atlanta, GA 30322

Dekalb Stroke Club
Dekalb Medical Center, 2701 N. Decatur Rd., Decatur, GA 30033

North GA Aphasia Conversation Group
Hudgens Professional Bldg., Community Education Center, Suite 140, Rm. A,
3855 Pleasant Hill Rd., Duluth, GA 30096

Stroke Support Group
Glancy Rehab Center, 3215 McClure Bridge Rd., Duluth, GA 30096

Regain Aphasia Group
NE Georgia Health System, Regain Prog.
743 Spring Street, Gainesville, GA 30501

Strive From Stroke
Coliseum Medical Center, 350 Hospital Dr., 1st Floor Classroom, Macon, GA 31217

Hawaii
University of Hawaii Aphasia Group
University of Hawaii, Department of SPA, 1410 Lower Campus Rd., Honolulu,
HI 96822

Maui Aphasia Support Group
J. Walter Cameron Center, 95 Mahalani St., Wailuku, HI 96793

Idaho

ISU Communication Support Group
Idaho State University – Boise Center, Speech & Language Clinic, 12301 W. Explorer Dr., Suite 102, Boise, ID 83713-1571

Life After Stroke
St. Joseph Regional Medical Center - Outpatient, 1250 Idaho St., Lewiston, ID 83501

South East Idaho Stroke Club
Quail Ridge Assisted Living Center, 797 Hospital Way, Pocatello, WA 83201

Illinois

After Glow Stroke Support Group
Resurrection Professional Bldg., Day Rehab Dept., First Floor, 7447 W. Talcott Ave., Chicago, IL 60631

RIC Stroke Club
Rehabilitation Institute of Chicago, 345 E. Superior St., Chicago, IL 60611

Candi Bone Stroke Club
Jayne Shover Easter Seals, 799 McLean Blvd., Elgin, IL 60123

Conversation Support Group for People with Aphasia and Apraxia
Alexian Rehabilitation Hospital, 935 Beisner Rd., Elk Grove Village, IL 60007

Aphasia Communication Support Group
Northwestern University Aphasia Research Program, Northwestern University, Speech & Language Clinic, 2240 N. Campus Dr., Evanston, IL 60208
(meets 2nd Saturday of every month)

Young Adult Stroke Survivors Program
Northwestern University, Speech & Language Clinic, 2240 N. Campus Dr., Evanston, IL 60208

Stroke Support Group
Little Company of Mary Hospital, 2800 West 95th St., Evergreen Park, IL 60805

Stroke Support Group
MedCare, 3633 West Lake Ave., Suite 102, Glenview, IL 60025

Southern Illinois Stroke/Brain Injury Support Group
Herrin Hospital, Acute Rehabilitation Center, Activity Room, 201 South 14th St., Herrin, IL 62948

Stroke Support Group
Hinsdale Hospital, 120 N. Oak St., Hinsdale, IL 60521

"What's Aphasia?"
Johnsburg Public Library, 3000 W. Johnsburg Rd., Johnsburg, IL 60051

Aphasia Support Group
Condell Day Center for Intergenerational Care, 700 Garfield Ave, Libertyville, IL 60048

Advocate Christ Medical Center Stroke Support Group
4440 W. 95th St., Percy Hopkins, Oak Lawn, IL 60453

Lutheran General Stroke Club
Lutheran General Hospital, 1775 W. Dempster, Rm. 1043 C, Park Ridge, IL 60068

The Illinois Communication Activities Network
Carle Foundation Hospital, 602 W. University, Urbana, IL 61801

Marianjoy Aphasia Support Group
Marianjoy Rehabilitation Hospital, 26 W. 171 Roosevelt Rd., Wheaton, IL 60187

Indiana
Indiana University Aphasia Support Group
Robert L. Milser Speech-Language and Hearing Clinic, 200 S. Jordan Ave., Bloomington, IN 47405
Website: www.indiana.edu/~aphasia

Northside Aphasia Group
Community Health Pavilion North, 11911 North Pennsylvania, Carmel, IN 46032

Elkhart Area Aphasia Support Group
Elkhart Hospital, 600 East Blvd., Elkhart, IN 46516

SouthWestern Indiana Aphasia Support Group
750 S. Kenmore, Evansville, IN 47714

Goshen Community Aphasia Group
1212 Wilson Ave., Goshen, IN 46526

Brainwaves
M.D. Steer Audiology & Speech Language Clinic, 1353 Heavilon Hall, West Lafayette, IN 47907

Iowa
Aphasia Support Group
Genesis Medical Center, Genesis Plaza, Suite 8, 2535 Maplecrest Rd., Bettendorf, IA 52722

Stroke Support Group
Genesis Medical Center, Genesis Plaza, Suite 8, 2535 Maplecrest Rd., Bettendorf, IA 52722

Stroke Club
New Hope Methodist Church, 4525 Beaver Ave., Des Moines, IA 50309

The Aphasia Group
Mercy Capitol, 603 E. 12th St., Des Moines, IA 50309

The Stroke Club
Easter Seals Society of Iowa, 2920 30th St., Des Moines, IA 50310

Kansas

Northwest Kansas Stroke Support Group
First Presbyterian Church, 2900 Hall St., Hays, KS 67601

Conversation Group
University of Kansas, Schiefelbusch Speech-Language Clinic, 1200 Sunnyside Dr.,
2101 Haworth Hall, Lawrence, KS 66045-0239

Stroke Support Group
Lawrence Memorial Hospital, Conference Room, 325 Maine St., Lawrence,
KS 66044

MARH Motivators
Mid America Rehabilitation Hospital, 5701 W. 110th St., Overland Park,
KS 66211

American Stroke Foundation Activity Center
5960 Dearborn St., Mission, KS 66202

Young Stroke Support Group
Mid America Rehabilitation Hospital, Speech, Language Pathology Dept., 5701 W.
110th St., Overland Park, KS 66211

Community Group
Antioch Library, 8700 Shawnee Mission Pkwy., Shawnee Mission, KS 66202

Kentucky

Stroke Support Group
King's Daughters Medical Center, 2201 Lexington Ave., Ashland, KY 41101

Aphasia Support Group
Gateway Rehabilitation Hospital, 5940 Merchants St., Florence, KY 41042

Stroke Support Group
Jewish Hospital, Frazier Rehab Center, Speech Pathology Dept., 220 Abraham
Flexner Way, Louisville, KY 40207

Stroke Support Group
Pattie A. Clay Regional Medical Center, 795 Eastern Bypass, Richmond, KY
40475

Louisiana
The Stroke Support Group of Baton Rouge
YMCA, 350 S. Foster, Baton Rouge, LA 70806

Stroke Support Group
Christus St. Patrick's Hospital, Garber Auditorium, 1770 Engleside St.,
Lake Charles, LA 70601

The Adult Communicative Disorders Support Group
BrentHouse, 1512 Jefferson Hwy., New Orleans, LA 70121

Maine
Portland Aphasia Support Group
The New England Rehabilitation Hospital of Portland Maine, 335 Brighton Ave.,
Unit 201, Portland, ME 04102

Maryland
Annapolis Stroke Club
Glenwood High Rise Senior Center, 701 Glenwood Ave., Annapolis, MD 21401

Good Samaritan Stroke Club
Good Samaritan Hospital, 5601 Loch Raven Blvd., Baltimore, MD 21239

Loyola College Adult Communications Disorders Clinic
Loyola College, 4501 N. Charles St., Baltimore, MD 21210

Stroke Survivors Support Group
Kernan Hospital, Conference Center, 2200 Kernan Dr., Baltimore, MD 21027

Stroke Support Group
Colony South Hotel, Hospital Dr., Clinton, MD 20735

Howard County Stroke Club / Speak Easy
Florence Baines Senior Center, 5470 Ruth Keeton Way, Columbia, MD 21045

Rose Hill Stroke Support Group
Frederick County Health Dept., Montevue Ln., Frederick, MD 21701

Stroke Folks - Aphasia Community Group
Gaithersburg Upcounty Senior Center, 80-A Bureau Dr., Gaithersburg,
MD 20878

Stroke Support Group
Padussis Conference Center, North Arundel Hospital Dr., Glen Burnie, MD 21061

Stroke Support Group
Charles County Adult Day Services, 10200 La Plata Rd., La Plata, MD 20646

Adult Communication Therapy Groups
Summerville Assisted Living, 11215 Seven Locks Rd., Potomac, MD 20854

Communication Enrichment Program
Adventist Rehabilitation Hospital of Maryland, 9909 Medical Center Drive,
Rockville, MD 20850

Stroke Support Group
Upper County Chapter of the Montgomery County Stroke Assoc. (MCSA), Shady
Grove Adventist Nursing/Rehab Center, 9701 Medical Center Dr., Rockville,
MD 20850

Young Stroke Group (30s-60s)
Ring House, 1801 East Jefferson St, Rockville, MD 20852

Leisure World Stroke Support Group
Leisure World Chapter of the Montgomery County Stroke Association (MCSA),
Leisure World, Georgia Ave. & Norbeck Rd., Club House #2, Silver Spring, MD
20906

**Speech, Language Therapy Group, Silver Spring Chapter of the Montgomery
County Stroke Assoc. (MCSA)**
Margaret Schweinhaut Senior Center, 1000 Forest Glen Rd., Silver Spring, MD 20901

Stroke Survivors Group
Towson University, Administration Building, 7720 York Rd., Towson, MD 21252

Massachusetts
Aneurysm Group
Massachusetts General Hospital, Brain Injury and AVM Center, Vincent Burnham
Bldg., BBK710, Fruit Street, Boston, MA 02114 Attn: Deidra Buckley

Aphasia Community Group
Spaulding Rehabilitation Hospital, 125 Nashua St., Boston, MA 02114

Aphasia Community Group
HealthSouth Braintree Rehab Hospital, Conference Room A, 250 Pond St.,
Braintree, MA 02185-9020

The Cape Cod Aphasia Community Group
Rehab Hospital of the Cape and Islands, 311 Service Rd., East Sandwich, MA 02537

Holyoke Hospital Aphasia Therapy Group
Speech and Hearing Center, Holyoke Hospital, 575 Beech St., Holyoke,
MA 01040

Weldon Rehab Hospital Aphasia Support Group
Weldon Rehabilitation Hospital, 233 Carew St., Springfield, MA 01102-9012

Michigan
Communication Recovery Support Group
The Physical Rehab Building, 328 E. Warwick Dr., Alma, MI 48801

Language Enrichment Group
University of Michigan, University Center for the Development of Language and Literacy, 1111 East Catherine St., Ann Arbor, MI 48109-2054

Bay Area Support Group
Bay Medical Center for Rehabilitation, West Campus, 3190 E. Midland Rd., Bay City, MI 48708

New Beginnings Aphasia Group
St. Joseph's Mercy of Macomb, 15855 Nineteen Mile Rd., Clinton Township, MI 48038

GOTCHA (Group Organized Together to Compensate for Having Aphasia)
John D. Dingell VAMC, Dept. of Speech Pathology, 4646 John R., Detroit, MI 48201

Lansing Area Aphasia Support Group
Hope Network, Children and Adult Outpatient Bldg., 2700 East Lansing Dr., East Lansing, MI 48823

First Step Stroke Group
Farmington Hills Senior Center, 28600 Eleven Mile Rd., Suite 111, Farmington Hills, MI 48336

Cerebral Aneurysm & Stroke Club
Garden City Hospital, Rehab Services, 6245 N. Inkster Rd., Garden City, MI 48135

Aphasia Maintenance Group
St. John North Shores Hospital, Macomb Center, 26755 Ballard Rd., Harrison Township, MI 48045-2458

Aphasia/Language Maintenance Groups
Van Riper Speech/Language & Hearing Clinic, Western Michigan University, Unified Clinics, 1000 Oakland Dr., Kalamazoo, MI 49008

Kalamazoo Stroke Club
Senior Services Center, 918 Jasper, Kalamazoo, MI 49001

Stroke Support Group
Marlette Community Hospital Center for Rehab, 2770 Main St., Marlette, MI 48453

Central Michigan Stroke Support Group
CMC Hospital, 1221 South Dr., Mt. Pleasant, MI 48858-3234

The Happy Hour Stroke Club
Palmer Park Recreation Center, 2829 Armour St., Port Huron, MI 48060

Port Huron Hospital Stroke Support Group
Port Huron Hospital, 1221 Pine Grove Ave., 1st Floor, Port Huron, MI 48061-5011

Luke's Aphasia Group
St. Luke's United Methodist Church, 3980 Walton Blvd., Rochester Hills, MI 48309

Beaumont Hospital - Group Treatment Programs
Beaumont Health Center, Adult Speech, 4949 Coolidge Hwy., Royal Oak, MI 48073

Royal Oak Aphasia Group
The Senior Center, 3500 Marais Ave., Royal Oak, MI 48073

Communication Enhancement Group
Lakeland Health & Healing, Upton Education Center, 1234 Napier Ave.,
St. Joseph, MI 49085

N.W. MI Stroke Survivors & Caregivers Group
Scottville Area Senior Center, 140 S. Main St., Scottville, MI 49454

Cane & Able: Stroke Recovery Group
William Beaumont Hospital Troy, 44300
Dequindre Rd., Sterling Heights, MI 48314

Grand Traverse Bay Area Stroke Club
Bethlehem Lutheran Church, 1050 Peninsula Dr., Traverse City, MI 49686

Friend's, B'Nai Moshe Synagogue
6800 Drake Rd., West Bloomfield, MI 48322

Minnesota

Fairview Ridges Stroke Support Group
Fairview Ridges Hospital, 201 E. Nicollet Blvd., Burnsville, MN 55337

The Rivers Education & Support Group
The Rivers, 1st Floor Conference Room, 11111 River Hills Dr., Burnsville, MN
55337

Crosby Stroke Group
Cuyuna Regional Medical Center, Crosby, MN 56441

Fairview Southdale Stroke Group
Fairview Southdale Hospital, 6401 France Ave., S, Edina, MN 55435

The Aphasia Support Group
800 East 28th St., Minneapolis, MN 55407-3799

Strive to Thrive
Communication and Caregivers Groups, MN Stroke Association, 13705 26th Ave.
N, Suite 106, Plymouth, MN 55441

Headwaters Stroke Support Group
Park Rapids City Library, Hwy. 34, Park Rapids, MN 56470

Strive to Thrive
Communication and Caregivers Groups, The Pines Senior Residence, 400 W.
67th St., Richfield, MN 55423

Strive to Thrive Communication and Caregivers Groups
The Pines Senior Residence, 400 W. 67th St., Richfield, MN 55423

"Speak Easy" Communication Group
North Memorial Medical Center, Stroke Center, 3300 Oakdale Ave. N.,
Robbinsdale, MN 55422

"Let's Talk Again" Group Communication Program
Whitney Senior Center, 1527 Northway Dr., St. Cloud, MN 56303

Lucky Stroke Support Group
Whitney Senior Center, 1527 Northway Dr., St. Cloud, MN 56303

Beyond Words
Methodist Hospital, 6500 Excelsior Blvd., 6th Floor Dining Room,
St. Louis Park, MN 55426

East Metro Stroke Support Group
Regions Hospital, 640 Jackson St., St. Paul, MN 55101

The Dream Team
St. Anthony Park Home, 2237 Commonwealth Ave., St. Paul, MN 55108

Mississippi
Stroke Support Group
VA Medical Center, Speech Pathology Services (126), 400 Veterans Ave.,
Biloxi, MS 39531-2410

Baptist De Soto Stroke Support Group
Baptist - De Soto Rehab, 7601 Southcrest Pkwy., Southaven, MS 38671

Missouri
Aphasia Conversation Connection
Barnes – Jewish Extended Care, 401 Corporate Park Dr., Clayton, MO 63105

Conversations With Aphasia
Central United Methodist Church, 5144 Oak St., Kansas City, MO 64112

Barnes – Jewish St. Peters Aphasia Support Group
#6 Jungermann Circle, Healthwise – 1st Floor, St. Peters, MO 63376

Nebraska
Stroke of Luck Club
Mary Lanning Memorial Hospital, 715 N. St. Joseph Ave., Hastings, NE 68901

Madonna Outpatient Aphasia Group
Madonna Rehabilitation Hospital, 5401 South St., Lincoln, NE 68506-2134

Univ. of NE - Lincoln Aphasia Therapy Group
Barkley Memorial Center, East Campus, Lincoln, NE 68583-0731

Northeast Nebraska Stroke Support Group
Faith Regional Health Services - East, 1500 Koenigstein, Norfork, NE 68701
(Evening Group)

Northeast Nebraska Stroke Support Group
Faith Regional Health Services, 1500 Koenigstein, Norfork, NE 68701
(Afternoon Group)

Nevada
TouchPoint Stroke Support Group
St. Rose Dominican Hospital, Conference Room #2, 102 E. Lake Mead Dr.,
Henderson, NV 89015

Stroke Support Group
10085 Double R Blvd #325, Reno, NV 89521
Meetings Second Wednesday of Each Month @ 2:00 P.M. Currently located @
Washoe Medical Center 77 Pringle Way, Reno, NV, Neurosciences Unit

New Hampshire
Brain Injury Association of New Hampshire
109 N. State St., Suite 2, Concord, NH 03301

Stroke Support Group
Cheshire Medical Center, Conference Room #3, 580 Court St., Keene, NH 03431

Aphasia Support Group
Catholic Medical Center, Rehabilitation Medical Unit, 100 McGregor St.,
Manchester, NH 03102

Talk It Out
Easter Seals of NH, 555 Auburn St., Manchester, NH 03103

Seacoast Aphasia Support Group
Community Campus, 100 Campus Dr., Newmarket, NH 03801

New Jersey
Stroke Support Group
Ocean Medical Center & Shore Rehabilitation Institute, 425 Jack Martin Blvd.,
Brick, NJ 08724

Somerset Medical Center Stroke Club
Bridgewater Library, 1 Vogt Dr., Bridgewater, NJ 08807

Stroke Club
Our Lady of Lourdes Medical Center, Rehab Solarium, 1600 Haddon Ave.,
Camden, NJ 08103

JFK Stroke Wives Support Group
JFK Hospital, Outpatient Conference Room, James St., Edison, NJ 08820

North Jersey Stroke Discussion Group
Grace Episcopal Church, 4 Madison Ave., Madison, NJ 07940

Aphasia Support & Discussion Group
Adler Aphasia Center, 60 W. Hunter Ave., Maywood, NJ 07607

Caregivers of Stroke Survivors Support Group
Montclair, NJ

Newton Memorial Stroke Club
Newton Memorial Hospital, Rehab Dept., 175 High St., Newton, NJ 07860

NJ Aphasia Community Support Group
The Kip Center, 55 Kip Ave., Rutherford, NJ 07070

Stroke Support Group
Kessler Institute, 375 Market St., Saddle Brook, NJ 07663

Stroke Support Group
Senior Care of Totowa, 120 Commerce Way, Totowa, NJ 07512

NJ Stroke Activity Center
725 Joralemon St., Suite 191, Belleville, NJ 07109-1483.

Kean University Aphasia Support Group
Kean University Speech & Hearing Clinic, CSI 104, 1000 Morris Ave., Union, NJ 07083-0411

New York
Selfhelp Clearview Senior Center Stroke Club
208-11 26th Ave., Bayside, NY 11360

Aphasia Support Group (for Veterans Only)
VA Medical Center, 130 West Kingbridge Road, Bronx, NY 10468

Lehman College Aphasia Community Group
Lehman College/CUNY, Speech and Hearing Center, 250 Bedford Park Blvd. West, Bronx, NY 10468

Stern Stroke Center Club
NW-1, Montefiore Medical Center, 111 East 210th St., Bronx, NY 10467

Lehman College Aphasia Community Group
Lehman College/CUNY, Speech and Hearing Center, 250 Bedford Park Blvd. West, Speech & Theatre Bldg., Rm. B-50, Bronx, NY 10468

Aphasia Therapy & Support Group
Brooklyn College, 2900 Bedford Ave., Brooklyn, NY 11210

Aphasia Therapy Group (for Veterans and Family Members)
Veterans Administration Medical Center, 15th Floor, 800 Poly Pl.,
Brooklyn, NY 11209

Aphasia Support Group
Long Island University: CW Post, Ladge Speech & Hearing Center, 720 Northern
Blvd., Brookville, NY 11548

Aphasia Support Group at Buffalo State College
1300 Elmwood Ave., Buffalo, NY 14222

The Aphasia Group
University of New York at Buffalo, 3435 Main St., 82 Bio-Medical Education
Building, Buffalo, NY 14214

U.B. Aphasia Support Group for Family Members
University of New York at Buffalo, 3435 Main St., 82 Bio-Medical Education
Building, Buffalo, NY 14214

Buffalo Hearing and Speech Center
50 East North St., Buffalo, NY 14203

Deer Park Library Speech Group
Deer Park Public Library, 44 Lake Dr., Deer Park, NY 11729

Aphasia Group
Hy Weinberg Center for Communication Disorders, Room 103, Adelphi
University, Garden City, NY 11530

Glens Falls Stroke Support Group
Glens Falls Hospital, The Rehabilitation Center, 100 Park St., Glens Falls, NY 12801

Stroke Support Group
Catskill Regional Medical Center, 2nd Floor Board Room, Bushville Rd.,
Harris, NY 12742

Tompkins County Stroke Support Group
Finger Lakes Independence Center, 215 Fifth St., Ithaca, NY 14850

North Shore Stroke Club
North Shore University Hospital, Volunteer Office, 300 Community Drive,
Manhasset, NY 11030

Stroke Group
Winthrop University Hospital, Conference Room, 200 Old Country Rd., Suite 125,
Mineola, NY 11501

Aphasia Group
N.Y.U. Speech, Language & Hearing Clinic, 719 Broadway, Suite 200,
New York, NY 10003

Aphasia Community Groups
Rusk Institute of Rehabilitation Medicine, Speech-Language Pathology Dept.,
400 E. 34th St., New York, NY 10016
(Reserved for former Rusk Institute patients)
(Group conversation, Current Events conversation & Board games &
conversation)

Aphasia Support Group
Columbia Presbyterian Medical Center, 622 West 168th St., Vanderbilt Clinic,
10th Floor, Area D, New York, NY 10032

Aphasia Support Group
New York Harbor Health Care System, 423 E. 23rd St., New York, NY
10010

New York Aphasia Group
St. Peter's Church, Lexington Ave. & 54th St. (Citicorp Building),
New York, NY 10022

Speech Language Therapy Services
Marymount Manhattan College, 221 E 71st St., New York, NY 10021

STAS—"Surviving & Thriving After Stroke"
Dept. of Rehab. Med./Therapeutic Recreation, 2nd Floor, Rm. 269, Mt. Sinai
Hospital, 1450 Madison Ave., New York, NY 10029

Post Stroke Communication Treatment Group
Plattsburgh State University, Sibley Hall, Plattsburgh, NY 12901

Sound Shore Aphasia Support Group
Rye Recreation Center, Girl Scout Room, 281 Midland Ave., Rye, NY 10580

Staten Island University Hospital Stroke Self Help Group
475 Seaview Ave., Staten Island, NY 10305

Stroke Communication Group
New York Medical College, WIHD/Cedarwood Hall, Westchester Medical Center,
Valhalla, NY 10595

Stroke Club & Support Group of Bloome County
Vestal Public Library, Rt. 434, Vestal, NY 13850

Aphasia Support Group
Helen Hayes Hospital, Route 9 W, West Haverstraw, NY 10993

Aphasia Group
Burke Rehabilitation Center, 21 Bloomingdale Rd., White Plains, NY 10605

Stroke Support Group
White Plains Hospital Medical Center, Davis Ave. at East Post Rd.,
White Plains, NY 10601

North Carolina

Asheville Area Aphasia Support Group
Thoms Rehabilitation Hospital, 68 Sweeten Creek Rd., Conference B Room,
Asheville, NC 28803

University of North Carolina Conversation Groups for Adults with Aphasia
UNC Hearing and Communication Center, 6015 Farrington Rd.,
Chapel Hill, NC 27517
(919)493-7980

Stroke Support Group
Alamance Regional Medical Center, Rehab Services, 1240 Huffman Mill Rd.,
Burlington, NC 27215

Charlotte Mecklenburg Stroke Support Group
Charlotte Institute of Rehabilitation, 1100 Blythe Blvd., Charlotte, NC 28203

Positive Steps Support Group
Lake Norman YMCA - Health Center, 21300 Davisdon St., Cornelius, NC 28031

Aphasia Support Groups
Triangle Aphasia Project
3131 RDU Center Dr., Suite 100, Morrisville, NC 27560

Durham VA Medical Center Stroke Support Group
Audiology/Speech Pathology Service (126), 508 Fulton St., Durham, NC 27705

Stroke Support Group
Teer House, 4019 N. Roxboro Rd., Durham, NC 27704

Fayetteville Stroke Club
Southeastern Regional Rehabilitation Center, 1638 Owen Dr., P.O. Box 2000,
Fayetteville, NC 28302-2000

Guilford County Stroke Support Group
Moses H. Cone Hospital Rehab Services, 1200 N. Elm St., Greensboro, NC 27401

Regional Rehabilitation Stroke Support Group
University Health Systems, Rehab Center Classroom, 2100 Stantonsburg Rd.,
Greenville, NC 27858

Vance County Stroke Support Group
Maria Parham Hospital, Doctors Lounge, Henderson, NC 27536

Frye Regional Stroke Support Group
Frye Regional Rehab Center, Outpatient Lobby, 420 N. Center St., Hickory,
NC 28601

Moore County Stroke Club
Moore Regional Hospital Auditorium, P.O. Box 3000, Page Rd., Pinehurst, NC 28374

New Hanover Stroke Club
Coastal Rehab Hospital at New Hanover Regional Medical Center, 2131 S. 17th St., Wilmington, NC 28402

North Dakota
Suvivors of Stroke
MeritCare HealthSystem, 1720 S. University Dr., Fargo, ND 58103

Ohio
Stroke Support Group
Edwin Shaw Rehabilitation Hospital, 1621 Flickinger Rd., Akron, OH 44312

Aphasia Support Group
Mercy Franciscan Hospital - Mt. Airy, 2446 Kipling Ave., Cincinnati, OH 45239

Deaconess Hospital Stroke Recovery Group
4 West Rehab Day Room, 311 Straight St., Cincinnati, OH 45219

Cleveland Stroke Club
Euclid Avenue Christian Church, 3663 Mayfield Rd., Cleveland Heights, OH 44121

Miami Valley Hospital Aphasia Support Group
R10 - Speech Pathology Dept., 1 Wyoming St., Dayton, OH 45409

Aphasia Support Group
Panera's (private dining room), 9587 Mentor Ave., Mentor, OH 44060

The Lucky Strokes
Mercy Medical Center North Cantan, 6200 Whipple Dr., NW, North Canton, OH 44720

Miami Speech and Hearing Stroke Support Group
Department of Communications, Miami University, 162 Bachelor Hall, Oxford, OH 45056

Stroke of Luck Club
Trinity East, 380 Summit Ave., Steubenville, OH 43952

Toledo Aphasia Support Group
Alternative Physical Therapy, 330 S. Reynolds Rd., Suite 16, Toledo, OH 43615

Oklahoma
The Bob McVay Aphasia Support Group
Jim Thorpe Rehab - Cancer Center West, 4219 S. Western Ave., Oklahoma City, OK 73109

Survivors of Stroke Support Group
Rehabilitation at Mercy Hospital, 1st Floor Rehab. Conference Room, 4300 West Memorial Rd., Oklahoma City, OK 73120

Tulsa Aphasia Group
University of Tulsa, Mary K. Chapman Center for Communicative Disorders, 600 S. College, Tulsa, OK 74104

Oregon
Rogue Valley Stroke Club
Rogue Valley Medical Center, 2825 East Barnett Rd., Medford, OR 97504

Men's Only Caregiver Support Group
Legacy Good Samaritan Hospital Medical Center, Goos Samaritan Medical Bldg., 2nd floor conference room, 1040 NW 22nd Ave., Portland, OR 97210

Pennsylvania
Stroke Re-entry Group
Good Sheperd Rehab. Hospital, 501 St. John St., Allentown, PA 18103

Altoona Hospital Stroke Support Group
Altoona Hospital Center for Nursing Care, 1020 Green Ave., Altoona, PA 16601

Cumberland Valley Stroke Club
Chambersburg Hospital, 112 N. 7th St., Chambersburg, PA 17201

"One-Step-at-a-Time" Stroke Club
Mercy Fitzgerald Hospital, Outpatient Center Community Room, 1500 Lansdowne Ave., Darby, PA 19023

Stroke Support Group
HealthSouth Rehab Hospital, 143 E. 2nd St., Erie, PA 16507

Stroke Support Group
Penn State Milton S. Hershey Medical Center, 500 University Dr., Hershey, PA 17033

Stroke Survivors Club
Homestead Village, 1800 Village Cir., Lancaster, PA 17603

Magee Aphasia Community Support Group
Magee Rehabilitation Hospital, Clinical Outreach, Six Franklin Plaza, Philadelphia, PA 19102

Voices of Moss Rehab Aphasia Center (VOMAC)
Moss Rehabilitation Aphasia Center, 1200 W. Tabor Rd., Korman Bldg., Suite 114, Philadelphia, PA 19141

Aphasia Support Group of Western
Pennsylvania, UPMC Passavant, Speech Therapy Dept., 200 Nineteen North Drive, #6, Pittsburgh, PA 15237

Aphasia Therapy Program
Duquesne University, Speech-Language-Hearing Clinic, 406 Fisher Hall, 711 Forbes Ave., Pittsburgh, PA 15282-2231

Stroke Survivors Support Group
VA Medical Center, 7180 Highland Dr. (132A-H), Pittsburgh, PA 15206

VNF Stroke Survivors Connection Groups
Visiting Nurse Foundation, 2 Parkway Center, Suite 101, Pittsburgh, PA 15220-3702

Marywood University Adult Aphasia Group
Marywood University, Dept. of Communication Sciences & Disorders, 2300 Adams Ave., Scranton, PA 18509

Stroke Support Group of Allied Rehab Services
475 Morgan Hwy., Scranton, PA 18501

Community Stroke Support Group
John Heinz Institute, 150 Mundy St., Wilkes-Barre, PA 18702

O.U.R. (Outreach, Understanding, Recovery) Stroke Club
2510 Maryland Rd., Suite 195, Willow Grove, PA 19090

Rhode Island
Newport Hospital Stroke Support Group
Newport Hospital, Dept. of Social Work, 11 Friendship St., Newport, RI 02840

Social Communication Group
Newport Hospital, 11 Friendship St., Newport, RI 02840

Our Lady of Fatima Stroke Support Group
Our Lady of Fatima Hospital, 4 South Rehab, 200 High Service Ave., North Providence, RI 02904

South County Stroke Club
25 St. Dominic Rd., Wakefield, RI 02879-1878

South Carolina
Aphasia Support Group
South Carolina State University, SCSU Speech-Language-Hearing Clinic, 300 College St., NE, Orangeburg, SC 29117

Stroke Recovery Groups
University of South Carolina, Speech & Hearing Center, 1601 St. Julian Place, Columbia, SC 29204

South Dakota
Sioux Empire Stroke Club
Avera McKennan Hospital, 800 E. 21st St., Sioux Falls, SD 57117

Tennessee
Jackson Communication Disorders Support Group
Jackson Madison County General Hospital, 4th Floor - W. TN Rehab. Center,
Forest Ave., Jackson, TN 38303-3855

The Mountain Empire Stroke Support Group
Quillen Rehabilitation Hospital, Cafeteria, 2511 Wesley St., Johnson City, TN 37601

Life After Stroke
HealthSouth - Cane Creek Rehabilitation Center, 180 Mt. Pelia Rd., Martin, TN
38237

Stroke Club of Memphis
Raymond F. Skinner Center, 412 Tanglewood (at Central and Tanglewood),
Memphis, TN 38104

Aphasia Group
HealthSouth Rehabilitation Center, 1282 Union Ave., Memphis, TN 38104

Caregivers Support Group
Christ United Methodist Church, 4448 Poplar Ave., Memphis, TN 38117

Stroke Support Group
3920 Titwiler, Memphis, TN 38122

Caregiver Support Group
ALPS Adult Day Care Services, 600 N. Daisy St., Morristown, TN 37814

Stroke Support Group
Lakeway Regional Hospital Rehab Center, 726 McFarland St., Morristown, TN 37814

Aphasia Community Group
Vanderbilt Stallworth Rehab Hospital, 2201 Capers Ave., Nashville, TN 37212

Texas
PAL DOGS (People with Aphasia & Language Difficulties of the Golden Spread)
BSA Health Systems, Outpatient Clinic, 5111 Canyon Dr., Amarillo, TX 79110

Aphasia Support Group
Wellness Center, Columbia Professional Bldg. C, Omega Dr., Arlington, TX 76015

Aphasia Center Stroke Club
TWU Aphasia Center, 1810 Inwood Rd., Dallas, TX 75235

North Texas Stroke Survivors Toastmasters Club #5079
C.C. Young Home, 4829 West Lawther Dr., Dallas, TX 75214

Different Strokes
Harris H.E.B. Hospital, Physical Medicine & Rehabilitation, 251 Westpark Way,
Euless, TX 76040

Aphasia Support Group
Harris Methodist Fort Worth Hospital, 1301 Pennsylvania Ave., Fort Worth,
TX 76104
(Family and Friends welcome)

V.B.M.C. Stroke Support Group
V.B.M.C. Inpatient Rehab, 2101 Pease St., Harlingen, TX 78550

Stroke Support Group
Memorial Hermann Northwest Hospital, 1635 N. Loop West, Houston, TX
77008-1693

Texas Tech Aphasia Group Therapy Program
3601 4th St., Suite 2A-300
Lubbock, TX 79430

McKinney Stroke Support Group
Senior Center, McKinney, TX 75070

West Texas Aphasia Center
3301 Sinclair Ave., Midland, TX 79707

Stroke Survivors & Aphasia Club of East Texas
First Baptist Church, 301 E. Lane St., Quitman, TX 75783
(survivors and caregivers welcome)

Utah
Salt Lake City Aphasia Support Group
University of Utah, Social & Behavioral Sciences Bldg., 12th Floor, 390 S. 1530
East, Salt Lake City, UT 84112

Young Stroke Survivors Support Group
University of Utah Sugarhouse Health Center, 1138 E. Wilmington Ave.,
Salt Lake City, UT 84106

Vermont
Post - Stroke Communication Group
University of Vermont, E.M. Luse Center for Communication, UVM - Pomeroy
Hall, 489 Main St., Burlington, VT 05450

Virginia
Speech Directions
268 Murtha St., Alexandria, VA 22304

The Northern Virginia Brain Injury Association
c/o Chairman of Support Groups, Falls Church High School, 7521 Jaguar Trail, Falls Church, VA 22042

Shenandoah Valley Stroke Club
Augusta Medical Center, Wellness Center, 96 Medical Center Dr., Fisherville, VA 22939

Helping Hands Aphasia Group
Patrick Henry Library, 101 Maple Ave., Vienna, VA 22180

Aphasia Group
Old Dominion University, Speech & Hearing Clinic, Child Study Center, Norfolk, VA 23529-0136

Halifax County Stroke - Aphasia Support Group
YMCA Cardinal Community Center, 650 Hamilton Blvd., South Boston, VA 24592

Helping Hands Stroke Club
Patrick Henry Library, 101 Maple Ave., Vienna, VA 22180

Aphasia Support Group
Southeastern Physical Therapy
5301 Providence Rd., Suite 80, Virginia Beach, VA 23464

Washington
Stroke/Aphasia Group
Communication Plus, Inc., 1407 116th Ave., NE, Suite 106, Bellevue, WA 98004

Everett Stroke Support Group
Providence Center for Outpatient Rehabilitation, 2940 W. Marine View Dr., Everett, WA 98201

Brain Injury & Stroke Education Group
Good Samaritan Hospital, Mt. Rainier Room, 407 14th Ave., SE, Puyallup, WA 98372

"Communication Groups" of the University of Washington
Speech & Hearing Clinic, 4131 N.E. 15th Ave., Seattle, WA 98105

Northwest Hospital Stroke Group
Northwest Hospital, Center for Medical Rehabilitation, 1550 North 115th St., Seattle, WA 98133

Aphasia Conversation Group
Group Health Cooperative, Speech, Language & Learning Services, Central South Building, 1st Floor, Room 101/102, 125 16th Ave., East, Seattle, WA 98112

Stroke Support Group
Silverdale Rehabilitation, 1800 NW Myhre Rd., Silverdale, WA 98383

Tacoma Area Stroke Support Group
c/o TACID Building, 6315 S. 19th, Tacoma, WA 98466

Aphasia Community Group
Vancouver Division V.A., 1601 E. Fourth Plain Blvd., Vancouver, WA 98661

West Virginia
Stroke Education Program
HealthSouth MountainView Regional Rehabilitation Hospital, 1160 Van Voorhis Rd., Morgantown, WV 26505

Ohio Valley Stroke Support Group
Peterson Rehabilitation Hospital, Homestead Ave., Wheeling, WV 26003

Tri-State Aphasia Support Group
Peterson Rehabilitation Hospital, Homestead Ave., Wheeling, WV 26003

Wisconsin
Chippewa Valley Aphasia Group - Bloomer Chapter
Bloomer Medical Center, 1501 Thompson St., Bloomer, WI 54724

St. Joseph's Community Aphasia Group
St. Joseph's Hospital, 2661 County Hwy. I, Chippewa Falls, WI 54729

The Chippewa Valley Community Aphasia Group
Luther Hospital - Neurosciences, 1221 Whipple St., Eau Claire, WI 54703

Aphasia Group
University of Wisconsin Speech & Hearing Clinic, 1975 Willow Dr., Madison, WI 53706

Living with Aphasia, Inc.: Conversation Group
Bowling Group and Theater Group, Madison Senior Center, 330 W. Mifflin St., Madison, WI 53703

Madison Area Stroke Support Groups
Meriter Hospital, 2 North (Evening Group), Atrium (Day Group), 202 S. Park St., Madison, WI 53715

Aurora Sinai Aphasia Group
Aurora Sinai Medical Center, 4th Floor Rehabilitation Dept., 945 N. 12th St., Milwaukee, WI 53201

St. Luke's Aphasia Support Group
St. Luke's Hospital, 2900 Oklahoma Avenue, Milwaukee, WI 53215

Stroke Support Group
Lakeview Medical Center, 1100 N. Main, Rice Lake, WI 54868

Canadian Resources

Alberta

The Young Survivors
(A support group for stroke survivors under the age of 60 and their families), call for information on meeting places. (403) 948-2965. *Mailing Address:* Janel Nadeau, 2107 Morris Rd., Airdrie, AB T4A 1V9, Canada
Website: **www.geocities.com/youngsurvivors**

Stroke Recovery Association of Calgary
(Various Locations - Call for Information) (403) 289-7520. *Mailing Address:* 21 Moreuil Ct. SW, Calgary, AB T2T 6B1, Canada
Website: **www.geocities.com/sracalgary**

Neighborhood CHAT
Duggan Public Health Center, 5035 108 A St., NW, Edmonton, AB T6H 2Z9, Canada

British Columbia

The British Columbia Aphasia Centre #212-5021 Kingsway, Burnaby, BC V5H 4A4, Canada
Website: **www.bcaphasia.org**

Life Enhancement Aphasia Program (LEAP)
23 Adanac Services, 2355 Richmond Rd., Victoria, BC V8R 1J8, Canada

Newfoundland

St. John's Stroke Survivors Support Group
100 Forest Rd., St. John's, NL A1A 1E5, Canada

Nova Scotia

Communication Strategies Group
Interact Program, Dalhousie University, School of Human Communication Disorders, 5599 Fenwick St., Halifax, NS B3H 1R2, Canada

Ontario

The Halton Aphasia Centre
Georgetown & Burlington sites, Burlington, ON, Canada

Nottawasaga Bay Stroke Recovery Network
250 Erie St., Collingwood, ON L9Y 1P7, Canada

Living With Stroke
Halton Hills Speech Centre, 211 Guelph St., Suite 5, Georgetown, ON L7G 5B5, Canada

Aphasia Program
Guelph Services for Persons with Disabilities, 238 Willow Rd., Guelph, ON
N1H 8H1, Canada

Aphasia Centre of Ottawa
Heartwood House, 153 Chapel St., Ottawa, ON K1N 1H5, Canada

York-Durham Aphasia Centre
12184 Ninth Line, Stouffville, ON L4A 4T8, Canada

The Aphasia Institute
73 Scarsdale Rd., Toronto, ON M3P 2R2, Canada

Quebec
Hamel - French Speaking
Association Des Personnes Interessees A L'Aphasie
525, boulevard, Hamel, CDN QC G1M 2S8, Canada

Association Quebecoise des Personnes Aphasiques
4565 Queen Mary Rd., Montreal, QC H3W 1W5, Canada

Other Sources of Information

National Organizations That Offer Information About Groups:
American Heart Association
7272 Greenville Ave., Dallas, TX 75231. Call (214) 373-6300 or
(800) 242-8721. Local offices in many parts of the United States.
Website: www.americanheart.org

National Easter Seal Society
230 West Monroe, Suite 1800, Chicago, IL 60606-4802. Call (800) 221-6827 or
(312) 726-6200
Website: www.seals.org

National Family Caregivers Association
10400 Connecticut Ave., Suite 500, Kensington, MD 20895-3944.
Call (800) 896-3650 or (301) 942-6430.
Website: www.nfcacares.org

National Stroke Association
9707 E. Easter Ln., Englewood, CO 80112-3747. Call (800) 787-6537 or
(303) 649-9299.
Website: www.stroke.org

Glossary

A

Addition   In speech articulation, a sound placed in a word where there should not be one.

Agnosia   A perceptual disorder in which a person has trouble interpreting and appreciating information coming from the senses.

Agrammatism   Loss of the ability to know and use the grammar of a language.

Aneurysm   A ballooning or swelling in a weakened area in the wall of an artery.

Anoxia   Lack of oxygen to the brain.

Aphasia   The loss of the ability to use language due to damage to the speech and language centers of the brain. The loss includes verbal expression, understanding the speech of others, reading, writing, using gestures, and the ability to do simple arithmetic. *Dysphasia* means partial loss of language.

Aphonia   Loss of the ability to vibrate the vocal cords to produce voice. *Dysphonia* means partial loss of voice.

Apraxia   Loss of the ability to plan and sequence voluntary body movements due to a stroke or other neurological disorder. This loss is not due to paralysis or weakness. *Dyspraxia* means some ability to make these voluntary movements remains.

Apraxia of speech   Loss of the ability to plan and sequence speech due to a stroke or other neurological disorder. *Dyspraxia* of speech means that some ability to produce speech remains.

Artery   A tube that carries blood from the heart to other parts of the body.

Articulation   Shaping compressed air from the lungs into individual speech sounds. The tongue, for example, is an articulator or "shaper" of speech sounds.

Aspiration   When food or liquid gets into the lungs or the airways leading to them.

Ataxia   Loss of the ability to engage smoothly in motor activities.

Atrophy   When a body structure, such as the tongue, withers, shrinks in size, and becomes weak.

B

Bilabials   Sounds produced with both lips, such as *b* and *p*.

Bilateral   Referring to two sides of a structure. The opposite of *unilateral*.

Brainstem The widened upper part of the spinal cord located where the neck meets the skull.

Breathy Voice quality created by excessive leakage of air when the vocal cords vibrate.

Broca's area The part of the left side of the brain important to expressive communication.

C

Cardiovascular The body system that includes the heart, lungs, and blood vessels.

Carotid artery A major blood artery that comes from the heart and goes up through the neck to the brain.

Catastrophic reaction An overwhelming feeling of anxiety and the reaction to it.

Central nervous system (CNS) The brain and spinal cord.

Cerebellum The part of the brain responsible for muscle tone, balance, and coordination.

Cerebral vascular accident (CVA) A disruption of the flow of blood to the brain; a stroke.

Circumlocution Using a substitute word for the one that cannot be remembered or spoken.

Cognition Higher mental functions that include reasoning and information processing.

Computerized axial tomography (CAT) A brain scan.

Confabulation Giving answers to questions with no regard for their truthfulness; making up false stories.

Content words Words that carry the most meaning, such as nouns and verbs.

Continuants Speech sounds such as s and v that do not have stops or gaps in the airstream.

Cortex The outer layer of the brain also known as the grey matter.

D

Decode The process of breaking down and analyzing a signal, such as speech and language, into its component parts.

Deficit A lack of or a reduction in something.

Denasality Reduced nasality. Also called *hyponasality*.

Distortion In speech articulation, the indistinct production of a sound.

Dysarthrias A group of neuromuscular speech disorders often caused by a stroke. *Anarthria* means complete loss of speech due to neurological and muscular deficits.

Dyscalculia Problems with simple arithmetic. *Acalculia* means total loss of the ability to do simple arithmetic.

Dysfluency A breakdown in the rhythm and flow of speech caused by repetitions, prolongations, and/or pauses.

Dysgraphia Problems with writing. *Agraphia* means total loss of the ability to write.

Dyslexia Problems with reading. *Alexia* means total loss of the ability to read.

Dysnomia Word-finding problems, particularly with nouns. *Anomia* means complete loss of the ability to remember words.

Dysphagia Problems with the ability to swallow.

E

Echolalia Automatically repeating or "parroting" something that has been heard.

Edema Swelling due to too much fluid in cells, tissues, or cavities.

Egocentric Self-centered.

Embolism A plug that develops in one part of the vascular system and ends up in another. *Emboli* means more than one plug, as in a "shower of emboli."

Empathy Feeling the emotions of another person.

Encode The process of putting an idea or thought into a signal system, such as speech and language.

Esophagus Tube leading from the throat to the stomach.

Etiology The cause of something.

Expiration During breathing, the process of letting air out of the lungs.

Expressive aphasia A type of neurologically based language disturbance in which the person has problems with the expressive components of language: speaking, writing, and gesturing.

F

Flaccid A weak or limp muscle; can be due to paralysis.

Fluent speech Smooth and effortlessly produced speech without hesitations, interjections, or repetitions.

Fricatives Speech sounds made by forcing air through a constricted area, such as *f* and *v.*

Functional communication The ability to express and understand basic ideas, needs, and wants.

Function words Words that are important grammatically, such as conjunctions, articles, and prepositions.

G

Glide In speech articulation, a sound requiring movement of the articulators from one position to another, such as *w* and *l.*

Glossal Pertaining to the tongue.

Glottal fry   A gravelly sound produced by the vocal cords, usually low pitched.

Glottal opening   The space between the vocal cords.

Grey matter   Grey-colored tissue of the brain made up of primarily cell bodies.

Gustatory   Related to the sense of taste.

H

Habitual pitch   The pitch that a person uses most often.

Hard palate   The bony roof of the mouth.

Harshness   Voice quality caused by excessive force of vocal cord vibration.

Hematoma   An area filled with a blood clot.

Hemiparesis   Weakness of the muscles on one side of the body. *Hemiparalysis* means complete loss of the ability to move the muscles on one side of the body.

Hemorrhage   Escape of blood from a vein or artery; bleeding.

Hoarseness   Raspy voice quality; a combination of harsh and breathy voice qualities.

Homonymous hemianopsia   Defective vision in one-half of the fields of both eyes.

Hydrocephalus   Too much fluid in the cavities of the brain; also known as "water on the brain."

Hyperkinesia   A disorder characterized by excessive movement that the person cannot control.

Hypernasality   Too much nasal resonance.

Hypokinesia   A disorder characterized by reduced and/or slowed movements.

Hyponasality   Too little nasal resonance; denasality.

I

Incidence   The frequency of occurrence.

Infarct   The sudden death of tissue due to a lack of blood supply.

Inflammation   Swelling of a part of the body due to injury.

Inspiration   During breathing, the process of taking air into the lungs.

Intelligibility   The degree to which a person can be understood by others.

Intubation   Insertion of a tube into the body.

Ischemic   Inadequate flow of blood to a part of the body.

J

Jargon   Fluent but unintelligible speech; fluent speech that makes no sense.

K

Kinesthesia   The perception of one's body movement.

L

Labial   Having to do with the lips.

Language   The multimodality ability to encode, decode, and manipulate symbols for the purposes of verbal thought and/or communication. Modes of language include speaking, writing, listening comprehension, reading, and gestures.

Larynx   The voice box.

Lingual   Having to do with the tongue.

Linguistics   The study of language.

Localization   In neurology, the idea that all brain functions can be discovered and mapped.

M

Magnetic resonance imaging (MRI)   A brain scan.

Mandible   The lower jaw.

Maxilla   The upper jaw.

Midline   The center point or line.

Morpheme   The smallest unit of meaning in language.

Motor unit   A muscle and the nerve closest to it.

Mutism   Completely without speech.

N

Nasal emission   Air flowing out through the nose.

Naso-oral   Pertaining to the nose and mouth.

Neuron   In the nervous system, those cells that transmit electrochemical impulses. They contain the cell body, dendrites, and an axon.

Neuroscience   The interdisciplinary science that studies the brain and behavior.

Nonverbal communication   Communication without using words.

O

Occlusion   An obstruction or plugging of a blood vessel.

Olfactory   Related to the sense of smell.

Omission   In speech articulation, the lack of a sound in a word where one should be expected.

Optimal pitch   The pitch that is most efficient for a given person to use.

Organic   In medicine, the physical basis for a disorder.

P

Paralysis   When a muscle loses its ability to contract or move.

Paraphasia   Aphasic naming problem characterized by choosing an incorrect word that either rhymes or has a semantic relationship to the correct one.

Perception   Realizing the significance of sensory information.

Peripheral   Away from the center.

Peripheral nervous system (PNS)   The part of the nervous system made up of the cranial and spinal nerves.

Perseveration   The automatic continuation of a speaking or writing response seen in some stroke patients.

Phonation   Any voiced sound that occurs at the level of the vocal cords.

Phonology   The study of the sounds of a language and the way they are combined into words.

Plosive   A speech sound characterized by the release of a puff of air during its production, such as *p* and *t*.

Posterior   Toward the back, or behind.

Prevalence   The extent a disorder occurs in a population or a group.

Prognosis   An educated guess or prediction about how well a patient will recover.

Propositionality   The meaningfulness and amount of content in an utterance.

Prosody   Fluency, melody, cadence, inflection, and emphasis aspects of speech.

Psychology   The study of human consciousness and methods of measuring, explaining, and changing behavior in humans and other animals.

Q

Quadriplegia   Paralysis or weakness of all four limbs.

R

Receptive aphasia   A type of neurologically based language disturbance in which the person has problems reading and understanding the speech and gestures of others.

Reinforcement   The consequence or response to a behavior; can be positive or negative.

Respiration   Breathing.

S

Schedules of reinforcement   The duration and frequency with which reinforcements are administered.

Schwa sound   The sound *uh* as in *understand.*

Seizure   A spontaneous excessive discharge of cortical neurons.

Semantics   The meaning of words. The relationship between a symbol and what it represents.

Sibilant High-pitched speech sounds produced by pushing air through a constricted area, such as *s* and *z*.

Soft Palate The soft part at the back of the roof of one's mouth. The muscle at the back of the hard palate; the velum.

Sound discrimination The auditory ability to perceive the difference between two sounds, especially similar ones. Also called *auditory discrimination*.

Spastic A form of paralysis in which a muscle is contracted due to a stroke or other neurological injury.

Stop consonant A speech sound produced by momentarily stopping the air flow, such as *p*, *t*, and *k*.

Stroke Sudden interruption of the flow of blood to the brain.

Subcortical The areas of the brain below the cortex.

Substitution In speech articulation, replacing the correct sound with another one.

Syndrome A combination of symptoms that usually occur together.

Syntax The grammatical structure of language, especially word order.

T

Tactile Relating to the sense of touch.

Telegraphic speech Speech with the fewest words possible to get the meaning across. So called because it sounds like a telegram. Such speech is usually high in content words.

Tempo The rate, as in the speed, of speaking.

Thorax The chest.

Thrombosis A plug that stops the flow of blood. Unlike an embolus, it does not form elsewhere and migrate.

Tone Background tension of a muscle.

Trachea The windpipe.

Transient ischemic attack (TIA) Like a stroke, but does not result in permanent damage to the brain and lasts less than 24 hours.

Trauma Injury or shock to the body.

Traumatic brain injury (TBI) Injury to the brain caused by an outside impact or a penetrating object.

Tremor Vibration of a muscle or structure of the body; or a waver in the voice.

U

Unilateral One side.

Unilateral neglect Problems attending to one side of the body.

Unvoiced A sound produced with no vibration of the vocal cords, such as *sh* and *h*.

Uvula The muscle that hangs down at the back of the soft palate.

V

Veins   Blood vessels carrying blood to the heart.
Ventricles   Interconnected, fluid-filled cavities in the brain.
Voice   Any sound in the voice box produced by vocal cord vibration.

W

Wernicke's area   The part of the left side of the brain important to receptive communication (understanding).
White matter   The part of the brain that is white in appearance because it contains
more nerve fibers, located below the cortex.

Index

Note: Page numbers with *f* indicate figures.

Blindness, 155, 214–215
Blockage type of stroke, 15–16
Blood clots, 15
Blood pressure, 15
Blood supply, to the brain, 14–15
Body image
  improving, 105–106
  self-esteem and, 103–104, 105
Body jerks, 55, 56
Body language, 142–143
Braille method, 214–215
Brain, 92
  approximate sites of Broca's and
    Wernicke's areas of, 12f
  blood supply to, 14–15
  Broca's area of, 12, 13
  complex capabilities of, 43
  general boundaries of lobes of, 10f
  gray matter of, 8f
  holistic operation of, 6–8
  left hemisphere of, 7f, 7–8
  lobes of, 9
  looking down at right and left
    hemispheres of, 8f
  power of speech and, 5–6
  right hemisphere of, 6–7
  scientific inquiry into functioning of, 5–6
  speech and language centers of, 11–14
  Wernicke's area of, 12, 13
Brain cancer, 17
Brain damage
  depression-anxiety in patients with,
    228–229
  understanding nature of, 171
Brain injuries, recovery from and location
    of, 184
Brain mapping
  goal of, 13
  studies, 13, 62
Brain research, understanding complete
    aphasia and, 26
Brain scans, purpose of, 176
Brainstem, 11
  human, 11f
Breathing, 45
Breathing muscles, dysarthric patients and,
    189

Breathing strength and coordination,
    testing for dysarthria and, 180
Breathing system, speech-programming
    computer and, 46–47
British Columbia, aphasia support groups
    and associations in, 269
Broca, Pierre Paul, 11, 12, 13, 32
Broca's aphasia, 32–33, 44, 127, 208
  automatic utterances in, 33–34
  communication problems with, 35
  gender and, 38
  panic attacks and, 62
Broca's area of the brain, 12, 13
  approximate site of, 12f
Burst type of stroke, 16

C
Calendar dates, awareness of, 76
California, aphasia support groups and
    associations in, 242–244
Canada, aphasia support groups and
    associations in, 268–270
Cancer of the brain, 17
Catastrophic reactions, 60
Cerebellum, 11, 12, 54
  human, 11f
Cerebral vascular accident, 15
Certificates of clinical competence, in
    speech-language pathology and/or
    audiology, 173
Change
  in communication disorders, over time,
    177–178
  unwanted, accepting, 151–169
Character, stroke survivor, denial and, 159
"Charades," 205
Checkbook balancing, 145
Chemical imbalances, anxious feelings
    related to, 116
Chewing problems, 45
  swallowing therapy and, 197–198
Child-rearing decisions, coping with
    depression and, 100
Children
  echoed speech in, 63–64
  meanings of words understood by,
    23–24

Memory notebooks, 212
Memory problems, 77–84, 225–227
  amnesia before and after stroke, 83
  attention, 78
  recall, 79–80
  storage, 78–79
Memory tests, 83
Men
  stroke and depression in, 99
  Wernicke's aphasia and, 38, 39
Meningitis, 6
Menninger, Karl A., 73
Mental sets, fixed, echoed speech and, 64
Michigan, aphasia support groups and
    associations in, 253–255
Mild communication disorders, 2
Mind, 92
Mind's eye, problem-solving in, 92–93
Minnesota, aphasia support groups and
    associations in, 255–256
Mirrors, use of, for feedback purposes,
    175
Mississippi, aphasia support groups and
    associations in, 256
Missouri, aphasia support groups and
    associations in, 256
Mixed dysarthria, 56
Mobility, Bill of Rights for aphasic patient
    and, 200
Money, communication and, 145–146. *See
    also* Financial management
Moods
  color words and, 131
  swings in, 220
Moon circle, in Peyote Healing Ceremony,
    224
Mortality, awareness of, 74
Mother Teresa of Calcutta, 135
Motivation, considerations related to, 185
Motor speech disorders, 43–56, 155
  aphasia and, 194
Mouth
  creation of a word and, 47
  stroke survivors with apraxia of speech
    and, 192
Movement, cerebellum and coordination
    of, 11, 54

MRIs. *See* Magnetic resonance imaging
    (MRI) scans
Multi-lingual persons, effects of aphasia
    on, 41
"Murphy's Inner World of Aphasia," 1,
    160, 161
  "Beth's Story," 234–240
Muscle movements
  forms of paralysis and, 52–53
  in speech, 48
Muscle-regulating computers, 53–54
Muscles
  flaccid, 54
  spastic, 53–54
  tremors in, 56
Muscle tension, reducing, 132–133
Music, 112
  reducing anxiety levels with, 131

N

Naming problems or errors, 40, 108
  awareness of, 42
  confusion *vs.,* 77
  types of, 40–41
Nasality, 54
  testing for dysarthria and, 180
Nasalization, 47
Nasogastric tubes, 69
National Easter Seal Society, 270
National Family Caregivers Association,
    270
National Stroke Association, 270
Native American Church, 223
Navajo Indian Reservation, 224, 225
Navajo Indians, Peyote Healing Ceremony
    and, 223–225
Navajo language, 223, 224
Neal, Patricia, 217
Nebraska, aphasia support groups and
    associations in, 256–257
Negative stress, depression and, 229
Negative thoughts, 101
  countering, 111
Neurological factors, grieving process
    and, 158
Newfoundland, aphasia support groups
    and associations in, 269